Richard Bright, G. Hilaro Barlow

Clinical Memoirs on abdominal Tumors and Intumescence

Richard Bright, G. Hilaro Barlow

Clinical Memoirs on abdominal Tumors and Intumescence

ISBN/EAN: 9783337118129

Printed in Europe, USA, Canada, Australia, Japan

Cover: Foto ©ninafisch / pixelio.de

More available books at **www.hansebooks.com**

CLINICAL MEMOIRS

ON

ABDOMINAL TUMOURS

AND

INTUMESCENCE.

BY THE LATE
DR. BRIGHT.

Reprinted from the 'Guy's Hospital Reports.'

EDITED BY
G. HILARO BARLOW, M.D., M.A. CANTAB.,
PHYSICIAN TO GUY'S HOSPITAL.

THE NEW SYDENHAM SOCIETY,
LONDON.
MDCCCLX.

EDITOR'S PREFACE.

There has been no English physician—perhaps it may be said none of any country—since the time of Harvey, who has effected not only so great an advance in the knowledge of particular diseases, but also so great a revolution in our habits of thought, and methods of investigating morbid phenomena and tracing the etiology of disease, as has the late Dr. Richard Bright.

To those who have received the knowledge of the connections of dropsy, albuminous urine, and disease of the kidney, among the first rudiments of medicine, the facts which establish that connection may appear so simple and so easily ascertained, that the amount of labour, the accuracy of the observation, and the rigid adherence to the inductive method which characterised the whole of Bright's researches, may hardly have been suspected, still less adequately appreciated.

For some time after the commencement of the present century, dropsy was regarded as in itself a primary disease, dependent upon a deficient action of the absorbents, though it was by no means proved that they were mainly, if at all, concerned in the removal of fluid from the serous membrane and cells of the areolar tissue; the cause, then, which was commonly assigned for dropsical effusion was in the first place not a *vera causa;* since, as the function ascribed to the absorbents could not be proved, thus, a defect of function must also be a gratuitous assumption. The favorite notion, also, of referring every disease to the liver was not without influence, and since, when morbid anatomy began to be more carefully prosecuted, the liver was found structurally changed, the internal lesion upon which dropsy depended was supposed to have hence been satisfactorily demonstrated. But, though disease of the liver was so far a *vera causa* as that its existence was apparent in many instances, yet it was not one which could be shown to be capable of producing the effects ascribed to it, neither could it really be said to be a *vera causa*, since in many instances of dropsy it was wanting.

A great advance towards the true pathology of dropsy was made by Blackall, who pointed out that in a great number of cases the urine coagulated upon the application of "heat or nitrous acid;" and those which were for the most part cases of general dropsy, he called inflammatory dropsies. It is, however, remarkable that Blackall, although he availed himself of all opportunities of inspection after death, never succeeded in connecting the coincidence of these two remarkable phenomena, dropsy and albuminous urine, with disease of any internal organ. Dr. Wells, too,—a name scarcely less illustrious than Bright or Blackall,—investigated the subject in a most philosophic spirit, but missed, though narrowly, the discovery of the disease of the kidney. Such was the state of knowledge upon this subject when the inquiry was taken up by Dr. Bright.

And here we may pause, to observe the character of mind which was then brought to bear upon one of the most important investigations within the whole range of medical science.

Dr. Bright was, indeed, a man of naturally clear judgment; and, as far as such a virtue can be said to have been a natural gift, of great industry. But the strongest powers of intellect languish and become feeble, if not matured by exercise, and industry which is not consistently exercised upon some definite object degenerates into a fitful restlessness.

Now it is to be remembered, that Dr. Bright brought not only these gifts to the study of his profession, but that his clear and vigorous intellect had been rendered more discriminating by the strict discipline of a sound and extended education, by which, too, he had learned to exercise his industry upon objects worthy of his energetic pursuit. He had also what might be considered as a natural gift, and by no means a common one—a singular power of observation, which had, perhaps, by constant exercise, become so habitual that the most trifling circumstance rarely escaped him; and he was in the habit of recording facts and observations in disease or morbid anatomy apparently the most trifling; saying, that if he did not at the time perceive their importance, they might be available to himself or others at some future period.

It is not a little remarkable that this faculty of observation displayed itself before Dr. Bright devoted himself, as he subsequently did, to his acquiring distinction in his profession, by the honorable course of, at the same time, advancing that profession. This faculty of observation made the opportunities of travelling which he enjoyed a real advantage to Bright, and he produced a work upon Hungary which was at the time considered a most valuable acquisition to the knowledge of the natural history, the statistics, and the social condition of that country.

There was one other quality by which Bright was eminently distinguished, and that was his philosophic truthfulness. He was, indeed, in all the relations of life, a man without guile, and as he would have scorned an untruth, so would he not endure that the slightest bias should be given to any observation, in order to favour any particular views or opinions. This rigid and self-denying honesty in scientific investigation is no ordinary virtue; but in Bright it reaped its reward, for there have been few, if any, who have observed and recorded so much, and have reasoned so extensively upon those observations, who have subsequently been required to correct or retract so little.

The first volume of the 'Select Medical Reports' was published in 1824, and in this work, which includes observations on the morbid anatomy of continued fever, and of phthisis, which for their carefulness and accuracy would alone have established his reputation as a morbid anatomist and pathologist, Dr. Bright investigates the pathology of dropsy; we say advisedly *pathology*, for Dr. Bright valued anatomy only in so far as he could connect structural changes with symptoms during life, and was not satisfied unless he could establish the connection by a rational etiology.

Observations upon diseased liver in dropsy are also detailed; and these, whilst they point out the connection of ascites with obstructed portal circulation, show also that the necessary connection with diseased liver is limited to that particular form of dropsy. The most important series of cases consists of fatal cases of it in which the urine was albuminous, and by these observations was the connexion of diseased kidney, albuminous urine, and dropsy established. It is but just to Dr. Bright, as well as to those who have followed him in the same path of discovery, to state that he described three, or, at the most, four forms of disease, with which the train of symptoms constituting what is now generally known as Bright's disease were associated; and that, having done this, he has left the investigation of the minute structural changes to be worked out by others, whilst he devoted himself mainly to the completion of the clinical history.

It was not enough that the urine was found to be albuminous; it was also examined as to its difference from the healthy secretion in other respects. This led to the discovery that, not only was there a continual abstraction from the system of a most important constituent of the blood in the form of albumen, but also that there was a non-elimination from the system of the natural ingredients of the urine, particularly of urea; and this led to the examination of the blood by Drs. Bostock and Babington, and the discovery of the urea in the circulation of those patients from whose system it was not eliminated, owing to the disease in the kidney. It was this that perhaps constituted the most important part of the discovery, and which produced so great a change in the whole science of pathology. For it was argued, and with reason, by Dr. Bright, and still more earnestly by his disciples, that this inquination of the blood was the cause of many of the morbid phenomena, such as cerebral disturbance, and inflammation of the serous membranes; and thus was introduced a modified and rational humoral pathology. The doctrines of the solidists, as they were termed, were, however, in the ascendant; and it was not till after much opposition, that the whole theory of the effects of retained secretion and consequent toxæmic poisoning was generally adopted. The facts upon which it was established were, however, not to be shaken, and the doctrines of Bright are now universally received.

They naturally, however, gave rise to inquiries as to the analogy of the disease of other excretory organs, and toxæmic poisoning, owing to inquination of the blood by impurities from other sources; and thus, not only was the possibility of bile poisoning recognised, but also was opened a wide field of investigation—blood-disease.

We must not here pursue this subject, but simply point out that although the investigations connected with what is called κατ' εξοχην, "Bright's Disease," were going on through so large a proportion of his professional life, his active mind was frequently directed to other points of pathology. Diseases of the brain, of the liver, and of the pancreas received from him much attention and elucidation. Disease of the abdominal viscera was, perhaps, always a favorite object of research with Dr. Bright, and accordingly we find that his last contributions to the literature of his profession was the following series of monographs upon Abdominal Tumours; which, however, want of health and time did not allow him to finish.

These papers require little or no comment; they do not, indeed, suggest any new doctrine; but, besides abounding in important suggestions as to diagnosis and function, they are especially valuable as examples of care and accuracy in observing and in recording observations. It is but due to the memory of Bright to state, though without any design of imputing plagiarism to more recent continental pathologists, that the description of acephalocyst hydatids, at page 18, *et seq.*, is altogether original, and certainly an anticipation of similar observations which have since been published in Germany.

The papers in question being essentially clinical, and consisting chiefly of well-grouped examples of the diseases under consideration, it has been considered better to reprint them almost exactly as they were originally published. The memoirs themselves had no pretension to constitute a complete monograph on the subjects which they illustrate. To have attempted to make them such by the addition of notes or interpolated material from other sources, would have been to wholly change the character of the work. It would have taken it beyond the scope of what was contemplated by the Council of the Society, and would also in some degree have deprived it of its greatest merit—that, namely, of being clinical portraits, fresh from the hand of a master. The task of editing has, therefore, as far as the body of the work is concerned, been restricted to the careful correction of verbal errors and obscurities of expression, and the rearrangement of the plates, so as to bring them into juxtaposition with the cases to which they belong. In the original papers most of the illustrations were on stone, and were appended at the end of the volume; in the present reprint they have been reproduced in wood (by Mr. Tuffen West), and are incorporated with the text, so as to facilitate reference. The addition of the List of Cases, which is given at page xii, and of the Index at page 323, will doubtless be found useful.

In a few subjects, such, for example, as the histology of the acephalocyst hydatid, great advance in knowledge has been made since the publication of Dr. Bright's papers. It has been thought best, however, even in these matters, to adhere to the rule stated above, of not making any additions to the original statements.

5, UNION STREET:
September 15th, 1860.

CONTENTS.

CHAPTER I.
On the Exploration of the Abdomen . . . 1

CHAPTER II.
On Tumours dependent upon Acephalocyst Hydatids . 11

CHAPTER III.
Ovarian Tumours . . . 57

CHAPTER IV.
Disease of the Spleen . . . 148

CHAPTER V.
Renal Disease . . . 198

CHAPTER VI.
Diseased Liver 239

LIST OF CASES.

HYDATID TUMOURS.

		PAGE
Case 1.	Hydatids in the abdomen, of many years' standing, showing the acephalocysts in almost every stage of their existence	13
Case 2.	Hydatids extensively occupying the abdomen. Autopsy	23
Case 3.	Hydatids developed in the abdomen. Death from peritonitis	30
Case 4.	Tumour of the abdomen supposed to depend on the presence of hydatids	36
Case 5.	Hydatid cyst connected with the liver. Death from suppuration of the sac and its consequences	37
Case 6.	Hydatid cysts in the liver ossified	38
Case 7.	Tumour in the pubic region from an hydatid cyst situated behind the bladder	39
Case 8.	Tumour in the pubic region from an hydatid cyst behind the bladder	40
Case 9.	Hydatid cyst connected with the liver, emptied by paracentesis	41
Case 10.	Hydatid connected with liver emptied by paracentesis	42
Case 11.	Hydatids in the spleen bursting into the abdomen, and causing death very speedily	44
Case 12.	Hydatid of the liver suppurating and bursting into the abdomen, causing death	45
Case 13.	Supposed hydatid of the liver bursting into the cavity of the abdomen	47
Case 14.	Hydatids in the liver, supposed to have passed off by the intestines	49
Case 15.	Hydatid cyst in the liver, discharging itself externally; and death from hæmorrhage	50

OVARIAN TUMOURS.

Case 1.	Small simple cyst hanging from the uterine appendages, discovered after death	70
Case 2.	Small simple cyst in the ovary	70
Case 3.	Incipient ovarian dropsy, probably of a malignant character	71
Case 4.	Diseased ovary with cysts in a case of extensive malignant disease of other organs	75

CONTENTS.

		PAGE
Case 5.	Ovarian dropsy of eleven years' standing. Death probably from inflammatory changes going on in the interior of the cyst	76
Case 6.	Ovarian dropsy, anasarca, and ascites. Death from peritonitis, after the fluid was partially drawn from the cyst	81
Case 7.	Ovarian dropsy of many years' duration, showing several cysts in different conditions; with the analysis of the fluids they contained	85
Case 8.	Malignant tumour in abdomen, probably ovarian; discharging constantly from the wound made by paracentesis	95
Case 9.	Compound ovarian cyst. Death from exhaustion	96
Case 10.	Compound ovarian cyst; the fluid never removed. Slow exhaustion and death; adhesions of the tumour to the parietes discerned during life	98
Case 11.	Compound ovarian cyst; the fluid never removed. Death from irritation and exhaustion	101
Case 12.	Ovarian dropsy, fatal from peritonitis after the partial abstraction of the fluid	103
Case 13.	Cyst, probably a diseased Graafian vesicle, communicating by ulceration with the colon. Death from irritation of the mucous membrane of the large intestines	104
Case 14.	Ovarian cyst, probably a diseased Graafian vesicle; fluid partially removed; inflammation of cyst and peritoneum	106
Case 15.	Ovarian dropsy; paracentesis. Death from peritoneal inflammation	170
Case 16.	Cyst in the broad ligament of the uterus. Death sudden	109
Case 17.	Ovarian tumour, partly fluid, partly fungoid; paracentesis rendered necessary from the great pain experienced. Death after several operations, from peritoneal inflammation	110
Case 18.	Ovarian dropsy, possibly enlarged Graafian vesicle, rupture of the cyst internally. Death from inflammation of the cyst and neighbouring parts; the cyst tympanitic	115
Case 19.	Malignant ovarian cyst ruptured internally; subsidence of the tumour. Death in about two years, from increase of the disease	118
Case 20.	Ovarian cyst ruptured internally. Death after three years, with emaciation	121
Case 21.	Compound ovarian cyst, ruptured internally; followed by death from peritonitis	121
Case 22.	Malignant disease of the ovary; fibrous tubera in the uterus; paracentesis, subcutaneous tubera in the abdominal wall. Death from extensive scirrhous disease	124
Case 23.	Ovaries affected with a modification of the malignant disease; the peritoneum extensively involved in a similar affection	129
Case 24.	Ovarian tumour, with extensive growth of pendulous malignant tumours from the peritoneum	130
Case 25.	Malignant ovarian tumour, with ascites, communicating disease by contiguity to the sigmoid flexure and rectum	131

xiv CONTENTS.

PAGE

Case 26. Ovarian dropsy, cerebriform disease, communicating to contiguous organs 133
Case 27. Hysterical distension of the bowels, mistaken for ovarian tumour; operation to attempt its removal . . 137
Case 28. Ascites complicated with ovarian cyst . . . 140
Case 29. Ovarian tumour. Diagnosis complicated by pregnancy . 141

TUMOURS OF THE SPLEEN.

Case 1. Simple enlargement of the spleen connected with intermittent fever 159
Case 2. Enlarged spleen cured by tonics and purgatives . . 162
Case 3. Enlarged spleen in a child 163
Case 4. Remarkable distension of the spleen without disorganization. Death from the effects of diseased liver . . . 165
Case 5. Enlarged spleen, occurring in a case of fatal diarrhœa . 169
Case 6. Enlarged and fleshy spleen, with chronic disease of the liver . 171
Case 7. Enlarged and fleshy spleen, with chronic disease in the abdomen, mottled kidneys, and albuminous urine . . . 172
Case 8. Abscess in the spleen opening into the colon . . 173
Case 9. Sloughing abscess of the spleen 176
Case 10. Jaundice from general enlargement of the liver. Spleen greatly enlarged, and studded with small, hard, opaque bodies. The glandular and absorbent system much diseased . 177
Case 11. Spleen reduced nearly to a fluid state, connected with extensive disease of the absorbent system . . . 179
Case 12. Tuberculated spleen, in a case where the tubercular diathesis greatly affected the glands 180
Case 13. Tubercles in the spleen in a case of phthisis where the glands were greatly affected 180
Case 14. Tubercles in the spleen in a case of phthisis where the glands were greatly affected 181
Case 15. Tubercle in the spleen, lungs, and liver . . . 181
Case 16. Suppurating tubercles in the spleen, in a case of fever, with ulceration of the mucous membrane of the intestines . 182
Case 17. Tuberculated spleen in a case of fever . . . 183
Case 18. Spleen pervaded by malignant matter. The absorbent glands very extensively affected 184
Case 19. Spleen pervaded by malignant matter. The absorbent glands very extensively affected 186
Case 20. Malignant disease of a scirrhous character affecting the spleen, together with many other organs of the body . . 187
Case 21. Malignant disease of a cerebriform character affecting the spleen, in common with other organs 188
Case 22. Bony deposit in the spleen and mesenteric glands . . 189
Case 23. Cysts in the cellular membrane of the spleen . . 189
Case 24. Peculiar appearance of the peritoneal coat of the spleen . 191

	PAGE
Case 25. Tubercular deposit on the peritoneum of the spleen .	192
Case 26. Spleen with the peritoneal covering studded with flat scirrhous growths .	192
Case 27. Laceration of the spleen	194
Case 28. Abscess in the fibrine left after the extravasation of blood in the spleen .	195

RENAL TUMOURS.

Case 1. Tumour of the kidney from numerous cysts formed in its substance .	208
Case 2. Suppuration of the kidney from stricture of the urethra attended with perceptible tumour .	210
Case 3. Tumour formed by the kidney, the pelvis being distended with pus .	212
Case 4. Tumour from puriform collection in the kidney, first perceived after parturition, but apparently depending on the presence of a calculus .	217
Case 5. Large tumour formed by the left kidney, supposed to be uterine, the pelvis being distended with grumous matter, and the substance of the organ suffering, together with the liver, from malignant disease .	220
Case 6. Tumour formed by the kidney dilated with puriform fluid .	223
Case 7. Tumour of the kidney with copious puriform discharge through the urethra, and probably through the bowels .	224
Case 8. Tumour formed by the left kidney, discharging pus copiously both by the urethra and the rectum, depending on a large renal calculus .	227
Case 9. Cerebriform tumour of the right kidney, supposed to be a tumour arising from the concave surface of the liver .	229
Case 10. Tumour of the kidney from fungoid disease mistaken for the spleen. Death by rupture into the peritoneal cavity .	232
Case 11. Fungoid tumour of the kidney, affording the appearance of two tumours .	233
Case 12. Fungous tumour of the mesentery, resembling enlarged kidney	235

TUMOURS OF THE LIVER, &c.

Case 1. Accumulation of fæces in the sigmoid flexure of the colon, imitating organic tumour .	242
Case 2. Fæcal accumulation in the colon, imitating hepatic enlargement .	243
Case 3. Fæcal accumulation in the colon, imitating fungoid tumour .	244
Case 4. Fæcal accumulation in the colon, imitating malignant disease of the liver .	246
Case 5. Malignant disease of the peritoneum resembling hepatic tumour .	251

	PAGE
Case 6. The liver pushed down by fluid in the right side of the thorax	255
Case 7. Apparent tumour of the liver, owing to that organ being pushed down by pleuritic effusion	256
Case 8. Abscess situated between the diaphragm and the liver, producing apparent enlargement of the liver	257
Case 9. Small intestines situated anteriorly to the liver	259
Case 10. Malignant tumour confined entirely to the left lobe of the liver, and ascending towards the thorax	260
Case 11. Liver enlarged and altered in its structure from frequent congestion	264
Case 12. Tumefaction of the liver from retention of bile	271
Case 13. Tumefaction of the liver from retention of bile. The gall-bladder distended with its own secretion	277
Case 14. Gall-bladder forming a tumour. The liver not gorged with bile	279
Case 15. Liver and gall-bladder distended with bile	280
Case 16. Hepatic tumour from chronic hypertrophy of the organ	281
Case 17. Hepatic tumour from chronic change in the liver	283
Case 18. Fatty liver descending below umbilicus	285
Case 19. Fatty change in the substance of the liver	286
Case 20. Liver large from the fatty change in its substance	289
Case 21. Malignant disease producing a regular, smooth enlargement of the liver	291
Case 22. Chronic abscess presenting great difficulties in its detection	294
Case 23. Deep cicatrices in the liver from former abscesses	296
Case 24. Tumour in the abdomen from cerebriform tubera in the liver	299
Case 25. Tumour in the abdomen from cerebriform growth in the liver	301
Case 26. Tumours in the abdomen from cerebriform growths in the liver	303
Case 27. Tumour in the abdomen from scirrhous tubera in the liver. Peritoneum and other organs affected	305
Case 28. The small, hard, scirrhous tumour of the liver nearly confined to the left lobe. Peritoneum affected	307
Case 29. Liver converted into a scirrhous mass, so contracted as to form no external tumour. Uterus scirrhous	310
Case 30. Scirrhous tubera of the liver. Mamma and ovaria diseased	313
Case 31. Large irregular tumour from melanosis of the liver	313
Case 32. Melanosis occupying the liver very extensively. Very slight jaundice before death	315
Case 33. Extensive malignant disease very rapidly implicating the organs both of the chest and abdomen	318

LIST OF WOODCUTS.

FIG.		PAGE
1.	Outline of abdomen, showing division into regions (male)	4
2.	,, ,, ,, (female)	5
3.	,, ,, ,, position of malignant tumours	8
4.	,, ,, ,, hydatid tumours	9
5.	The abdomen of Ann W— (Case 1), hydatid tumours	15
6.	The same, after the removal of the integuments	16
7, 8, 9, 10, and 11.	Microscopic appearance of hydatids	18—21
12 and 13.	Interior of hydatid cysts	28—29
14.	A cluster of hydatid cysts	26
15.	Hydatid tumours in abdomen (Case 3)	30
16.	The same, eight years after the previous one	32
17.	The same, laid open at the post-mortem examination	33
18.	Ovary and Fallopian tube, showing pendulous, cystiform bodies	58
19.	Cyst in the broad ligament	58
20.	,, ,,	59
21.	Compound ovarian cyst	61
22.	Stencilled outline of an abdomen, in a case of ovarian tumour	65
23.	Diagram showing gradual enlargement of an ovarian cyst	66
24.	Incipient stage of a malignant ovarian tumour	72
25.	The same, a vertical section	73
26.	Malignant disease of the ovary	75
27.	Malignant intra-cystic growth	79
28.	Intra-cystic growths	80
29.	Secondary cysts in a larger one	83
30.	Internal surface of a malignant ovarian cyst	84
31.	Portrait from a case (Case 7) of large ovarian cyst	87
32.	The same, laid bare at the post-mortem	89
33.	The same—the abdomen after the removal of the cyst	90
34.	Sketch of a large ovarian cyst taken at the post-mortem examination	99
35.	Internal view of an ovarian cyst	103
36.	Post-mortem appearances in a case (Case 21) of rupture of an ovarian cyst	122
37.	Section of an ovarian tumour	141
38.	Ovaries containing solid tumours	147
39.	Section of spleen, showing deposits of bone	153
40.	,, ,, ,, cysts in the cellular membrane	154
41.	Stencilled outline showing enlarged spleen	160
42 and 43.	The same, showing gradual diminution of the enlarged organ	161, 162

FIG.		PAGE
44 and 45. Enlarged spleen, in successive stages of the complaint, in the same patient		168, 169
46. Abdominal tumour produced by enlarged spleen		170
47. Section of a spleen affected with tubercle		182
48. Section of an enlarged spleen from a case of fever		184
49. Section of spleen, with malignant growths		186
50. ,, ,, ,,		187
51. Section of spleen which had probably been lacerated		194
52. ,, ,, ,,		194
53. Outline of abdomen, from a case of cystic disease of kidneys		209
54. ,, ,, suppuration of kidneys		211
55. Appearance of abdomen in a case of purulent distension of the kidney		212
56. Diagram showing the situation of the tumour in the same case as fig. 55		213
57. Post-mortem appearances from the same case		215
58. The same, after further dissection (on a larger scale)		216
59. External appearance of the abdomen in a case of purulent distension of the kidney		218
60. Diagram showing the situation of an enlarged kidney		219
61. The same, from another case		222
62. Diagram showing the position of a large kidney in relation to the colon		228
63. Diagram of a fungoid tumour of the kidney		231
64. Diagram of a tumour of the kidney crossed by the colon		234
65. Appearance at a post-mortem of a case of enlarged kidney		235
66. Diagram showing tumour caused by accumulation of fæces		247
67, 68, and 69. Diagram showing varieties in the position and natural extent of the colon		248, 249, 250
70. Post-mortem appearance in a case of malignant disease of the peritoneum		251
71. Diagram showing the position of a malignant tumour in the right lobe of the liver		261
72. Sketch showing the relative positions of the heart and liver in a case of congested liver from diseased heart		267
73. Sketch showing enlargement of the liver from biliary congestion		271
74. Diagram showing position of tumour depending on distended gall-bladder		278
75. Sketch showing the liver enormously enlarged by malignant deposit		292
76. Diagram showing the situation of a tumour depending on chronic abscess of the liver		295
77. Sketch showing malignant disease in the liver		303
78. Diagram showing a portion of a tumour in a case of malignant disease of the liver		308
79. Sketch showing melanotic tumours in the liver		313

CLINICAL MEMOIRS

ON

ABDOMINAL TUMOURS

AND

INTUMESCENCE.

CHAPTER I.

ON THE EXPLORATION OF THE ABDOMEN.

As it is my intention to devote the following pages to the consideration of Abdominal Tumours and Intumescence, it will be well, in the first place, to give a general outline of the subjects which may probably be included in such a survey; although it is not proposed to adhere closely to the line marked out, but rather to take up the various points, as circumstances may render most convenient, or the hospital afford me the requisite means of illustration. The topics which naturally present themselves admit of being arranged under the following heads:—1. The integuments. 2. The peritoneum. 3. The stomach. 4. The intestines. 5. The liver. 6. The spleen. 7. The pancreas. 8. The mesenteric glands. 9. The kidneys. 10. The bladder. 11. The uterus. 12. The ovaries. 13. Extra-uterine bodies. 14. Aneurism.

1. The integuments; including various cutaneous changes, polysarcia—anasarca—malignant deposits—abscesses—protrusions.

2. The peritoneum—the various results of inflammatory action; as, effusion, including ascites—adhesions, and various depositions of adhesive matter—tubercular deposits—malignant diseases—hydatids.

3. The stomach; including flatulent distension—chronic diseases—malignant changes.

4. The intestines; including flatulent distensions—retained fæces, and other matters—mechanical obstruction—malignant strictures.

5. The liver; enlarged from congestion—forced down by the lungs or by effusion—distended with bile—enlarged by various changes of the structure generally—enlarged by malignant or other adventitious growth.

6. The spleen; enlarged by congestion—changed in structure.

7. The pancreas; enlarged or hardened.

8. The mesenteric glands; simple enlargement—scrofulous, malignant, and osseous changes.

9. The kidneys; enlarged by vesicles—by abscess—by malignant disease—distended ureter.

10. The bladder; distended—thickened—forced forward.

11. Uterus enlarged from pregnancy; chronic increase—scirrhous disease, and other changes.

12. Ovaries; enlarged by simple cysts—by malignant growths.

13. Extra-uterine fœtation.

14. Aneurismal tumours; cœliac—aortal—iliac.

The sources to which we turn for evidence respecting the existence and nature of abdominal tumours, are, the form and appearance presented to the eye; the form still further discovered by the touch; the resistance ascertained by pressure; the sounds elicited by percussion; and, in a few instances, the sounds perceptible to the ear, either alone or by the aid of the stethoscope: and besides these local and physical signs, we look to the general condition of the system, and of the various excretions, as rendering us most important assistance, and being frequently indispensable towards the formation of a tolerably correct diagnosis.

In studying the local indications of disease, the first object is, of course, to learn, and fix in our minds, the exact normal position of each viscus, and the modifications of form, appearance, and resistance which the muscles of the parietes are capable of impressing upon the different parts of the abdomen. There is, however, one circumstance connected with the abdominal viscera, which must always throw a certain degree of doubt upon all physical diagnosis, as directed to this part of the body; and this is the diversity which sometimes takes place in the organs themselves, and that more particularly with regard to the colon; the arch and the sigmoid flexure of which not unfrequently form extensive convolutions, which render any inferences derivable from its natural position somewhat doubtful. The liver, likewise, occasionally deviates from its ordinary situation and form; and, in rare instances, an anomalous position of the kidney, or other organs, may be a source of fallacy: still, however, these deviations are not sufficient to interfere materially with our probable conjectures, though they must, of course, place a bar to that perfect certainty which it would be desirable to obtain, and which, at all events, it would be very satisfactory to look forward to, in such an important research.

To facilitate our investigation, and to render our reference more exact, it has been found necessary to divide the abdomen into regions, by drawing imaginary lines, or passing imaginary planes, through the body. The divisions which have been proposed vary a little, on account of the irregular form of the abdominal cavity, and the difference of the fixed points assumed by various observers; but the following, which I venture to lay down with the assistance of my friend Mr. Edward Cock, will perhaps approach as nearly as any to a useful, though still an artificial and somewhat variable subdivision of this part of the body: and to render the subject still more obvious, I have drawn an outline of the male and female figure, with the divisions marked upon them. (Figs. 1 and 2.)

The first general division will be into three regions—the upper, the middle, and the lower; or, the epigastric, the umbilical, and the hypogastric.

The epigastric region is bounded above by the diaphragm; below, by a horizontal plane passing through the anterior extremities of the tenth rib of either side. In a well-formed chest, the cartilage of the tenth rib offers a projection on its convex or lower edge, just as it is leaving the bone, and rising towards the sternum; and this may generally be felt, without difficulty, on the living subject. It must, however, be observed, that the situation of the two points, which have thus been chosen to mark the lower boundary of the epigastric region, vary somewhat in different subjects, according to the size and shape of the chest; and in the female, more especially, are often found to have undergone considerable alteration from their original position, owing to the constriction produced by the long-continued use of tight stays. A horizontal plane, carried backwards, through these points, will pass between the bodies of the first and second lumbar vertebræ; and emerge posteriorly, just at the lower edge of the spinous process of the former.

The upper boundary of the epigastric region, being formed by the diaphragm, varies in its position, at each effort of respiration. Anteriorly, it corresponds with the junction of the ensiform cartilage with the sternum; but from this point it will be found to descend from before, backwards towards the spine, and on either side towards the ribs, until it reaches the lower boundary of this region.

The epigastric region is subdivided into the right and left hypochondria, or the spaces enclosed by the false ribs; and the scrobiculus cordis in the middle, covered in merely by the abdominal

Fig. 1.

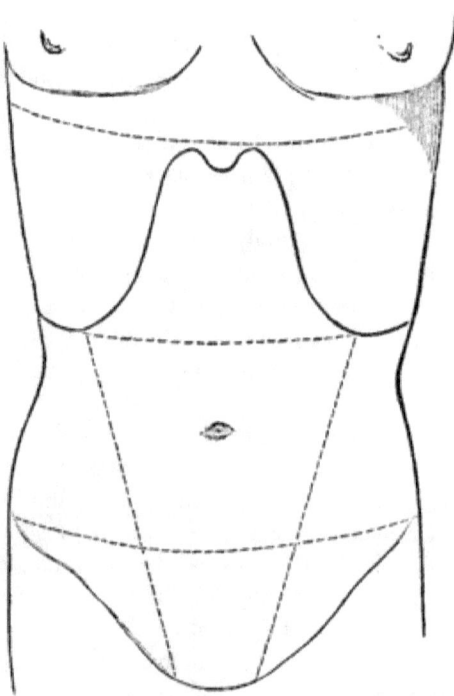

Figs. 1 and 2 present a general outline of the human abdomen, as seen in a front view, divided by dotted lines into its several regions:
The scrobiculus cordis, and the two hypochondriac regions.
The umbilical and the two lumbar regions.
The pubic and the two iliac regions.

Fig. 1 is intended to represent the outline of the male, and
Fig. 2 of the female, form.

muscles. This latter is much broader below than above; as may be seen by referring to the skeleton.

Fig. 2.

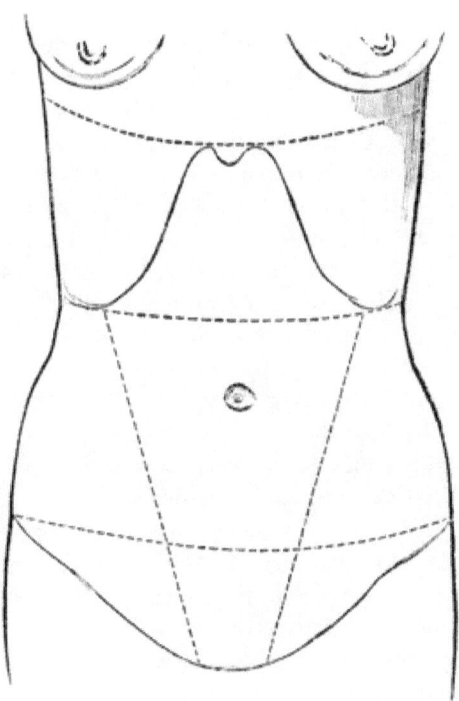

The umbilical region is bounded above by the lower epigastric plane; and below, by a horizontal plane passing through the anterior and superior spinous processes of the ilia. This plane, if produced backwards, will cut through the centre of the second portion of the sacrum, on the anterior or concave surface of that bone; and emerge posteriorly, between the second and third sacral spines. This region is likewise subdivided by imaginary planes, as will be shown hereafter.

The hypogastric region is bounded above by the lower umbilical plane, and below by the upper margin of the pubes in the centre, and Poupart's ligament on either side; the latter forming two divergent lines, extending from the spinous processes of the pubes, upwards and outwards, to the spinous processes of the ilia. This region may be said to be extended into the hollow of the true pelvis, occupying its whole cavity, and continued to its lower outlet. A horizontal line passed backwards from the upper edge of the symphysis pubis nearly corresponds with the extremity of the coccyx.

The umbilical and hypogastric regions are each divided into three, by two ascending planes passing directly backwards, and drawn through the spinous processes of the pubes and the points on the tenth ribs, already alluded to as marking the lower epigastric plane. These planes diverge from each other; and if continued over the chest, will pass rather to the outside of the nipple in the male, until they reach the clavicle, not far from its scapular extremity.

The umbilical subdivisions thus produced, consist of a central region, which retains the name of "umbilical," and two lateral regions. These last may be again divided into the iliac fossa below, corresponding with the venter of the ilium; and the lumbar region above and behind, comprising the space between the lower epigastric plane and the level of the crista of the ilium. The deep fossæ on either side of the bodies of the lumbar vertebræ have more particularly received the name of lumbar regions.

The hypogastric subdivisions consist of the middle or pubic, which descends into the cavity of the true pelvis; and the lateral or inguinal regions. These latter comprise but a small extent of surface; and are likewise exceedingly shallow, in consequence of the approximation which here takes place between the anterior and posterior abdominal walls, previously to their union at Poupart's ligament. Indeed, the serous cavity of the abdomen may be truly said to terminate at a line a little above Poupart's ligament, where the peritoneum becomes reflected, from the fascia transversalis before, on to the fascia iliaca behind; thus rendering the inguinal region of the belly smaller, from above to below, than its external boundaries would appear to indicate.

Assuming these, then, as the regions into which the abdomen may be divided, it is evident that they will not correspond exactly with the extent and form of the different viscera; but that one division will often contain portions of several viscera, and one viscus will occupy portions of several divisions. Generally speaking, however, the position of the different organs will be as follows:— The epigastric region will contain, in its whole length, the liver with the gall-bladder, the stomach, the contents of Glisson's capsule, the two angles and part of the arch of the colon, the duodenum, the spleen, the pancreas, the renal capsules, and a portion of each kidney; together with the aorta, the cava, the cœliac axis, and the commencement of the superior mesenteric artery.

The middle portion of the upper region, which is called the scrobiculus cordis, contains the whole of the left lobe of the liver, and a part of the right; together with part of the gall-bladder, the ducts and Glisson's capsule, the pyloric end of the stomach with the commencement of the duodenum, a portion of the colon, the pancreas, the aorta, and the cœliac artery with the cava and superior mesenteric artery.

The right hypochondrium contains nearly the whole of the right lobe of the liver, the angle of the ascending colon, the greater part of the duodenum, the renal capsule, and the upper portion of the kidney.

The left hypochondrium contains the rounded cardiac portion of the stomach at all times, but a very large part of that organ when distended, the left angle of the colon, the spleen, and a small portion of the left kidney, with the renal capsule.

The central subdivision of the umbilical region, which may be called the "umbilical region proper," is chiefly occupied by a portion of the arch of the colon, the omentum, and the small intestines; and contains, likewise, the mesentery and its glands, the aorta, and the vena cava.

The right lumbar region, again subdivided into the "lumbar region proper" and the iliac fossa, contains the cæcum, chiefly lodged in the iliac fossa, the ascending colon, the lower and middle portion of the kidney, a portion of the ureter; and, as it is bounded posteriorly by the lumbar and psoas muscles, these parts may be considered as entering into its composition.

The left lumbar region, also subdivided as the right, is occupied by the descending colon, and, chiefly in the iliac fossa, by the sigmoid flexure, the left kidney, and the ureter.

The small intestines likewise occupy the lumbar regions on either side, and cover the ascending and descending portions of the colon.

The lower or hypogastric division is the smallest of the three.

The central subdivision, termed the pubic region, contains the urinary bladder, with portions of the ureters, the rectum, and sometimes a projecting convolution of the sigmoid flexure of the colon; together with some portions of the small intestines, more particularly the lower convolution of the ileum, and, in the female, the uterus and its appendages.

The two lateral subdivisions of the hypogastric region, termed the inguinal regions, are very limited: the right sometimes contains the lowest part, or *cul de sac*, of the caput coli, and the vermiform process and the iliac vessels.

The left inguinal region contains a part of the sigmoid flexure, and the iliac vessels of that side.

Fig. 3.

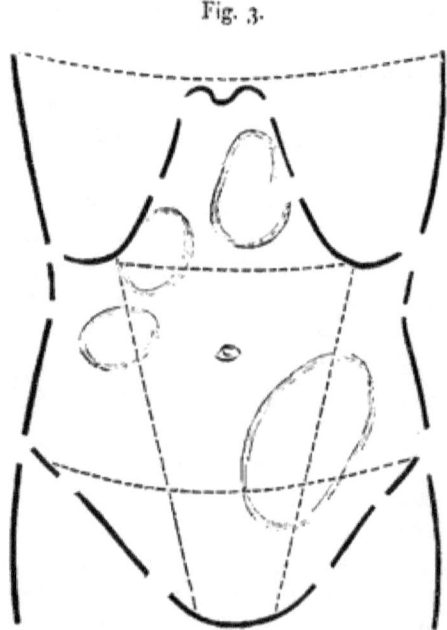

Such, then, is the distribution of the different parts and viscera, in their healthy and quiescent state: but they are subject, as I have said, to some variations, from anomalous formations; and besides this, many of the viscera, particularly those which are hollow, undergo considerable changes, as to form and extent, according to the state and progress of the operations in which they are destined to assist: and we must, of course, be prepared to appreciate and make allowance for such changes, when investigating the condition of the abdomen, or speaking of the natural contents of its different artificial subdivisions.

EXPLORATION OF THE ABDOMEN. 9

Fig. 4.

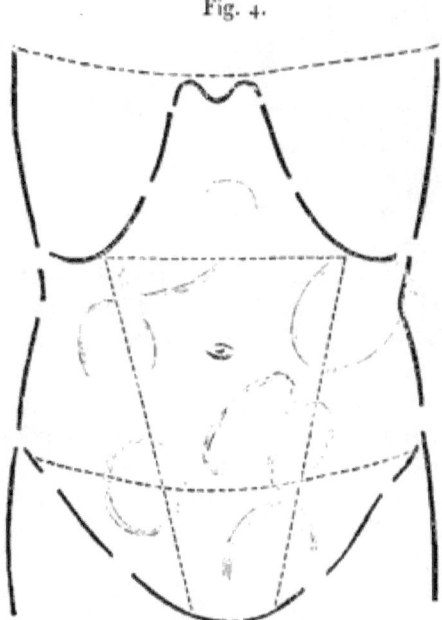

Figs. 3 and 4 present two outline figures of the male abdomen, as obtained by a brass plate properly prepared for stencilling; by means of which, such an outline may be transferred to the blank page of a note-book in a few seconds. The plate from which this outline was obtained, as likewise one of the female figure, was made, under my instructions, by Mr. Bentley, of High Holborn; and may be had, by any one, at an expense of two or three shillings.

Fig. 3 has had the marks drawn upon it, signifying the situation of abdominal tumours which occurred in a case of cerebriform malignant disease.

Fig. 4 is intended to mark the situation of several abdominal tumours in a case of hydatids.

With a view of assisting in registering facts, it appears very desirable that every one who is really anxious to make the most of the experience which comes within his reach—a duty which, unfortunately, from the time it occupies, we are all too apt to neglect—should provide himself with some ready mode of transferring to the corner or the blank page of his note-book an outline of the abdomen; upon which he may mark, as nearly as possible, the exact position of any tumour which he is called upon to treat: and, for this purpose, I have employed one or two different little contrivances, which it may not be amiss to mention. In the first place, having drawn on a thick sheet of paper the outline desired, we may, with a pin, make holes in a few prominent points; and pricking the note-book through these holes, the least-experienced draftsman will be enabled to make an intelligible sketch in a very short time. I have likewise had the figure cut in a brass plate, to use it in the mode of stencilling; and have thus procured, in a few seconds, upon any part of the page, such an outline as is represented in Figs. 3 and 4. Again, it would be a matter of a very few shillings' expense, to have a woodcut or type formed, which might be used like a seal, even with common ink. It is obvious that no one single sketch can serve for every case; because the relative proportions of the different parts of the abdomen are somewhat altered, as it becomes distended, and consequently thrown out of its natural form; but still, the convenience of some such mechanical contrivance is very great, and there is no difficulty in being provided with more than one form of outline; and perhaps a second, representing the moderately distended abdomen, would be quite sufficient for every purpose. It will be at once perceived, by a reference to the figures, how the situation and extent of tumours, whether visible to the eye or ascertained by the touch, may be traced on the outline; and thus remain a fixed record, by which to judge of the progress of the individual case, or afford a means of comparison with others.

CHAPTER II.

ON TUMOURS DEPENDENT UPON ACEPHALOCYST HYDATIDS.

It is intended to confine the present communication to the illustration of abdominal tumours derived from a single disease; which, though not strictly an affection of the peritoneum, yet, as most extensively occupying the peritoneal sac, or the parts immediately covered by that membrane, may be arranged, for convenience, amongst its diseases.

Of the origin of hydatids we are so completely ignorant, that it would be vain to hazard a conjecture on the subject. They are believed to be independent animals, existing without any vascular connexion with the body in which they are developed; but whence the ova are derived, or how introduced into the body, is altogether unknown. They are confined to no particular organ; having been found in the abdomen, the chest, and the pelvis, and various other parts: occupying, indiscriminately, the glandular, the muscular, and the cellular structure; but, undoubtedly, the most common situation is somewhere in the abdominal region: while, of the individual organs, the liver is most frequently affected by them; and, in many cases, it is probable, that when they have ultimately occupied a larger space, and spread more extensively through the abdomen, they have originally been situated in the liver only. Almost the only indication of their existence, at the commencement, is the occurrence of swelling, corresponding with the part in which they are situated; and the gradual increase of this is, for a time, the chief mark of the progress which the disease is making. Occasionally, when a rounded projecting elastic tumour has been observed and felt for a time, a sudden subsidence takes place, accompanied by more or less constitutional and local excitement; and then the tumour may never arise again; or, instead of one definite tumour which had before been observed, several may appear to develop themselves within a limited period: at other times, the sudden disappearance of such a tumour may be followed by symptoms indicating peritoneal inflammation, so severe, as quickly to lead to dissolution. In a few instances, the subsidence of such a tumour is attended by the evacuation of hydatids, through the lungs, or the intestines, or in some other way, attended by various results.

The tumour which presents itself externally is most commonly, at first, distinctly referable to the liver; and either occupies the right hypochondrium, or, protruding from beneath the ribs and their cartilages, encroaches upon the middle subdivision of the epigastric region, or descends into the right lumbar region, or approaches the umbilicus: its form is rounded, and its feel elastic; sometimes varying a little in the resistance it presents, being occasionally hard and even bony in some parts, and often indistinctly fluctuating on percussion. When situated in the right hypochondrium, it is sometimes accompanied by jaundice. When situated in other parts, the derangement of the functions of the particular organs upon which pressure is made will afford collateral indications not to be neglected. This form of disease is not confined to any age, or either sex; and the length of its continuance is not ascertained, though it is certain that it may exist for a great number of years without destroying life, as will be shown by some of the cases I am about to state.

Neither the situation, nor the sensation yielded to the touch, will be found to afford a complete means of diagnosis, in cases of hydatids: for, as I have said, they may occupy any part of the abdomen, and may arise from, or encroach upon, any organ: and this source of difficulty will be well illustrated by Figs. 3 and 4; in which Fig. 3 represents the sketch I took in a case of cerebriform disease of the abdomen; while Fig. 4 is a similar sketch from a case of hydatids. In these cases, the liver was, in both, the seat of elastic tumours; and so likewise was the space corresponding to certain convolutions of the intestines. There was, it is true, an appreciable difference in the feel: in the case of the hydatids, the elasticity was greater; but as the tumours in the other case were full of soft cerebriform matter, they were by no means devoid of a degree either of elasticity or of imperfect fluctuation. It is therefore quite necessary, in all cases, to call to our aid the concomitant circumstances. Thus, in the present instance, the greater constitutional affection, the general irritability of the system, the sallow and unhealthy complexion of malignant disease, and, on the other hand, the slowness with which hydatid tumours develop themselves when compared with cerebriform disease, would be amongst the most decisive marks, modifying or confirming the conclusions to which situation and feel had led.

Case 1.—*Hydatids in the abdomen, of many years' standing; showing the acephalocysts in almost every stage of their existence.*—Ann W——, æt. 54, was admitted into Guy's Hospital, under my care, August 15th, 1827, with a peculiar swelling of the abdomen; her health at that time suffering so far, as to make her feel all exertion irksome. It appeared, from her account, that she had given birth to her first child, which was still living, about fourteen years before;—that, about two years after, she bore a second healthy child, which was her last. She never thought that she returned completely to her natural size, after her first confinement; but it was not until nine or ten years ago that she suspected any unnatural condition of the abdomen; and the enlargement was so gradual, that she was unable to say whether it began in one part more than another; nor was it till about three years ago, that the swelling, gradually assuming its present appearance, very decidedly attracted her attention. At the time of her admission, the whole abdomen was greatly enlarged; the upper two thirds occupied by an irregular tumour, indistinctly fluctuating, and, in various parts, somewhat tender on pressure: the lower part of the abdomen was also occupied by a fluctuating tumour, apparently a large cyst arising from the pelvis. The intervening space was soft; and was the only part which gave a clear or tympanitic sound on percussion. She complained chiefly of constipated bowels and loss of flesh, although her appetite continued good. During the first months that she was in the hospital, she remained chiefly in bed, sitting up but little; not so much from any feeling of positive illness, as from the uneasiness produced by the weight of the tumour. She lay down without suffering any inconvenience, or any additional dyspnœa. Her urine was clear, and not in the least coagulable; and there was no anasarcous swelling at any time. In October, she complained, on several occasions, of increased pain and tenderness in various parts of the abdomen, which were always much relieved by the application of ten or twelve leeches: she at the same time took gentle bitter and tonic medicines, and occasional purgatives; amongst which I found none more efficacious than five grains of the Hydrarg. c. Cretâ, followed, in four hours, by castor-oil. On the 29th of October, she complained much of uneasy sensations in the abdomen, which she spoke of as throbbing, starting, and jumping, and was apprehensive that suppuration was taking place; and at two or three separate periods, in November and December, she was affected with faintness and cold perspiration, continuing for half an hour, and followed by a sense of lowness, and a feebleness of pulse, which lasted for a day or two. The breathing all this time was strong and clear, and the bowels regular.

December 31st, a dull aching pain came on, in the lower part of the abdomen, with slight tenderness on pressure. This was followed by a diarrhœa; which continued, in some degree, for ten days, with occasional attacks of sickness and vomiting. She again returned to a more comfortable state; but in the middle of February, suffered some pain in the abdomen, which she sometimes compared to the formation of an abscess, and, at other times, to something suddenly running through her. In the latter part of this month, the urine became high coloured and very scanty, with pain in the loins: and on the 27th, hæmaturia took place, the urine throwing down a brown flaky coagulum on exposure to heat. The countenance was now beginning to lose the healthy appearance it had hitherto maintained, becoming sallow. The hæmaturia continued for several days. Throughout the months of March, April, and May, she suffered occasionally from rigors, which continued for two or three hours; and her stomach became so irritable, that she often rejected her food almost as soon as it was swallowed, or experienced pain if it was retained. Diarrhœa returned in the beginning of June; and on the 10th of that month she expired.

I have not thought it necessary to detail the various remedies which were administered during this protracted illness: they were throughout directed rather with a view to relieve symptoms, than with any expectation of curing the disease, which, from the first day of her admission, I plainly perceived to be beyond the reach of medicine. The tumour of the abdomen had already existed for several years; and from its peculiar and irregular forms, and its obscure fluctuation, I concluded that it consisted either of hydatids extensively distributed, or was an ovarian tumour; and if the latter, —which, from its very singular form, and more particularly from the existence of the upper portion so separated from the lower, I could scarcely believe,—I supposed that it must be one of those complex and malignant forms of disease which could afford very little prospect of permanent relief from paracentesis. This remedy, however, I proposed to the patient, who was a remarkably sensible and well-educated woman, shortly after her admission, and again when the irritability of the stomach became urgent, probably from the pressure of the tumour; but I was obliged fairly to confess, that I considered it an experiment of doubtful issue, and only likely to give temporary relief.

The day subsequent to her decease, the body was examined, in pursuance of her own particular request, made to me during life, and likewise left in writing on her death.

Sectio cadaveris.—The body was extremely emaciated. The abdomen presented two large tumours, the one occupying the lower, the other the upper part, projecting greatly, and divided by a soft, yielding portion. (Fig. 5.) When the integuments were turned

Fig. 5.

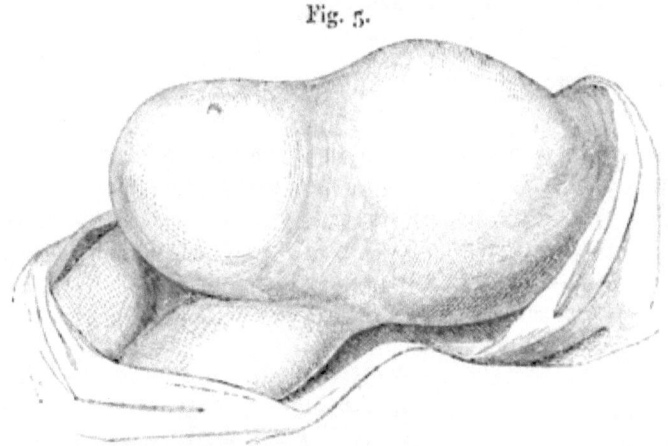

Figs. 5 and 6 represent the abdomen of Ann W— (Case 1, p. 13).

Fig. 5. A view of the abdomen during life, seen on the left side.

Fig. 6. A view of the abdomen, seen on the right side, after the integuments had been removed; showing the two large hydatid cysts. The upper one is seen incorporated with the liver, from which it arose; and which it has forced upwards, encroaching on the thorax. The lower is obliquely traversed by one of the Fallopian tubes, attached to the angle of the uterus. Part of the small intestines are seen occupying the right lumbar and iliac regions; while the contracted arch of the colon is stretched across the abdomen, between the two large hydatid cysts.

back, two large cysts came into view; between which, the arch of the colon was seen, in a very contracted state, passing across the abdomen; while the small intestines, likewise greatly contracted, chiefly occupied a triangular space in the right lumbar region. (Fig. 6.)

Fig. 6.

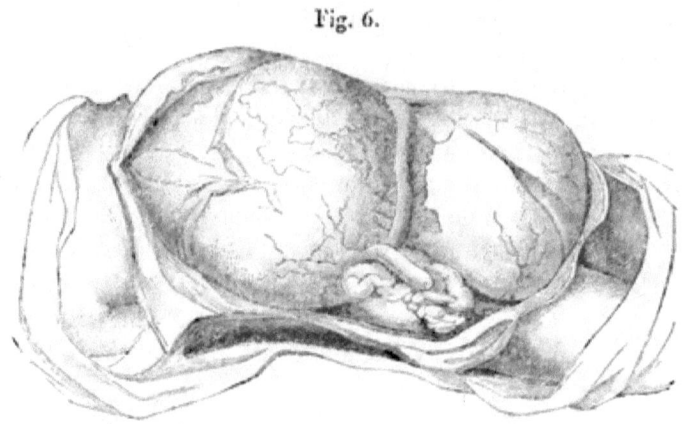

The lower cyst was nearly spherical; and on its anterior surface, to the right of the centre, was seen a flat triangular body, from which a long line extended upwards towards the left; and besides this, several nerves and vessels were stretched on its surface. On further examination, this triangular body proved to be the uterus, compressed to half its natural thickness, and proportionably extended in surface; and the line from it was one of the Fallopian tubes, closely united to the cyst. On making a small incision into the tumour, nearly a gallon of perfectly limpid fluid escaped; and then several hydatids, each of the size of a hen's egg, presented themselves at the opening. It now appeared that the whole of this enormous cyst was closely lined by one hydatid, the thickness of which was as great as tolerably thick wash-leather. It was transparent, and easily torn, and fitted, in all parts, closely to the sac in which it was contained; but was so slightly attached, that it might have been torn away perfect, by the application of very slight force. The sac itself had its inner surface of a bright pink colour, and appeared very vascular.

Behind, and to the left of this large cyst, a smaller one was discovered, of the size of a very large hen's egg, which was attached to the left ovary, and proved to be of the same nature as the large cyst; but in this, the hydatids, instead of being entire and spherical, were all burst; and that which appeared to have served at one time as a lining to the sac, was found, when taken out and examined, to be at least four times as large as the whole superficies of the present cavity.

The superior tumour of the abdomen was attached to the liver, in the substance of which it was partly imbedded. The upper part, where it had come in contact with the integuments, was completely cartilaginous; and a very singular appearance was discovered by raising the body of the tumour. There were a great number of enlarged absorbents, filled with a puriform fluid: they were quite varicose, of the size of the iliac artery after its division. One of these was seen of the length of two or three inches; while others were convoluted, and assumed a cellular appearance. Owing to the weakness of their coats, they were mostly flattened, collapsing like veins. When an incision was made into this tumour, the fluid which escaped was turbid, and of a yellowish-white colour; and it was chiefly filled with hydatids, in all their different states and stages; but by far the greater number were compressed and broken, the shreds and empty cysts being compacted together; while several, even of the size of an egg, were unbroken; and from this cyst, again, nearly a gallon of fluid and of hydatids was collected.

To the left of the gall-bladder, which was itself seen in a tolerably natural condition, was another cyst, about a third part as large as the one we had just opened: and in this case, the bile had communicated with the cyst, and the fluid it contained was green and turbid; while the hydatid cysts floating in it, and chiefly broken down, were deeply tinged of the same colour; and the internal surface of the general cavity, to which probably an hydatid had formerly been attached, was now scabrous to the feel, and covered with yellow and dark olive-coloured particles, apparently inspissated bile.

With regard to the viscera, the stomach was greatly compressed by the tumour appended to the liver; and the contracted condition of the intestines bespoke the scanty supply of nutriment which had passed into them during the last weeks of life. The kidneys had suffered most materially from the pressure made upon the ureters, and were almost reduced to the state of membranous sacs. The right was the larger of the two, and was distended with grumous, bloody urine. The inner surface of the pelvis approached, in one or two parts, to a condition of ulceration, or sphacelus. The liver was granulated, of a light colour and soft texture. The lungs were healthy, with the exception of some œdematous effusion. The heart was flabby, and of a light colour.

As to the hydatids themselves, they seem to have varied from the size of the large cyst in the lower part of the abdomen to the minutest object capable of being seen by the eye: many of them were of the size of a hen's or a thrush's egg; and these were often studded internally with little rounded bodies of an opaque white

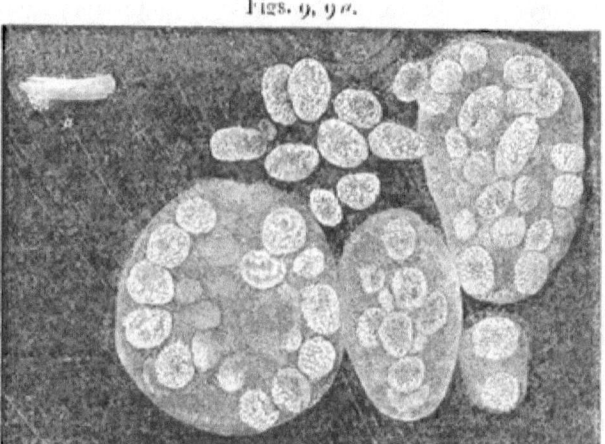

Figs. 9, 9 a.

Figs. 7 to 11 represent different appearances of minute hydatids, from Case 1, as seen through Amici's microscope. Figs. 12 and 13 are representations of the natural size, from Case 2.

 Fig. 7. A very small portion of an unbroken hydatid, as seen through Amici's microscope (p. 19).
 Fig. 8. Internal surface of a portion of hydatid, as seen through the microscope (p. 21).
 Fig 9. A cluster of very minute hydatids, as seen through the microscope (p. 19). Fig. 9 a. The natural size of the cluster of hydatids.
 Fig. 10. A cluster of small hydatids, seen through the microscope (p. 20).
 Fig. 11. A collection of minute hydatids, as seen through the microscope (p. 20). Fig. 11 a. The natural size of Fig. 11.
 Fig. 12. Appearance presented on the internal surface of some hydatids; natural size (p. 29).
 Fig. 13. Another peculiar appearance occasionally seen on the inner surface of an hydatid; natural size (p. 29).

colour, which, when separated from the surface, floated for a little while in the fluid, and then gravitated to the bottom. It was observable, that the coats of the hydatids were elastic, and admitted of an almost indefinite division into smooth and even lamellæ.

As, in this case, the hydatids were exceedingly numerous, and presented themselves in various forms, I availed myself of my friend Dr. Roget's kindness, and submitted many specimens to observation under the microscope he had lately obtained from Amici; and I procured, at the same time, the assistance of Mr. Say, of whose talents as an artist I need say nothing, in delineating some of the appearances they presented.

An hydatid, of about the size of a pigeon's egg, taken from the lower cyst, having been carefully ruptured, was found to contain almost innumerable small hydatids, scarcely visible to the eye: and a little group of them, not exceeding in size, altogether, a few grains of sand, being examined by the third power of Amici's microscope (Figs. 9, 9 a), was found to consist of simple hydatids, and of such as, having generated others within themselves, might be considered as pregnant or prolific. The single minute hydatids generally inclined to an oval form; and all of them appeared to be studded within by innumerable points or inequalities, giving them a spotted appearance; the specks being light or dark, according to the direction in which the light fell upon them. These single hydatids seldom completely touched, and never compressed each other as they lay. The pregnant minute hydatids contained from two to twenty, or more, within them: they were exceedingly thin and transparent, so as but little to obscure the appearance of the contained hydatids, by the projection of which they frequently seemed to be changed from their regular ovoid or spherical shape.

Another hydatid, of the size of a thrush's egg, but exceedingly

Fig. 7.

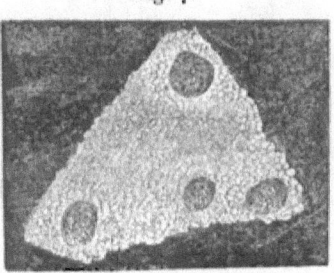

transparent, was examined, without being broken, through Amici's third glass. (Fig 7.) It appeared as if it were covered internally with innumerable small projections, hardly larger than those seen within the small single hydatids I have just described; while, at the same time, a few vesicular bodies were seen within; but whether floating in the fluid, or adhering to the sides, could not be determined.

A portion of an hydatid, about the size of a pigeon's egg, being taken so that a part of the internal surface was seen at the edge, as the membrane coiled upon itself (Fig. 10), groups of single

Fig. 10.

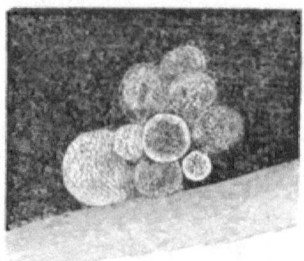

small vesicles were seen attached, almost like clusters of grapes closely set upon a branch; an appearance which I had several times an opportunity of seeing and drawing. (Figs. 11, 11 a.)

Figs. 11, 11 a.

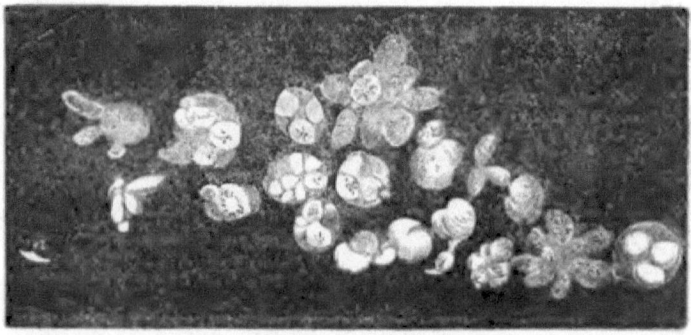

A similar portion of another hydatid being examined, it was

observed, that over a considerable part of its surface a botryoidal appearance prevailed (Fig. 8), from the elevation of oval bodies

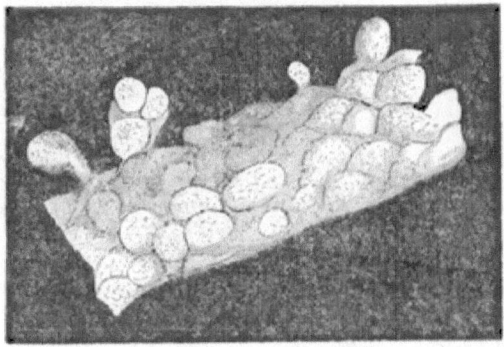

Fig. 8.

like compressed single hydatids, transparent and spotted as the other minute single hydatids had been; and some of these hemispheres projected more than the rest, either forming little clusters, or apparently attached to the surface by a footstalk formed of a portion of lining membrane drawn out from the parent hydatid: and on examining some portions of the internal surface, an appearance of a number of very minute rents and oval depressions was seen, not improbably left by the escape of hydatids from their nidus.

There is every reason to believe that the disease in this case had existed ten, or probably twelve years, before it proved fatal; for to that period could the patient trace the gradual enlargement of her abdomen. The progress of the symptoms corresponded well with the appearances discovered after death: and from the condition of the various cysts, I think we are authorised in concluding that the hydatids had first developed themselves in the liver. The disease, perfectly local in its nature, had given rise to no urgent symptoms, till the tumour pressed upon the ureters, and thus mechanically produced irritation and absorption of the kidneys; and afterwards, by its pressure on the stomach, as well as by the sympathy of the stomach with the kidneys, it interrupted the function of that organ likewise. It is difficult to say what was the cause of those faintings, peculiar sensations, and rigors, which were frequently experienced from the month of October. They might possibly have been connected with changes taking place within the cysts; and I was, at the time, inclined to consider them in that light, thinking it not improbable that something analogous to the constitutional impressions which have appeared to take place when the cysts of ovarian tumours successively burst might be thus produced: but I believe that the operations and changes of the hydatids themselves would have very little influence on the patient; it is rather those diseased actions, and that absorption, which takes place from the cavity in which the hydatid is contained, that may be looked upon as the sources of the serious and distressing symptoms which attended the concluding periods of this patient's life.

There can scarcely be on record a more instructive post-mortem examination, as regards the history of the disease; containing within itself, as has been seen, a most singular variety of the different states and conditions in which the hydatid presents itself. The four principal masses into which these were distributed each afforded its remarkable peculiarity. In the large inferior tumour, the whole economy of the hydatid was in its most flourishing and healthy state. The parent, or protecting cyst, accurately lined the cavity in which it was contained; and the numerous progeny might be supposed to exult in the uninterrupted prosperity of their prolific community, and the pellucid medium by which they were surrounded. In all the other masses, or communities, some of the accidents to which the hydatid existence is subjected, were illustrated and proved.

In the small inferior cyst, placed behind the cyst of which I have just spoken, we found the parent hydatid separated from the cavity, that cavity contracted, and the hydatids crushed by the diminution of the cavity, and exposed to the influence of the absorbents of the body.

In the large superior cyst, the hydatids had apparently multiplied till they had perished for want of space: the parent cyst had died, the cavity suppurated, and the few hydatids which remained entire were floating in a mixture of pus and the decomposing *débris* of other hydatids; and here, likewise, the absorbents seemed to have been distended by the fluid of the cyst, and probably impeded in their action.

In the fourth cavity, the secretion of the liver had insinuated itself behind the parent cyst, destroyed its vitality, forced it from its situation, and, mingling with its contents, proved a source of death and destruction to the greater part of the hydatids it contained. Thus, as I have said, does this single case illustrate many of the most important epochs and accidents which mark the progress of the hydatid.

The following case I find already detailed, somewhat at length, in the excellent volume of lectures lately published by my friend Dr. Hodgkin, who has selected it as a very illustrative example to which this affection occasionally goes; but as I had this patient frequently under my care, and was of course greatly interested in the post-mortem appearances, which afforded several varieties and modifications, I shall not hesitate to give a pretty full abstract of the notes I took at the time, though they may appear more minute than absolutely necessary for the elucidation of the subject.

CASE 2.—*Hydatids extensively occupying the abdomen.*—Edward C—, æt. 26, a dyer by trade, admitted February 22d, 1826. Has a large, firm, elastic tumour of the abdomen, which projects abruptly from the hypochondria, and soon attains its largest circumference, which, at present, measures forty-three inches, afterwards tapering downwards to about forty inches. It is not tender on pressure, and, when grasped, presents an irregular knotted surface, both above and below a margin which crosses the umbilicus, and seems to be that of the liver. The integuments of the abdomen exhibit a number of enlarged veins, running upwards, but are otherwise healthy. With this tumour he has considerable dyspnœa and cough. An attempt to lie on the back or on the left side is attended with a sense of suffocation, in consequence of which, he either sits during the night or reclines on the right side. He sleeps ill, is somewhat emaciated, complains of much weakness, and, towards evening, has a little œdema of the legs. Pulse 20, quick, and rather irregular; respiration 28, chiefly thoracic, and attended with some effort and wheezing. On percussion, the chest everywhere sounds well, except on the right side, throughout the lower half of which the sound is dull. Examined by the stethoscope, the respiration in the same region is inaudible, as likewise in the lower part of the left side, but in other parts of the chest natural. The complexion is pale; conjunctiva slightly tinged, and injected; tongue white and clammy, with reddish edges; some thirst, and little appetite, much flatulence. Small quantities of light animal food, with bread, agree best; but vegetables, liquids, or a large quantity of anything taken at a time, inflates and oppresses the stomach. The bowels are inclined to costiveness, which increases the dyspnœa. Urine reported to be scanty, high-coloured, and occasionally turbid. He can assign no other cause for his complaint than pressure of the abdomen on the edges of the vats used in dying, which, at an earlier period, apparently induced hernia in each groin. The abdominal tumour commenced, nearly three years ago, in the right hypochondrium, and has gradually grown to its present size, with the addition of the symptoms above described. He has been repeatedly a patient in Guy's, and was last week dismissed, after a year's residence in Luke's Ward; since which, the dyspnœa, cough, and flatulence have increased, and he is therefore again admitted into the hospital.

The daily observations, which were carefully made till the 16th of March, when he died, confirmed what has been already stated. The respiration was frequently embarrassed, more at one time than another, but was performed about 28 times in the minute. The pulse not unfrequently intermitted very much, and was irregular; sometimes varying, in the course of a few minutes, from 58 to 120; at other times small, weak, and indistinct, having the second beat sometimes nearly lost. The urine was scanty, high-coloured, and very turbid, and, on one occasion, of a deep mahogany colour, with a pinkish sediment, as if tinged by the purpurates. The bowels required to be frequently assisted in their action by purgatives, but the evacuations were often natural, and only on one or two occasions, and for a short time, deficient in bile. His legs, which had occasionally before been œdematous, became very much so a few days after his admission, and continued in that state as long as he survived.

Sectio cadaveris, March 17th, 1826.—Face purple; veins of neck distended; abdomen covered with marks of a network of veins, but not so much enlarged as in many cases of pressure on the cava; a great many parts of the body and thighs quite purple or lilac, as in one who has died a violent death; abdomen much distended, with the same knotty feel as during life.

On opening the abdomen, the liver was seen descending much lower than natural, having afforded that evident margin which was perceptible during life. Almost the whole lower part of the abdomen was full of rounded bodies, of the size of moderate potatoes, partially covered or intermixed with omentum, the vessels of which ramified over their surface. The small intestines were seen in the left iliac region, occupying a very small space of the whole. A large dark-coloured body was seen above them, in the left side, which looked at first like diseased spleen. On further examination, it appeared that the whole of this morbid mass was a collection of hydatids, situated in the omentum, to which they were attached, and seemed as if entangled amongst the meshes of a net. (Fig. 14.) The dark body on the left side was another of these hydatids, as large as the largest orange, casually coloured, apparently by blood, of a darker or blacker tint. The liver, though to appearance so much enlarged, was, in fact, not at all larger than usual, but was filled with hydatid cysts, some of which held at least a pint of the most limpid fluid imaginable, as pure as distilled water; and the substance of the liver was, in some parts, attenuated like a membrane. One very large hydatid occupied the right hypochondrium, and entered the substance of the liver, and one, situated just above the gall-bladder, and capable of containing at least half a pint, seemed to have opened into a biliary duct, so that it was full of a turbid yellow fluid, bearing so much the character of bile, that at first it was supposed to be the distended gall-bladder; however, on further observation, it appeared that this had been filled by one large hydatid, completely discoloured by the bile, and that the surface, from which this cyst had been detached, was scabrous and uneven, and of a dark-green colour, with black and yellow intermixed. The gall-bladder itself was found quite healthy, and not communicating with any preternatural cavity, but rather compressed by the surrounding hydatids. The semi-transparent or opalescent hydatid cysts which lined the cavities formed in the liver were very easily detached, and left a yellow semi-membranous pouch in the liver itself, quite incapable of being separated from the substance of the organ.

The cysts were most of them filled with other hydatids, almost all fully distended, floating in more or less water. In some of the cysts there were no hydatids of any size larger than millet-seeds, which either floated, almost like dust, in the water, or were attached, as frost, to the large hydatid cyst. Some of the hydatids in the omentum were much thicker than others, and, in general, the thickest appeared to contain the greater number of hydatids

Fig. 14.

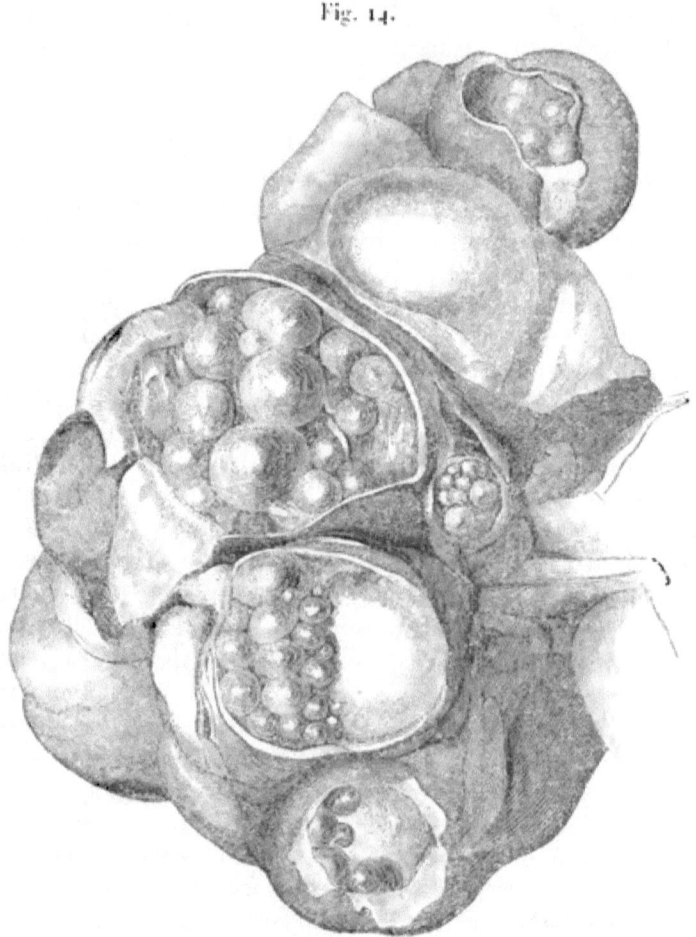

Fig. 14 represents a small portion constituting, perhaps, a twentieth part, of the large mass of hydatids which came into view when the abdomen of Edward C— (Case 2) was laid open.

The appearance of the hydatids in the omentum was that of sacs, not larger than moderate-sized potatoes; but, frequently, two, three, or four of them were found to communicate together, with a very imperfect septum between them, or only a depression in their surface; over which, in general, a vessel of the omentum was observed to pass, as if it had been in part the means of producing the form. On opening the sacs, they were found to be of a semi-cartilaginous consistence, so firm that, when completely emptied, they maintained their spherical form; and when all the hydatids had been removed, the sacs were lined with a somewhat scabrous, yellow structure, formed by an irregular coating of coagulable lymph. They were generally filled with a great number of pellucid hydatids, full of the most transparent fluid. The hydatids were of all sizes, from a pigeon's egg to a mustard-seed, spherical in shape; some of them were imbedded in the rough lining of the cartilaginous sac; and thus it appeared little pouches were sometimes formed, probably swelling afterwards into other subordinate sacs. Many, both large and small, appeared to have been burst by the pressure of the rest, so that they were squeezed quite flat; but it was remarkable that, in most of these instances, there was no fluid effused in the sac, but that it was quite full of the turgid hydatids, or the skins.

In a few instances, in which the hydatid to the right of the drawing was one, and which the space would not allow me to introduce in this figure, where a single hydatid had formed the lining of the cartilaginous sac, no others had developed themselves. In this instance, the single hydatid seemed to have been lately ruptured, and the sac was full of the water, in which the skin was seen curled up: the water contained thousands of little opaque white bodies, not much larger than sand, apparently of one shape and size, being all spherical; they were rather heavier than the water, and soon subsided to the bottom. They were not examined in a microscope, but were, probably, small hydatids.

within them; some were completely filled, and, when opened, poured forth one mass of globules, from the size of small shot to small marbles, only differing in degrees of transparency, scarcely at all in colour, except that some were quite transparent, some of an opaque white.

These numerous large cysts had forced the liver, forming one, as it did, with the cysts, very high up towards the thorax, so that the lungs only extended half way between the third and fourth ribs on the right side. In attempting to remove the liver by cutting through the diaphragm, two or three large hydatid cavities were opened. It is almost impossible to describe how the different cysts were placed in the abdomen. The spleen was surrounded and occupied, like the liver, with hydatid cysts, of the size of large oranges; two or three others had pressed upon the kidneys, particularly on the right one, so as to have completely deformed it, and produced some absorption, but, on the whole, the kidneys were rather large, and were quite healthy in structure. There were several small yellow calculi in the right, and the ureter of the left was distended, from the pressure of hydatids.

The pelvis was quite filled by two or three large hydatids, appended externally to the bladder.

The stomach was congested; and an hydatid of the size of an egg, not far from the pylorus, seemed as if it would have burst very shortly into the stomach. The small intestines were congested, but otherwise healthy. The colon was very much involved in the hydatids lying on every side in the omentum, but was itself quite healthy. The mesentery was altogether free from even any attached hydatids. The glands were slightly enlarged.

The lungs perfectly natural, but diminished in size, a few dilated air-vessels on the thin margin, on both sides extremely restricted for room—on the right by the liver, and on the left still more—by projections from the abdominal contents, and by the heart being much enlarged (probably nearly twice the natural size, but healthy in valves and structure). The lungs on neither side diseased.

The hydatids which lined the sacs in the liver and the spleen were rather opaque, as thick as wash-leather, and were very easily detached from the cavity in which they were contained, being entirely united, except by close apposition; yet their external surface, on being pulled out, was slightly shredded with lymph-like, transparent membrane. They tore easily, and had a strong tendency to curl up, whenever torn through, so that it was difficult to spread them out. Internally, they were slightly and

Fig. 12.

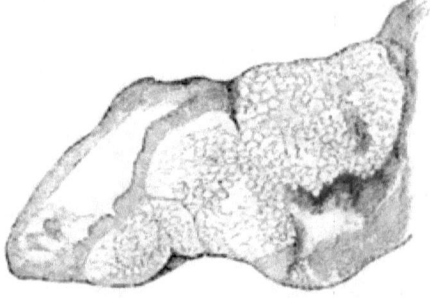

pretty evenly granulated, on every part; and in a large one, taken from the liver, a space about the size of a sixpence was very curiously marked with raised rugæ, forming semi-transparent waved lines, while in others, both small and large, irregular, but somewhat circular spots were, in two or three instances, seen, of the brightest white colour, studded with white tubercles, of the size of pins' heads (Fig. 12); and in a parent hydatid, lining a large cavity in the spleen, was a very singular mass of jelly-like substance, attached to the internal surface, and looking as if it were composed of a multiplicity of irregular transparent bodies, of the size of mustard-seeds, or larger, stuck together, so as partially to conceal their individual forms. Of this I procured a drawing (Fig. 13), and I observe that Dr. Hodgkin, speaking of this

Fig. 13.

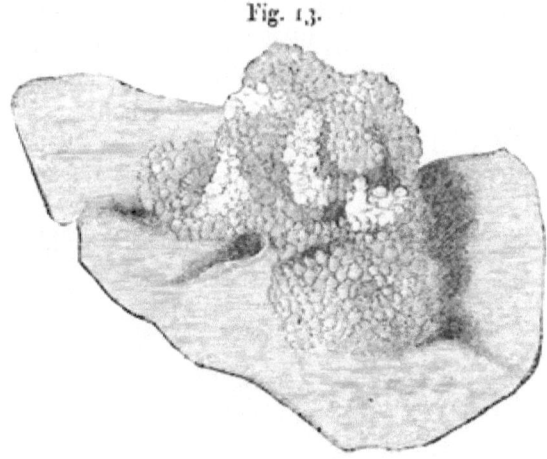

case, seems to consider these anomalous appearances in the light of diseases of the hydatids.

In the foregoing case the disease had certainly existed for several years, having begun, in all probability, in the liver; from which, at some unknown period, the hydatids had escaped into the cavity of the abdomen. The patient had distinctly observed the tumour in the right hypochondrium above three years before his death. The immediate cause of death in this case was probably connected with the very insufficient state of nourishment, which was the result of the pressure of the hydatids and their encroachment on the various organs of the abdomen, while the dilated condition of the heart favoured the tendency to internal congestion, and hastened death.

CASE 3.—*Hydatids developed in the abdomen. Death from peritonitis.*—Thomas D— was admitted, when at the age of 14, into Guy's Hospital, in June 1828; a slight-made boy, marked with the smallpox, the eldest of five children of a very poor family in the Borough. The account he gave of himself, as to the duration of his complaint, was not very satisfactory; for he stated, that he had observed nothing wrong about his abdomen till nine weeks previous to his admission, when he perceived a hard lump in the right side below the false ribs, and since that his abdomen had swollen to its present state. It was greatly enlarged; and over the whole might be felt, from the scrobiculus cordis to the pubes, a number of small round bodies, some of the size of walnuts, and others of large eggs, elastic to the feel, and scarcely leaving a doubt on our minds that they were of the hydatid character. In some instances, the projections occasioned by these bodies were sufficiently obvious to the eye; and a sketch, which was taken for me by Mr. Canton, at the time, will give a very fair idea of the appearance the abdomen presented, as the boy lay, inclining to the right side, on his bed. (See Fig. 15.) His general aspect was not unhealthy,

Fig. 15.

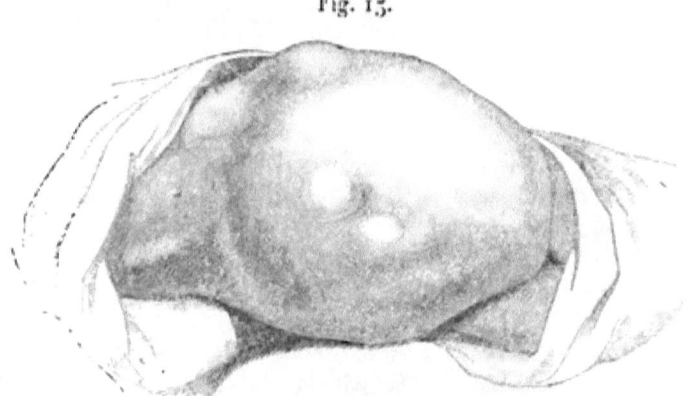

Fig. 15 represents the abdomen of Thomas D— (Case 3), as it presented itself in June, 1828, when the existence of hydatids was first discovered.

except from a certain degree of emaciation; his teeth were unusually white and regular, and his tongue clean. He experienced little or no uneasiness when pressure was made on any part of his abdomen.

He remained in the hospital several months, during which time he was generally able to go into the court-yard to walk, but suffered two or three febrile attacks, on which occasions his tongue became coated, his pulse accelerated, and the abdomen tender on pressure. On the whole, however, very little change took place, except in the gradual enlargement of the abdomen, and the general emaciation. He left the hospital after several months, and returned to his family. From that time he continued to be subject to all the hardships and irregularities to which his situation necessarily exposed him, and was chiefly employed in selling fish about the streets, in which occupation I frequently saw him, poor and miserable, but by no means so deficient in activity as might have been expected from his bulk.

On October 5th, 1836, he applied to be again admitted into the hospital. His symptoms were, at that time, those of an acute but neglected attack of peritonitis, accompanied probably by effusion into the abdomen. The fluctuation, however, was very indistinct, and the tenderness such as to preclude a very minute examination. The general size of the abdomen was greatly increased, and the surface was marked by numerous superficial veins. The lobulated form of the abdomen corresponded with the idea previously formed, that the disease depended on hydatids; but the rounded bodies were larger, and by no means so well defined or so elastic as they had been eight years previously. In two or three parts projections were obvious to the eye, and I had no doubt that one corresponded with a very prominent projection in the sketch taken on the former occasion, allowance being made for the greatly increased bulk, and consequent pushing upwards, of the whole mass. The enlargement of the abdomen had produced great dyspnœa, by the singular encroachment which had been gradually made upon the chest, as will be distinctly seen in the sketch made by Mr. Canton on this occasion. (See Fig. 16.) He survived in this state but a few days, and died on the 15th of October.

Sectio-cadaveris.—The abdomen was enormously enlarged, encroaching upon the thorax. In one part only, of small extent, was any clear or tympanitic sound elicited on percussion, and this was in the umbilical region, towards the left side, and in the left lumbar region. All the rest of the abdomen felt solid and lobulated, only slightly elastic, and was perfectly dull on percussion. The parietes adhered closely to every part of the contents of the abdomen, so that it was difficult to detach them, and one or two slight punctures of

Fig. 16.

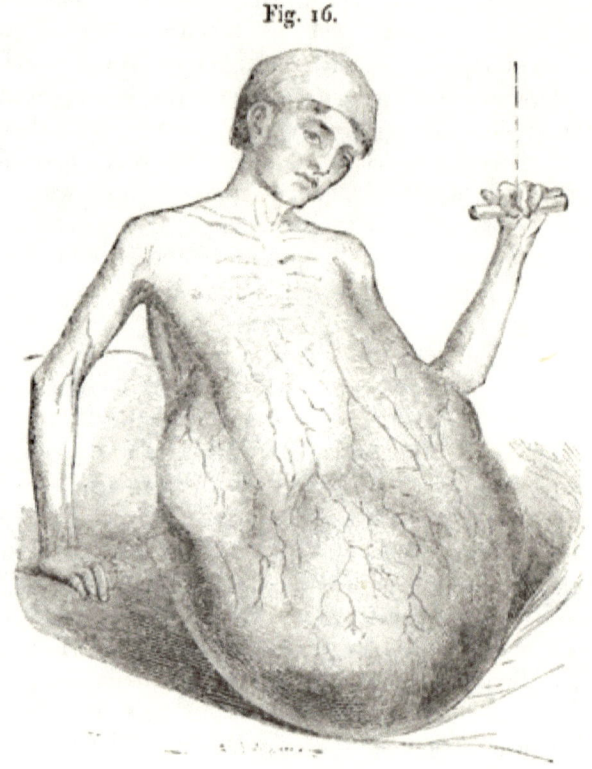

Fig. 16 represents the abdomen of Thomas D— as it presented itself in October, 1836; more than eight years after the sketch which is seen in Fig. 15 was taken.

The projecting tumour, a little below the right mamma, which contained a solitary hydatid, was believed to correspond with the lower of the two projecting tumours on the right side of the abdomen in Fig. 15.

the colon could not be avoided. When the integuments were at length carefully dissected off (Fig. 17), the whole, except the parts where the tympanitic sound had been elicited, proved to be one mass of cysts, covered with a firm dense membrane, which so closely bound them down that it looked like a large lobulated mass, rather than a collection of cysts. On opening the cysts, some of them were found to contain a solitary hydatid, having no others within it, while the greater part were full of small hydatids, presenting all the forms and peculiarities which are ever observable, and which have already been minutely described in the foregoing cases. In general, it might be remarked, that the skin and *débris* of the

Fig. 17.

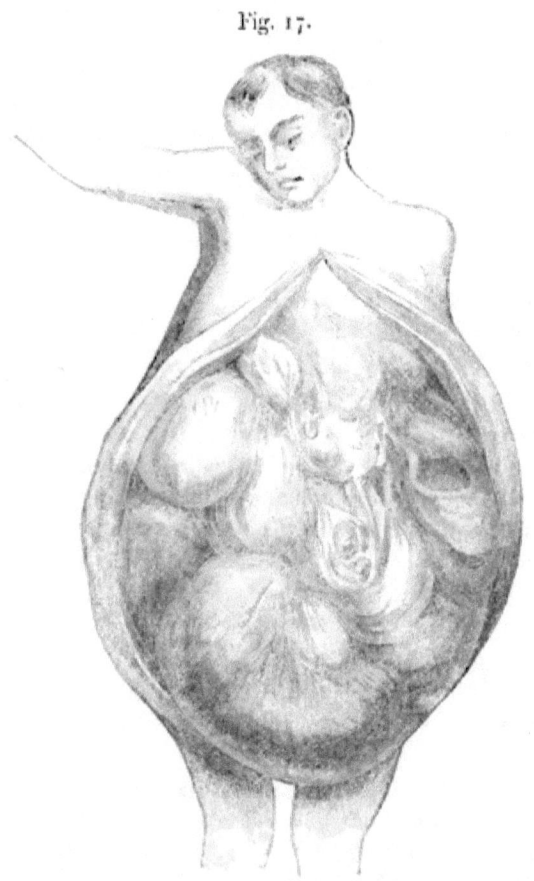

Fig. 17 represents the abdomen seen in fig. 16 laid open, and the integuments dissected carefully from the hydatids, to which the whole parieties were closely and firmly glued by thick deposits of adventitious structure. The disproportion between the abdomen and the thorax, encroached upon as it was by the disease, is very remarkable.

hydatids, which by compression had lost their vitality, bore a large proportion to those which were entire, spherical, and transparent. One particular cyst, which had been distinctly felt on the outside and had been obvious to the eye (and which I considered the same that I had observed and figured in the sketch made eight years before), contained a perfectly isolated hydatid, which formed the lining membrane of the cyst, and was filled with the most pellucid fluid. A very large cyst occupied the upper portion of the liver, and was full of hydatids, of different sizes and in various states, and another very large one, apparently communicating with the gall-bladder, was filled with a congeries of hundreds of small hydatids and innumerable broken fragments, with a large quantity of soft, broken-down biliary concretions, the whole of the contents being deeply stained with bile. One cyst encroached upon and was insinuated into the substance of the spleen, while a few smaller hydatids had apparently found their way amongst the fibres of the diaphragm, and occupied the lower part of the mediastinum.

The kidneys were healthy in structure; but the right was in a great degree absorbed, owing to the excessively distended state of its pelvis caused by the obstruction of the ureter. The bladder contained about half a pint of urine. The small intestines were found occupying the central part of the diseased mass; they had evidently been the seat of recent peritonitis, for wherever former chronic diseases had left them free, which was over a large part of their extent, they were now connected together by long bands of yellow friable lymph; there were also many flocculent tufts of fibrinous matter hanging about these portions of the peritoneum, the evident remains of former inflammation. The lungs were most exceedingly compressed, for the contents of the abdomen actually reached the second rib.

In this case, then, we have a distinct history of the disease having existed in its most characteristic form for a period little short of ten years, during which time comparatively little general derangement had been experienced; indeed, under the most unfavorable circumstances, this young man had continued to perform the avocations of life, with some interruptions, till within a few months of his death.

It seems probable, from all that can be gathered in this case, that the first development of the hydatids was in connexion with the liver; that for a period of considerable, though uncertain duration, the disease had been quite unobserved; and perhaps the attention was first called to its existence when some escape had taken place from the original seat, and probably the inflammatory action thus set up had produced the illness for which he first sought admission into the hospital. The hydatids, escaping from their original seat, soon enlarged, so as to be plainly felt over the whole abdomen, as round, well-defined, elastic tumours, although he clearly stated that nine weeks previously he had discerned nothing but the enlargement in the right hypochondrium. The hydatids thus poured out became fixed by inflammation in the various parts of the abdomen where they first lodged, and, according as they were single, or capable of multiplication, they remained either like simple sacs—as in one case, on the right side of the abdomen, was very well marked—or they became the source of those congeries of hydatids which were found in several parts; and the whole of them, owing to the repeated processes of inflammatory action to which they had given rise in the omentum and peritoneum, had changed their distinct elastic character for the more hard, lobulated, botryoidal substance discoverable by examination on his last admission. It was quite evident that the immediate cause of death was an extensive but accidental inflammation of the peritoneum, chiefly in those parts, amidst the convolutions of the small intestines, which had escaped the effects of chronic attacks and the gluing of adhesive inflammation, but it is very greatly to be doubted whether the disease in this case had not advanced almost to its natural or necessary termination, seeing that it had already greatly encroached upon the thorax, and compressed the lungs to such a degree that certainly these organs were no longer able to admit one fourth of the air requisite for the healthful discharge of the function of respiration.

There is one point deserving of remark in this and the two preceding cases. In each of them, but particularly the two last, it would appear probable, as I have said, that the hydatids were at first confined to the liver, but that, from some cause, they became diffused into the abdominal cavity; and yet it is observable that none of these bodies seem to have effected a lodgment, or to have been developed amongst the duplications of the mesentery and the convolutions of the intestines, and thus they have offered comparatively little interference to the peristaltic motions and the general functions of the alimentary canal. It is probable that the immediate cause of this immunity is the close apposition of the convolutions, and the tendency which the intestinal motions may have to propel the little bodies forward, but in the pelvis, particularly behind the bladder, where a good opportunity of lodgment is afforded, we often meet with the hydatid cysts.

Case 4.—*Tumour of the abdomen supposed to depend on the presence of hydatids.*—E—, æt. 42, a weaver, was admitted into the hospital, April 4th, 1832, on account of a great enlargement of the abdomen, under the care of Dr. Back, who afforded me an opportunity of examining the tumour very carefully. It appeared that the swelling was of a very irregular character, occupying the upper part of the abdomen, and that just below each hypochondrium a round, soft, and elastic projection was discoverable. The projection on the right side was the larger, and proceeded from immediately below the margin of the ribs, and, though it could not be traced decidedly under them, might well be supposed to arise from the liver. According to the statement of the patient, these two had been preceded by one or two nearer to the centre, and towards the umbilicus, which had appeared to disperse and move a little more to the right; but statements of this kind are always so doubtful, that little confidence can be placed in them. There was an umbilical hernia, of the size of a small egg, and several enlarged subcutaneous veins were seen passing longitudinally up the abdomen. In a sketch I made, a line, passing somewhat irregularly across the body, half way between the umbilicus and the pubes, had the whole tumour above it. He stated that, occasionally, when he neglected his bowels, his ancles swelled, but otherwise they did not. The motions were rather pale, and the urine high coloured. His own statement of the progress of the disease was, that about six years before he had a severe illness, which he believed to be scarlatina, and at that time his abdomen was enlarged. After about three months of active treatment, he became better; and though never quite well, he continued in tolerable health till three years ago, when his abdomen swelled, and a year after he first perceived the unequal tumours of which the swelling is now composed. He has never been decidedly ill in his feelings, nor has he been jaundiced. His eyes are clear and bright, and he has no pain on pressure of the abdomen, but the enlargement is such as to prevent his getting into the loom, on which he has always depended for his livelihood.

The extent of this irregular and lobulated tumescence, its being almost confined to the upper part of the abdomen, and the absence of that obvious fluctuation which could not fail to be present were so large an increase of the size to depend on fluid, distinguished this case from ascites, and its slow progress, together with the slightness of the constitutional derangement, rendered it very improbable that it should be a malignant growth. The inference therefore is, that it is a case of hydatids, which has now been at least three years in its progress.

CASE 5.—*Hydatid cyst connected with the liver. Death from suppuration of the sac and its consequences.*—Sarah T—, æt. 42, admitted into Guy's Hospital, March 25th, 1829, rather a bulky woman, with a dark sallow complexion. She states that, during the last twelve years, she has been at least twelve times the subject of jaundice; that about six weeks ago she became again suddenly jaundiced, and continued so for ten days, the stools being perfectly white, and the urine bilious. Three weeks ago, when the jaundice had gone off, she suffered a severe rigor, of four hours' continuance, and has not since recovered. At present, her pulse is 84, and sharp; tongue moist, but covered with a brown fur. There is great appearance of prostration, the bowels are relaxed, and the stools of a very dark colour. There is a tumour at the pit of the stomach, extending almost to the umbilicus, tender on pressure, elastic to the feel, and appearing to have a solid base. This tumour she says has been observed for three or four years, appearing larger or smaller, according to the degree of distension of the stomach.

The symptoms went on increasing; the sickness became more urgent; the tongue more dry and red at the edges; the abdomen more tender. On the 30th, she passed blood, by stool, two or three times, and falling into a state of insensibility, remained so about twenty-four hours, when she died.

Sectio cadaveris.—The tumour was very evident, projecting at the scrobiculus cordis. There was a considerable accumulation of yellow adipose matter in the integuments. The parietes of the abdomen were attached very firmly by old adhesions to the tumour, which occupied chiefly the right lobe of the liver; the tumour was of a membranous appearance and vascular, and contained nearly a washhand-basin full of hydatids, of all sizes, from that of a French walnut to a pea, but chiefly of about the size of a hazel-nut. The greater number were burst and opaque, but many retained their globular form. The fluid in which they were closely impacted was puriform, and the parietes of the large cavity were lined internally with a layer of thick pus-like matter, with shreds and cakes of a cheesy substance, adhering closely. The cyst itself, owing to the suppuration that was going on, had assumed a worm-eaten appearance.

The liver seemed healthy, but was thrown out of its shape by the large cyst, which had likewise encroached upon the thorax. The gall-bladder contained about an ounce and a half of yellow fluid, almost entirely mucus, with a slight bilious tinge. The whole peritoneal surface of the abdomen showed marks of severe recent inflammation, having on it shreds of yellow lymph and a considerable quantity of puriform serum. The intestines were highly vascular.

With regard to the hydatids themselves, they differed in no respect from what have been already described; many of them had a number of small holes within them, and some of them presented that peculiar appearance of the inner surface which resembles a heap of transparent granulations arising from their inner surface, such as is represented in Fig. 13.

In this case there can be no doubt that the irritation produced in the system by the unhealthy suppuration going on in the cyst, and afterwards the diffused inflammation of the peritoneum, were the immediate causes of death. The strong adhesions which subsisted between the cyst and the parietes suggest the probability that, had this cavity been evacuated by an operation before the inflammation had been set up, the result might possibly have been favorable. But the time when such an operation could have been useful must have been long antecedent to her admission into the hospital, before her system had suffered from the slow suppuration of the sac, and still more, before this general peritoneal inflammation was set up, which, from the actively vascular appearance of the tumour, was, no doubt, a consequence of the local disease.

CASE 6.—*Hydatid cysts in the liver ossified.*—Lydia S— was admitted into Guy's Hospital, October 8th, 1813, labouring under slight jaundice and mania. It appeared that constipation of the bowels, attended with sickness and pain, had occurred about ten days before, and that two or three days after jaundice came on, with occasional derangement of the intellect, which had been constant for the last two days. She frequently lay in a state of insensibility, approaching to coma; at other times she was raving in mania; her motions were very dark. She died on the 16th.

The liver was found to contain hydatid cysts, of which one, about the size of an orange, was completely ossified throughout more than half its extent; and there were two or three smaller ones imbedded in the liver, which were not larger than a pea, but were also ossified, and all of them were filled with the remnants of hydatids pressed together, and in some parts the convoluted laminæ were capable of being separated and unrolled. The dura mater was in this case spotted over its whole internal surface with a great number of bloody points from ruptured vessels.

In each of the two following cases the only hydatid cyst which was discovered had developed itself in the space between the bladder and the rectum.

CASE 7.—*Tumour in the pubic region from an hydatid cyst situated behind the bladder.*—W. S——, æt. 54, was admitted into Guy's Hospital, labouring under serous effusion, with dyspnœa, and coagulable urine. He died after remaining in the hospital some weeks; and on examining the body a tumour was found, about the size of a very large orange, situated between the bladder and the rectum, so that it had pushed the bladder forwards, and, together with the bladder, presented a projection which was quite obvious before the abdomen was laid open. This proved to be a cyst, containing a number of hydatids about the size of marbles and smaller, with a large collection of the broken remnants of other hydatids. The cyst was in some parts nearly a quarter of an inch in thickness, and internally many patches of bony matter had been deposited; grasped in the hand it gave, when emptied, the elastic feel of an India-rubber bottle. The mucous membrane of the bladder was quite free from any inflammation. The rectum was a little irritated. The kidneys were rather small, their tunics adhered firmly, their external surface was coarse and granulated, and they were not easily broken down by pressure.

Another case had previously come to my knowledge of a very similar character; and as I was present at the post-mortem examination, and I believe the preparation is in the Museum at Guy's, I will state the facts nearly as I collected them.

CASE 8.—*Tumour in the pubic region from an hydatid cyst situated behind the bladder.*—The patient, who had been labouring under other disease, complained of the difficulty he had in retaining his water; and when an examination was made, it appeared that the urine was continually passing away, and that a tumour bearing all the characteristics of a distended bladder presented itself at the pubic region. This at once suggested the idea that the patient was suffering from retention of urine produced by enlarged prostate or some such mechanical cause. A catheter was introduced by a skilful surgeon, and a few drachms of perfectly healthy urine drawn off, without producing any diminution in the bulk of the tumour. As it was still supposed that urine was retained, more than one medical man attempted to draw it off, and at length the catheter became obstructed by the passing of small hydatids. When this was discovered a sucking-pump was applied to the catheter, and thus a considerable quantity of the *débris* of hydatids were removed; however, the symptoms of this disease remained, his other complaints increased, and ultimately the patient died.

Sectio cadaveris.—The tumour which appeared on opening the body, filling the whole pubic region, proved to be a large hydatid cyst, attached to the posterior part and the fundus of the bladder, and pressing so much forwards as to prevent entirely the bladder from being filled with urine; and this was the source at once of the tumour and of the constant escape of urine. The bladder itself was quite healthy, nor had the catheter passed through it to reach hydatid cyst, but on the contrary, had passed by an opening from the urethra behind the bladder. The cyst which contained the hydatids was in some parts about one sixth of an inch in thickness, and irregularly converted into a cartilaginous substance, with a rough internal surface. It contained at least a quart of the shreds of burst hydatids, with a few of the size of small marbles, which were quite perfect and transparent, the whole contents being of the thickness and consistence of a paste. The tumour made pressure on the orifices of both the ureters, which were consequently very much distended with urine; and the pressure which had been made upon the kidneys by the fulness of the pelves had produced a very extensive absorption of the substance of both. The fluid contained in the ureters was puriform, and there were some small clots of blood in the infundibula.

In cases of so doubtful a kind we might derive diagnostic marks from the history of the tumour, if the patient had sufficient intelligence to assist us in the inquiry; so likewise from the feel of it, which would probably be harder or less regular than the bladder, but on this no perfect reliance could be placed. The character of the urine which is drawn off would almost be sufficient to decide the question, for if the urine be retained any time in the bladder, it generally acquires a much darker hue, and all its sensible properties at once bespeak that it has been long secreted and concentrated or altered by retention.

CASE 9.—*Hydatid cyst connected with the liver, emptied by paracentesis.*—M. H— was admitted into Guy's Hospital with a large fluctuating tumour of the abdomen, occupying apparently almost the whole cavity. As she suffered much, both from constitutional irritation and from the pressure of this tumour, Dr. Cholmely, whose patient she was, thought it right to draw off the fluid by tapping, and a very large quantity of purulent fluid, mingled with shreds and portions of hydatids, came away. It was now discovered that she was pregnant, a circumstance which she had concealed. By perfect quiet she recovered somewhat after the operation, but, after two or three weeks, miscarried. Her bowels became obstinately costive, she had frequent vomiting, became deeply jaundiced, was unable to take any food, and died completely exhausted.

Sectio cadaveris.—A large cyst was found arising from the liver, descending quite to the pubes, adhering to the parietes of the abdomen on the whole of the right side and making pressure on the kidney. This cyst arose as high as the diaphragm, and had pushed all the intestines back into the left lumbar and iliac spaces, so that they did not occupy one third of the abdominal cavity; the stomach had likewise been completely displaced by its pressure. This cyst still contained about three pints of greenish-yellow pus, and a large quantity of the skins and remains of hydatids, but not one could be found in its entire or globular form. The cyst itself, which was of considerable thickness, was internally undergoing a process of suppurative softening, and was pulpy and irregular on its surface. The upper part of it near the diaphragm, where it seemed to have originated in the substance of the liver, contained a curd-like matter, almost cheesy in its consistence, apparently a mass of fibrine, pus, and the shreds of hydatids.

Exactly in the seat of a femoral hernia there was a small tumour, of the size of two large marbles, which proved to be a cyst, containing a number of hydatids.

The liver was soft throughout, and the left lobe very large, extending far towards the left side. The gall-bladder was much distended with bright green bile, and the obstruction to the passage down the ducts had probably been the cause of the deep jaundice which had occurred before death. The right kidney was to a great extent absorbed by the pressure of the tumour, and the pelvis much enlarged, containing some calculi. The left kidney was unusually large. The uterus was large, and imperfectly contracted; the ovaries were unhealthy, with vesicles.

In this case I am unable to say how long the disease had existed, but there could be no doubt, from the great extent of the cyst, and what we know of the general progress of such cases, that many years had elapsed; and as it had gradually encroached upon the right lobe of the liver and the liver and the right kidney, it was curious to observe the apparent compensation which had been established by the unusual increase of the left lobe of the liver and of the left kidney. In this case the inflammation and suppuration set up in the cyst seems to have been quite destructive of the organization and the validity of the hydatids, none of which were found in their globular and unbroken state.

CASE 10.—*Hydatid connected with the liver emptied, by paracentesis, with success.*—A young woman was admitted into Guy's Hospital, in December, 1828, under the care of Mr. Key, with an elastic swelling occupying almost the whole scrobiculus cordis, and inclining rather to the left side; it was not the least discoloured, and gave an evident sense of fluctuation. The swelling was divided into two lobes, of which that to the left was the largest, and the fluid seemed to pass from one to the other. Her health did not suffer; but of late the tumour had become rather painful, and, by its bulk, had interfered considerably with her comfort, having enlarged much more rapidly than when first perceived. She had been in the hospital two years before, when Mr. Key attempted without success to make an opening gradually by a caustic issue; he now thought it right to employ a small trochar; and, accordingly, on the 22d of December, four pints of a perfectly limpid fluid, with little or no smell, nor any appearance of lymph, shreds, or flocculent matter were drawn off. The operation afforded her great ease, and was followed by no symptoms of inflammation. For a time the cyst appeared to fill gradually; she lost her colour, and had frequent tendency to faint, and afterwards a little diarrhœa came on, which, however, was easily checked.

February 5th.—The tumour, though it has not entirely disappeared, is much less than before the operation, and presents no unequal or lobulated swelling, as it formerly did, but gives a slight appearance of fulness to the scrobiculus cordis.

Towards the end of the month she left the hospital: and I have heard from Mr. Key, within these few days, that she remains perfectly well, has since married, and enjoys excellent health, without any reaccumulation having taken place.

I examined the fluid very carefully, by means of Dr. Roget's microscope; but could detect nothing like minute hydatids, or other foreign matter. Mr. Key also allowed me to put a portion of it into the hands of Dr. Bostock, who was kind enough to undertake its analysis; and I shall give the communication I received from him a few days ago; observing, that, in one point, his account differs from what I find stated in my notes; the fluid having apparently lost a little of its pure and limpid character, when he undertook the investigation.

"My dear Sir,—I have revised my note-book, which contains the account of the experiments that were performed on the fluid from the hydatid, in December, 1828; and I have extracted what appear to be the most remarkable or characteristic circumstances respecting it. If you require any further explanation, on any of the points connected with the experiments, I shall be most happy to furnish you with it, as far as lies in my power.

"Most truly yours,
J. Bostock.

"Putney Heath; Aug. 28th, 1837.

"The fluid was homogeneous, somewhat opaque, of a light-brown colour; it had a slight but peculiar acrid odour, and a specific gravity of 1008. It scarcely affected the most delicate test-papers;

the uncombined alkali, if any, being in so minute a quantity, that one part of the acetic acid of the Pharmacopœia, added to 100 parts of the fluid, caused it to redden litmus. There was, however, a perceptible, although very slight, indication of alkalescence, when it was evaporated to one tenth of its bulk; a portion of it, also, became slightly alkaline, after being exposed for about three weeks to the atmosphere; at the same time, it had acquired a sharp, acrid odour, and was covered with a very thin, brown film; the fluid was somewhat more opaque and coloured, but there was no sediment. It was not affected by the boiling temperature; and the reagents for albumen indicated the presence of this substance in a minute quantity only. When evaporated by a heat not exceeding 150°, a residuum was obtained of 1·25 per cent., which evidently consisted, for the most part, of muriate of soda. Along with this there was a portion of an animal substance; which was soluble both in water and in alcohol, and which I should characterise as nearly related to the substance which forms the specific ingredient in the serosity of the blood. There were also indications of the presence of sulphuric acid and potash, but each of them in very minute quantity. No lime could be detected in it. It appears, therefore, that this fluid exhibited some decided peculiarities, when compared with other fluids which may be presumed to have a similar origin: 1. The absence, or at least the very minute quantity, of uncombined alkali. 2. The small quantity of albumen, compared with the total amount of solid contents. 3. The presence of a considerable quantity of extractive matter; and, 4. The large proportion of the muriate of soda which it contained. The composition of the fluid may be estimated as follows, in 1000 parts:

" Water . . . . 987·5
  Extractive, with a trace of albumen . . . 4·
  Muriate of soda, with minute quantities of sulphuric acid
    and potash . . . . . . 8·5
                                                         ———
                                                         1000·0"

CASE II.—*Hydatids in the spleen bursting into the abdomen, and causing death very speedily.*—In the month of February, 1821, a patient in Guy's Hospital, who had been under the care of Dr. Back, with obvious hepatic derangement, and a large tumour in the abdomen, became suddenly most alarmingly ill, and died within half an hour. On a post-mortem examination, it appeared that the immediate cause of death was the bursting of a large hydatid in the spleen, by which at least a pint of limpid fluid had been effused into the abdomen. The appearance of this large hydatid was rather peculiar; as it entered so much into the substance of the spleen, that over nearly half the cyst that viscus formed an external coat, gradually dying away into a tough leather-like substance, which formed the more protruding part of the membrane covering the hydatid, and which, in the present case, seemed to consist of a thickened portion of the peritoneum. Within this was situated the true hydatid cyst, like a lining of soft leather, having its external surface marked by numerous projections, which fitted into little cavities in the spleen—an appearance which probably depended on the cellular structure of the viscus which the hydatid occupied. The internal surface was smooth, as if covered with a thin transparent membrane. In the liver there was an hydatid, of the same size as that of the spleen; and there were smaller cysts in the kidneys. These hydatids were, as far as I remember—and the notes I made at the time do not contradict it—each formed of a single unproductive cyst.

CASE 12.—*Hydatid of the liver, suppurating and bursting into the abdomen, causing immediate death.*—In the year 1813, when I was attending the practice of the Bishop's-Court Dispensary, a very interesting case occurred, the hydatids taken from which I had a long time in my possession. Not being able to find the notes which I took on the occasion, I have applied to my excellent friend Dr. Laird, who during many years discharged the duties of physician to the institution at which the case occurred, and those of physician to Guy's Hospital, with singular diligence and success; and I shall give the case in his own words.

"Bognor, August 30th, 1837.

"I perfectly remember the patient to whose case you refer; and the interest you took in the examination, which you had the kindness to undertake at my request. But I think his death must have occurred in 1813; rather than in 1814, as you suppose.

"The patient was about five or six and twenty years of age, and was employed in the shop of Messrs. Laurie and Whittle, the mapsellers in Fleet Street, contiguous to whose premises he had fixed himself, on the west side of Fetter Lane. He suffered under obvious inflammation of the liver, attended with jaundice, indicating that the parenchymatous substance of the liver was affected. He was, at first, so much benefited by what was done for him, that I hoped a favorable issue in the case; but a visit which he most imprudently made to some friends at Vauxhall was immediately followed by a sad aggravation of his complaint; which then rapidly passed to its fatal termination in a few weeks, not more than two or three, to the best of my recollection. His death took place suddenly, on his getting out of bed; and I was the more anxious to know the immediate cause of death, because I had previously found, by a post-mortem examination, that the bursting of hepatic abscess had been followed by immediate failure of the vital energies. You will doubtless remember, in our Dispensary case, that you were obliged to remove much purulent effusion from between the folds of the intestines, I think to the amount of two or three pints, in order to follow your inquiry; and that a great number of small hydatids were found floating in the fluid. The source of this effusion you found in a ruptured cyst on the convex surface of the right lobe, the capacity of which must have been very great. In the left lobe there were several small independent abscesses; but I do not remember any appearance of hydatid origin in them. There was no appearance of recent inflammation in the peritoneum, death having so quickly followed the rupture of the cyst; the other viscera of the abdomen were, I think, in a healthy condition, as were those of the thorax."

In these two cases we find the sudden rupture of an hydatid cyst causing immediate death. There is every reason to believe, as I have before stated, that, under certain circumstances, the rupture of the cyst and the escape of the hydatid into the abdominal cavity is not followed by a fatal result; but where it happens suddenly, and by a large opening, we cannot but apprehend either immediate death or the occurrence of peritoneal inflammation. It is, however, no doubt, where suppuration has already gone on within the cyst, as in the last case, that we are to expect the more dangerous effects, both from the previous state of the constitution and from the condition of the part, as well as from the more irritating character of the fluid thrown into the abdominal cavity. In the following case it is believed that a large cyst burst suddenly into the abdomen, without being followed by a fatal result.

CASE 13.—*Supposed hydatid of the liver bursting into the cavity of the abdomen.*—June 13th, 1836. — —, a boy, æt. 14 years, was admitted into Barnabas Ward, under Dr. Addison, with the chest quite deformed by the protrusion of the lower ribs of the right side; but more particularly by the entire displacement of the false ribs, affording a sense of elasticity and almost of fluctuation in that part. At the same time the liver was pushed below its usual position, so that its margin was to be felt far down in the abdomen, below the umbilicus.

It appeared most probable from the projecting form of the tumour—from the way in which the false ribs were raised, and the degree in which, at the same time, the liver was pushed down, while the respiration was quite natural on that side of the chest—that the disease was situated below the diaphragm. At the same time, the absence of many symptoms and the want of any decided tendency to jaundice led to a belief that it was not an abscess of the liver; and it was therefore inferred as highly probable that the enlargement arose from an hydatid cyst situated in the convex surface of that organ.

His condition scarcely underwent any change while he remained in the hospital; and after staying about a couple of months he left it, and returned to his friends, who were in circumstances to maintain him comfortably. In the latter part of August he suffered from hæmorrhage, after having a tooth drawn; and while recovering from this, in the beginning of October, he was attacked with severe pain in the swelling of the right side, and was very ill for several days, but recovered from that attack; and in the middle of the same month he applied as an out-patient at the hospital. Till the 25th of October the fluctuation remained the same, and the swelling increased a little; but on rising from his bed on that morning he had a feeling of faintness, with a sudden sinking and a peculiar motion, as he stated, in the tumour, which from that time greatly diminished in bulk, giving the conviction to those who had seen him most, that the contents of the supposed hydatid tumour had escaped into the abdomen, without, however, producing any unpleasant symptom, except, perhaps, a little sickness at the stomach.

October 26th.—I saw him at his own house: the tumour had subsided; but there was evident fulness and fluctuation at the pubic region and below the umbilicus. He had taken two or three doses of calomel, followed by sulphate of magnesia; and had passed a tolerably healthy loose dejection. He had experienced a little pain that afternoon in the lower part of the abdomen, but very little tenderness. His chief pain was in the act of passing urine, as if from the contraction of the bladder. Pulse about 140, sharp; tongue slightly furred; countenance flushed.

27th.—No bad symptoms; bowels freely opened by the calomel, of which he had taken two grains three times a day, since the 25th. Pulse 120; no sickness; no tension of the abdomen.

28th.—I examined the abdomen very carefully, and found the margin of the liver much raised above its former position, descending only half-way to the umbilicus, and not apparently adhering to the diaphragm. The fluctuation at the lower part of the abdomen was diminished; there was neither tenderness nor pain. Bowels well open; he had scarcely moved from the same recumbent position, and had eaten nothing but a little gruel each day. Pulse 96. The ribs still bulged a little on the right side.

Rep. Pil. Hydrarg., gr. iij. Ext. Conii, gr. iij, bis die.

Mr. King, who observed this case very attentively from the first, has just now informed me that he soon began to manifest signs of amendment, to sit up, and to take food; and not long after, it was evident that the fluid in the peritoneum was decreasing in quantity. At that time, the displacement of the ribs was still great, and there was a considerable lateral curvature of the spinal column. He continued for some months in a very emaciated state. His present condition (September 7th, 1837), Mr. King says, is decidedly good. He is by no means thin, has some natural colour; the spine is straight; the abdomen not full, and the thorax is almost symmetrical.

He works for a printer; and has no complaint but that of a painful weakness in the left knee, which, as well as the right, seems to fall inwards, more than it has been wont to do.

If, instead of discharging into the peritoneal sac, the hydatids fortunately escape from the body, the event is occasionally favorable; though, as the organs through which the hydatids pass are liable to be inflamed and irritated, such a discharge may, at last, lead but to a more protracted fatal disease.

In the first volume of this work a case is related, which occurred under my care in the clinical ward, where an hydatid cyst in the liver opened into the lung; and a considerable number of the hydatids, mingled with bile, were evacuated, in their collapsed state, by expectoration; the patient ultimately doing quite well, and leaving the hospital without any obvious remnant of the disease.

Another case, almost precisely similar, has been stated to me by Dr. Babington, as occurring many years ago, under his observation, in the practice of his father. In that case it likewise happened to a young woman, who, after suffering a considerable time from symptoms of very serious hepatic derangement, with cough, began to expectorate hydatids, which she brought up to the number of several hundreds, and many of them unbroken; they were yellow, and deeply tinged with bile, leaving no doubt of their hepatic origin. After going on for some time, this expectoration ceased, and the young woman recovered completely.

CASE 14.—*Hydatids in the liver, supposed to have passed off by the intestines.*—In the spring of the year 1824, I was consulted by a shoemaker, about fifty years of age, whose abdomen was enlarged, almost like that of a man labouring under ascites, and the superficial veins were distended to a great size. On examining the abdomen more attentively with the hand, it appeared that a tumour, fixed in the right hypochondrium, occupied the whole of the right side of the abdomen, passing considerably beyond the linea alba, so as to encroach upon the left side also. To all appearance, this tumour was connected with the liver; it was elastic, and pretty smooth, though it varied in its hardness in different parts. He represented himself as having never possessed a very strong constitution, but having lived so temperate a life, that he was never but once intoxicated; he had always been able to work hard at his trade. About a year and a half ago, he had begun to feel out of health, with lassitude and drowsiness. About a year ago, while walking along, he was suddenly seized with a very acute pain in the right hypochondriac region; which lasted, in spite of remedies, for a few days, and then subsided gradually, leaving a dull, aching pain; and at that time he first perceived the enlargement, which had continued to increase to the present time, when his general health was beginning to suffer, and his respiration to be impeded. He was put upon a course of taraxacum and soda, and the camphorated mercurial ointment rubbed upon the abdomen till the gums were affected. In the month of July, three or four months after his first application, he was seized with a fit of vomiting, in which he brought up half a pint of what he called "matter;" and shortly after, passed, by stool, a large quantity of what, from his description, could have been nothing but hydatids: some were only skins or cysts, but others were full and round. This evacuation was attended with an immediate subsidence of the tumour; and when I saw him, on the 8th of August, the swelling had not increased again, and was very inconsiderable in comparison with what it was at first, though it was still to be partially detected.

It occasionally happens that hydatid cysts approach so near the surface, that, inflammation taking place, they discharge themselves externally; the result of which may be favorable or not, according to circumstances. I remember, some years ago, being taken by Dr. Stroud to visit a female, in whom, judging from her own minute account, this had taken place several years previously; but though one cyst had probably discharged in this way, her abdomen was still the seat of tumours, which had all the characters of hydatid cysts. The following case, however, in which there can be no doubt of the fact, was communicated to me by Dr. Babington; and I shall state it in his own words.

CASE 15.—*Hydatid cyst in the liver, discharging itself externally; and death from hæmorrhage.*—"It was during an attendance, two and a half years ago, on some other patient, with my friend, Mr. May, of Bow Lane, that he requested me to see Mrs. R—, a poor woman, whom he represented as labouring under visceral disease of a remarkable character. I found her in bed, much weakened by sickness and dyspepsia. Her skin was of a deep-yellow hue; and her secretions sufficiently demonstrated an obstruction to the natural course of the bile. This state of jaundice was described to have existed for many months. On examining the abdomen, a hard tumour, irregular in figure, and rising into roundish masses, was felt on the right ride, issuing from beneath the ribs, and extending to the pit of the stomach. Thus there seemed every reason for supposing an enlargement of the liver; but its precise boundaries could not easily be traced, in consequence of a further enlargement of the rest of the abdomen, dependent on an advanced state of pregnancy. In the tumour first mentioned there was no fluctuation. The whole presented a firm, solid growth, free from pain; and the symptoms to which its presence gave rise, were such as might proceed from any cause of hepatic obstruction. From time to time I learned from Mr. May the state of his patient. She gave birth to a healthy child; which she was able to suckle, notwithstanding her permanently jaundiced condition; and I may remark, by the way, that neither the skin of the child nor the mother's milk was in the slightest degree tinged with bile. Her general health must, indeed, have materially improved; for she again became pregnant, went her full time, and bore a living infant. After her first confinement, when I took an opportunity of examining her, the tumour was more distinct and larger than before; and I was subsequently informed that it continued to increase in size. In the beginning of December last, Mr. May again requested me to see Mrs. R——; and informed me, that, a day or two before, the parietes of the abdomen had spontaneously given way, and an enormous discharge of fluid had issued from the aperture. On removing a poultice and bandage, which had been subsequently applied, I found an ulcerated opening, rather less than an inch in length, situated immediately below the umbilicus. From this opening a portion of what, at first view, bore a general resemblance to intestine, protruded about half an inch. On closer examination, its collapsed and puckered form, its total insensibility, and its greater thickness, led to a belief that it was the empty cyst of an hydatid; and, by gradual and gentle traction, I succeeded in bringing it away. The part which passed last was thinner, and more gelatinous in appearance, than the rest; and was torn in coming out. The whole was nearly as large as a bullock's bladder; and would probably have contained, previously to its rupture, a gallon and a half of fluid. No pain was felt during its abstraction; and the patient expressed herself as relieved by its removal. We saw her on the following day, and found that she had passed a good night. A second cyst now presented itself at the aperture; but as it seemed, on gentle traction, to be adherent, no force was used to withdraw it. The bandage with which the abdomen had been bound was soaked by a constant drainage of serous fluid. On the day following my second visit, blood, instead of serum, began to make its appearance; and this was accompanied by such a degree of prostration, rigor, and faintness, as led to the apprehension that some serious internal hæmorrhage was taking place. This was verified, as the day advanced, by more alarming seizures of syncope; and one of these proved fatal, in the course of the night. That hydatids had caused all the mischief in this case, was demonstrated during life; and an examination, after death, proved that one of these had formed in the interior of the liver, near its under surface; forcing, as it grew, the substance of that organ upwards and forwards, and its posterior peritoneal coat backwards. A large cavity, lined with a false membrane, and filled with grumous blood, was found thus bounded. A second hydatid, the cyst of which remained, seemed to have occupied a portion of the same cavity; and a third, about the size of a walnut, appeared on the convex surface of the right lobe. Mr. King, of Guy's Hospital, has, I understand, succeeded in finding the mouth of an hepatic vein, whence the fatal hæmorrhage had its source. Mrs. R—'s age was about thirty-five. The tumour which caused her death was first observed by Mr. May, in March, 1833; and she died on the 9th of December, 1836."

I have thus brought together fifteen cases, occurring chiefly under my own observation; in most of which the existence of hydatids, in immediate connexion with the cavity of the abdomen, has been placed beyond a doubt, either by their discharge during life, or by examination after death; and they may be considered as forming a series, which includes a fair view, not only of the general history, progress, and result of such cases, but likewise of most of the particular facts, occurrences, and accidents which may be expected to present themselves to the practitioner during their course.

The history of this disease, when viewed attentively, is curious and interesting. The little hydatid first introduced, or generated in the structure of the human body, gradually increases in size; producing by its pressure, displacement and absorption of the surrounding parts; and leading to the deposit of lymph, and the gradual formation of a cyst, in which it becomes, as it were, insulated, interfering only by its bulk with the processes of the system. In some instances, it would appear that the principle of reproduction is not possessed by the individual hydatid; but, more generally, an indefinite multiplication takes place; and the new progeny may be traced arising again from the internal surface of many of the secondary and successive hydatids, and gradually increasing in size till they burst the cysts in which they have been generated. It is, however, remarkable, that while some, which have arrived at a very considerable size, still only appear to be producing the smallest offsets, others, when they seem but just to have separated from the internal surface of the parent, are pregnant with a new progeny, bearing so large a proportion to the whole dimensions of this young parent cyst, that they are already prepared to dilate it, or to escape from it, and mingle with those which float in the fluid contained within the older hydatid.

The first parent cyst, which now forms a lining to the cavity it has made for itself in the tissues of the body, continues to increase; but in vain can that increase be expected to keep pace with the internal multiplication of its offspring, which, pressing upon each other, are ruptured; and the fluid which escapes seems to form a pabulum for those which still retain entire the small degree of vitality with which they are endowed. It must likewise undoubtedly happen, that some are ruptured by the enlargement of those within them, when they attain a considerable size; but it is not very common to find those which have arrived even at a medium growth ready to give way, from the increase of their internal cysts; the multiplication generally taking place so rapidly, as to burst them before they arrive at that size. We do not know how long the original hydatid, which forms the lining to the whole cavity, is capable of existing, but probably for many years; and, as long as it does exist, it seems to serve as a complete protection to the whole of its contents, from the action of the absorbents of the organ in which it is developed: it often increases very much in thickness and firmness, and seems connected only by the juxta-position of its external surface with the interior of the cyst of coagulable lymph or thickened membrane, which belongs properly to the body, and not to the hydatid. As soon as, from circumstances, the protecting hydatid dies, it separates from the cavity, curls itself up, and falls down amongst the other *débris;* then, probably, the absorbents first begin to act upon the fluid; but whether they ever act on the more solid parts of the semi-membranous cyst of the hydatid itself, may be doubted; at all events, their action is very slow, so that the remnant of an hydatid, retaining all its usual character, was found in one of the cases related above, which must have belonged to a cyst three or four times larger than the cavity in which it was discovered; showing, that it must have remained unacted upon by the absorbents, while the cavity was contracting in that degree, and while the proportionate quantity of fluid was being absorbed. The absorbents do, however, gradually take away almost every drop of the fluid; reducing the contents of the cavity to a state of dryness, in which the original forms of the membranous structures become lost; and pressed together, and deprived of moisture, the mass assumes a paste-like, and almost cretaceous, consistence. I am inclined to believe, that as soon as the protecting cyst is separated from the cavity, there is no longer any security for the rest; for as the cavity contracts, which it does in proportion as the fluid is absorbed, it becomes a constantly opposing agency; and as quickly as, by its own contraction, or by the distension of the hydatids themselves, fresh hydatids are ruptured, the absorbents of the cavity take up the fluid; and nothing but the close application of another hydatid cyst to the whole absorbing surface, which is obviously almost impossible, can put a stop to the work of destruction.

With regard to the cyst in which the hydatid is placed, that undergoes such changes as an adventitious structure, formed from the vessels of the parts by the irritation of a foreign body, and itself often well supplied with vessels, may be expected to exhibit; and that it is capable, during some periods of the disease, of very active processes, may be inferred from the great vascularity sometimes observed; as was particularly marked by the diffused pink colour in one of the active and healthy parent cysts mentioned in the examination of the first case in this communication. Its vascularity is also marked by the occasional effusion of blood between the cyst and the hydatid; mentioned, in one case, as discovered after death, and itself bearing part in the fatal termination of another case. Suppuration, also, is not unfrequently established in the cyst; as is proved, by many cases, related above, to have taken place, as a source of great irritation to the system, and occasionally the more immediate cause of the fatal result. Morbid appearances are likewise impressed upon the containing cyst by the presence of bile, which has either found its way at once from the liver, or has been poured into the cavity by communication with the gall-bladder. Another alteration, which is very often observable in the cyst, is, a more or less perfect conversion of it, generally or partially, into cartilaginous or bony matter, which must interfere considerably with its power of distending; and how far this, or any of the other changes, take place antecedently to the separation of the hydatid lining its walls, may be matter of doubt; but certain it is, that some, at least, of these changes must necessarily lead to the derangement, if not to the disintegration, of the hydatid.

Of the treatment of this disease I have little to say. While confined to one cyst, whether formed by a solitary hydatid, or by one which is productive, and therefore contains within it a number of others, I believe that an opening, or a puncture, offers the best chance of cure; and if the cyst be solitary, it is not unlikely the result will be satisfactory. If, on the contrary, the cyst contain a great number, much risk will be incurred, lest some of the excessively minute bodies should find their way into the peritoneal cavity; where, in all probability, though they might not produce any intense inflammatory action, they would gradually develope themselves and multiply. On the other hand, there is great danger in the existence of such a cyst, lest it should burst suddenly into the abdomen; and then the extent of mischief is incalculable; so that, supposing our diagnosis quite certain, there would be the greatest justification in performing the operation. As, however, our diagnosis in a single cyst is infinitely more difficult than when the disease becomes diffused, it will be always right to employ an exploring needle, such as has been recommended by Dr. Davies in cases of empyema, before an opening is made. Should the operation be performed, the most careful treatment must afterwards be adopted, to prevent any portion of the fluid, which will almost certainly be left behind in the cyst, from passing into the abdomen.

In what way the puncturing of an hydatid cyst might be expected to prove useful, is a question worth inquiry. If the cyst contain numerous hydatids, it will be no easy matter to make such an opening as would allow the larger of these bodies to escape, without too great a risk to the patient's life; but perhaps this might not be necessary to the success of the operation. I imagine one of the best results which could arise from the operation, would be the destruction of the parent or protecting cyst. Whether a simple puncture would effect that purpose, I cannot say; but probably it would; more especially as, when a considerable portion of the fluid contents of the cavity was withdrawn, the cyst would be likely to fall in, and separate from the parietes of the cavity, and thus subject the whole contents to the influence of absorption; but this result would be more certainly obtained, if a more extensive rent or separation could be inflicted on the hydatid. In the cases which have been detailed, there are three instances of the external discharge of the hydatid, besides those discharges which have taken place by the intestines and the lungs. Of these cases, one was spontaneous, and was followed by hæmorrhage from the cyst, after the separation of the hydatid. In another case, suppuration was far advanced in the cyst, before recourse was had to the operation. In the third, the operation was performed upon an hydatid which proved apparently to be solitary and unproductive, and a cure was effected. Here, probably, the cyst was destroyed; and being separated from the walls of the cavity, which were healthy, the absorbents acted as far as was necessary, while the cavity contracted.

The chief good which it appears likely that medicine can effect, is to excite the action of the absorbents when the parent hydatid is dead or separated; for till that preliminary step is obtained, the absorbents may act upon the system, but are not likely to act upon the hydatid, or the fluid contained within it; and it would be a legitimate object, in the administration of medicines, to destroy the life of the parent hydatid; but, as yet, we know little upon this point of treatment. Whether repeated doses of turpentine, or other diffusible substances, might have any effect, or whether the more local agency of electricity might be applied directly to the part affected, is a subject of fair speculation; though so little is at present known of the agents which are able to destroy the hydatids, that such propositions must be classed as unsupported conjectures; and, amongst them, it might perhaps, be permitted to mention the assiduous application of ice to the tumour, as calculated to lower the animal temperature locally, and thus interfere with one of the conditions on which probably hydatid life depends, without at the same time inflicting such violence upon the containing cyst as is likely to induce suppuration, from which we have seen, in many of the foregoing cases, that very dangerous or fatal consequences will probably ensue.

CHAPTER III.

OVARIAN TUMOURS.

There are, unquestionably, no form of abdominal tumour, with the exception of that which is occasioned by the uterus in a state of pregnancy—if that natural enlargement deserves to be spoken of as a tumour—so frequent as those which arise from the uterine appendages; and which, as they often involve, and most frequently originate in, one or both of the ovaria, have acquired the name of ovarian tumours; and, when accompanied by the accumulation of fluid which often takes place within them, the denomination of ovarian dropsy. At the same time, it is right to bear in mind, that the analogy between these and other forms of disease, usually denominated dropsies, is very slight.

There are, perhaps, four distinct diseases which form pelvic tumours with fluid contents, and which are therefore spoken of as ovarian dropsies. The first presents itself as a simple bag, containing serum; whose external surface appears to possess all the attributes of the peritoneum, attached to the surface of the ovary or some neighbouring part, and supplied by blood-vessels from the point whence it arises; sometimes, sessile; more frequently attached by a longer or shorter neck; generally single; but occasionally presenting the appearance of being composed of more than one cyst. (Fig. 18.) This simple cyst, with a long footstalk, is not of unfrequent occurrence; and is sometimes congenital, or at least exists within a very few months after birth. The tumour is generally of small dimensions, from a size less than a pea, to that of an orange; and, though I have no case to adduce, it is not improbable that it occasionally attains to a considerable bulk. The sessile variety of the simple cyst often develops itself in the broad ligament; and appears still more decidedly placed beneath the natural fold of the peritoneum than the last variety, so as appa-

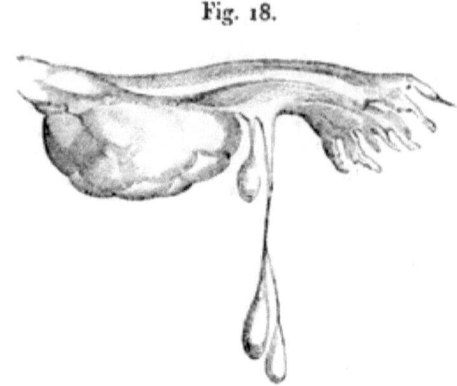

Fig. 18. Ovary and Fallopian tube, from which are seen arising three cystiform bodies, possibly the incipient state of the simple ovarian cyst.

rently to involve within it the Fallopian tube; which, however, is found passing round it, and not materially altered from its natural state, or slightly dilated, but not communicating with the cyst. Of this we have a specimen in the museum of Guy's (Fig. 19);

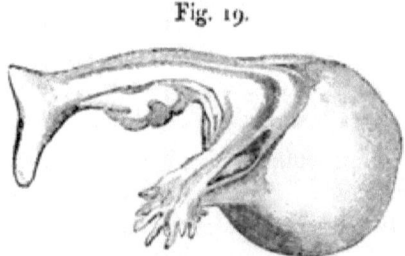

Fig. 19. A simple cyst in the broad ligament; which is evidently unconnected with the ovary, as that organ is perfect.

the ovary of that side being, at the same time, quite sound and healthy. In another specimen (Fig. 20), where a simple cyst of the size of an orange appears in a similar manner developed in the

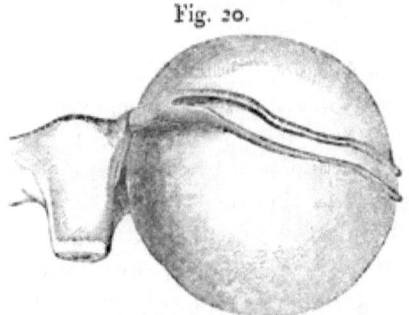

Fig. 20.

Fig. 20. A simple cyst, developed in the broad ligament of the uterus: the Fallopian tube, which is attached to it, has been laid open: it is doubtful whether this cyst may not depend on disease of the ovary itself, as that organ is not found in the preparation. The cyst, as preserved in the museum, is about four inches in its longest diameter.

broad ligament of the uterus, having the Fallopian tube on its outside; no ovary is discoverable, and therefore it is doubtful whether the cyst is not the product of a diseased condition of the ovary itself.

The second source of tumour containing fluid, connected with the uterine appendages, is found in a distended state of the Fallopian tube, which is not unfrequently seen obstructed and filled with serous fluid, so as to be much dilated, forming a pouch of considerable size, and often both of the Fallopian tubes are similarly affected. Whether, however, the dilatation is ever of such dimensions as to present a very distinct elevation above the pubes I cannot say from my own observation; I have much more frequently found these sacs capable of containing a few drachms, or at most an ounce or two, of fluid. One, which is preserved in the Museum of the College of Physicians, and of which a plate has been published in Dr. Seymour's excellent treatise on the diseases of the ovary, is five or six inches in length, and would probably contain half a pint of fluid.

It may not be altogether out of place to mention here the distended state of the Fallopian tube, which sometimes occurs from other causes, particularly from purulent and scrofulous deposits; this, however, is a disease which has never, in my experience, arrived at sufficient size to form a decided abdominal tumour, and is usually so complicated with scrofulous or inflammatory affections of the peritoneum as to form an undistinguishable portion of the original disease.

The third form of tumour, the existence of which, as a separate disease, distinct from others, appears to me very doubtful, consists of a simple vesicular body developed beneath the proper tunic of the ovary; supposed to be produced by an accumulation of fluid in one of the Graafian vesicles. Tumours said to be of this kind differ greatly in size; they are frequently not larger than a hazel-nut, sometimes of the size of an egg, and occasionally are believed to attain to a great magnitude, so as nearly to fill the abdomen. Yet, from the description which has sometimes been given of the contents of such supposed cysts and their glutinous quality, it is probable that they have often been no other than largely developed cysts of a malignant character. There is a state of the Graafian vesicle by no means uncommon, and of which we have several specimens in the Museum of Guy's, where a coagulum, more or less stained with blood, or of a somewhat glutinous character, is collected in the vesicle, distending it to the size of a hazel-nut, or sometimes larger; this, likewise, bears a doubtful relationship to the malignant forms of tumour; but from the circumstances of some of the patients and their youthful age, I suspect that they are, at least occasionally, unconnected with such disease. (See Case 2.)

The fourth is by far the most frequent form of ovarian tumour, and is essentially a specific disease, assuming all the varieties of structure which result from the numerous modifications of that morbid action called malignant. When speaking on this subject in a paper in 'Guy's Hospital Reports,' vol. i, p. 638, I endeavoured to point out, that the malignant disease was probably to be traced as originating more peculiarly in the cellular tissue of the body; first displacing, and then gradually involving and implicating, the proper structure of the organ in which it is developed. I need not, on the present occasion, repeat what I have already said; but having there mentioned ovarian tumours as affording some marked examples and very striking modifications of this fact, I shall refer to the cases and dissections I am about to state, as illustrating the extensive growth and propagation of malignant disease in the loose cellular tissue of an organ, the more essential parts of which seem to present, in their natural structure, a prototype of that involved system of cellular arrangement observable in malignant growths. But here I must observe, that the development of the disease in the ovary, owing to the decidedly cellular character of its various parts, seems, even in its early stages, to lay hold on the most important portions of the organ, as well as on the common cellular tissue; and it is often quite impossible to say whether it be the meshes of the cellular tissue, or the vesicles of De Graaf, which are become the seats of the morbid deposits, or to what extent new structures have been generated; for, looking at the innumerable cysts, vesicles, and cavities which display themselves in the various parts of these ovarian tumours, we may sometimes doubt whether they have all of them had a portion of the natural structure, complicated as it is, even as the commencing nidus of their growth; but are inclined to grant, that new vesicular bodies may probably have been added in the progress of the development, such as Dr. Hodgkin seems to consider almost essential to malignant disease; and yet, when we look to a portion of loose cellular tissue which has been distended with air or filled with serum, we find no apparent want of cellular cavities to bear out the possibility of the contrary supposition.

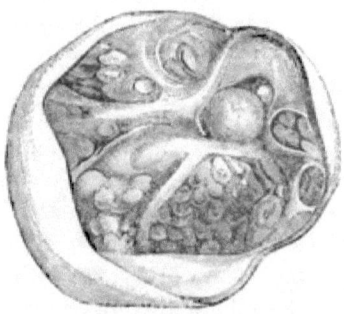

Fig. 21. A greatly diminished sketch of a large compound ovarian cyst, laid open. This is drawn with the design of giving a general view of the structure very frequent in this disease, where the whole diseased mass appears divided by septa; and in the compartments formed by them, when the mucilaginous secretion is removed, numberless small cysts display themselves. What part of this structure can be accounted for by the increase of natural cellular membrane, and what part is owing to peculiar growth, is no easy problem to solve. The preparation from which this sketch is taken is preserved in Guy's Museum, and is above a foot in diameter.

It is evident that a disease consisting of a simple cyst filled with a bland, inoffensive serum, apparently originating in some excess or irregularity of a comparatively healthy action, or arising from some inflammatory deposit, ought not to be confounded with any form of malignant disease, from which it must so essentially differ. Unfortunately, it is no easy matter to distinguish, with certainty, these two diseases; nor, indeed, does the subject often admit of perfect elucidation, either during life or after death. Still, however, we must endeavour to take as our guides the best indication we can find, in the age of the patient, the progress of the enlargement, or the feel of the tumour. I do not profess to be conversant with the history of the simple cyst; I believe that the only indication afforded is a tumour, more or less spherical, felt first in one of the inguinal regions of the abdomen, and very gradually, if at all, ascending. That this may take place very early in life—that its growth is slow—that the constitution suffers little or not at all—and that after the cyst has attained even a large size, it occasionally disappears, without any very evident cause, or under the action of remedies, or from being burst internally by some accidental occurrence—the fluid, in this last case, passing off by the Fallopian tubes, or taken up by the absorbents, and hurried very rapidly through the kidneys; and though this effusion of fluid may be accompanied by a certain degree of peritonitis, the symptoms are, in general, by no means so alarming as might be expected. I am not sure that I can recall to my memory a single dissection where the simple ovarian cyst has been the cause of death, or has even advanced to such a size as to be the subject of material inconvenience to the patient during life. In most of the cases—and they are pretty numerous—in which simple cysts have been discovered after death, they have been too small to have attracted notice during life, and have been casually detected. Their attachment has been even more frequently to the Fallopian tubes, or to their fimbriated extremity, than to the ovaries themselves; and they have seldom exceeded the size of a small plum. The subjects in which they have occurred have varied, as to age from children in arms, to women in the decline of life; and in these latter cases, though still small, they have often borne, in their structure, such evidence of having long existed, that I am inclined to believe their increase to be generally very slow; and that they frequently become stationary at a very early period.

With regard to the accumulation of fluid in a Graafian vesicle, leading to its gradual distension, this likewise cannot easily be detected; and, if detected, must with great difficulty be distinguished from other forms of ovarian tumour. As soon as it has acquired a sufficient size it will, of course, be felt rising from the pelvis; less spherical and less moveable than the simple cyst; less lobulated than the malignant disease; which circumstance, together with its more moderate growth, and the little inconvenience it produces, may afford a clue to our diagnosis, and guard us against an inordinate anxiety for the result. It is probable, however, that this form of tumour more frequently attains a larger size than the simple cyst; and that it more frequently affords those instances of sudden disappearance by accidental rupture of the cyst, or of gradual decrease, assisted by medicine, than any other form of ovarian growth. When rupture takes place, there is very often a more or less acute inflammatory action induced; and, according to the various circumstances arising from that inflammation, the succeeding history of the disease will be modified. Still it is a fact, that from a very early period of its history to the very end, we are not only unable to make any decided distinction between it and the malignant disease during life, but are seldom able to demonstrate, even after death, the precise nature of the tissue in which the cyst has been first developed.

With the history of the more ordinary form of ovarian tumour, we have, unfortunately, very frequent opportunities of becoming acquainted, and I will endeavour shortly to state the prominent points which it presents. This form of disease seldom shows itself much before the twentieth year of life, and generally much later, and is not, like the simple cyst, unexpectedly discovered during the examination of children or young persons who have died of other diseases. The first recognised symptom is usually a tumour, not altogether devoid of pain, in one of the inguinal regions; and which, on examination, evidently rises out of one side of the pelvis, and even at this early period is sometimes distinctly lobulated, or uneven in its form, and unequal in the resistance its different parts afford on pressure. The growth of this tumour is, on some occasions, so unperceived, that though it may have originated on one side, it has already risen into the pubic, and even the umbilical region; and when the medical man is first consulted, its lateral origin is with difficulty ascertained. At other times the enlargement is at first slow; and, after some indefinite period, the increase takes place suddenly, so that in a few months the whole abdomen presents, to a common observer, the size and appearance of pregnancy far advanced. From this time the patient often asserts that the abdomen does not increase, and she willingly deceives herself by measuring at some particular part, when it often happens that, with a little unconscious adjusting of the measure, no increase is discovered; but, in the mean time, there is no doubt in the mind of the medical attendant that the tumour becomes more and more tense—that the fluctuation bespeaks a further thinning of the parietes—that the functions of the abdominal viscera are interfered with—that the respiration is more embarrassed—and that increased pressure is made on the cava and other returning vessels, as evinced by the serum, which now begins to accumulate in the cellular membrane of the lower extremities, and the distension and turgescence of the subcutaneous veins of the abdomen; the important question of paracentesis presents itself, and to this operation, however unwillingly, he finds himself at length necessarily reduced.

When a physician is consulted, either at this or in any previous period of the disease, a careful examination of the state of the abdomen is necessary. In passing the flat hand cautiously and regularly over the abdomen, the extent of the tumour will often become at once manifest to the touch; at other times no limits will then be discovered, for the tumour occupies the whole of that part of the abdomen which is not formed by the concavity of the diaphragm, the recesses of the loins, and the hollow of the pelvis.

Casting the eye over the abdomen in the earlier part of the disease, the greater rotundity or projection of one part will often be most apparent; and the tumour will in this way immediately discover itself, as occupying the iliac and lumbar region on one side, and extending over half at least of the umbilical region, or beyond the umbilicus, so as to encroach on the opposite side; at other times its extent will be less; while, in the more advanced cases, no inequality will strike the eye, but the rounded form of the abdomen, while the patient lies on her back, will contrast it with the more ordinary ovoid appearance of ascites, as well as distinguish it in some degree from the form produced by the uterus distended in pregnancy. In many cases, moreover, the eye will be struck by a great enlargement of the subcutaneous veins, as I have just observed, and such as often takes place to a still greater degree in ascites.

On making more firm, though not violent pressure on the various parts of the abdomen, we often find at once the general sense of fluctuation, and ascertain inequalities which neither the eye nor the hand, when passed but gently over the surface, will enable us to detect; and then it sometimes happens, particularly if the abdomen be not very tense, that we discover considerable masses of unyielding matter, partaking of the general rounded feel of the whole disease, but conveying the impression of more or less flattened spherical bodies, attached to the inside of the fluctuating tumour; and these bodies are sometimes so large, and sometimes so variously placed, as to suggest to the inexperienced observer the idea that the liver, the spleen, or the kidneys are enlarged, and in some way involved in the disease. (Fig. 22.)

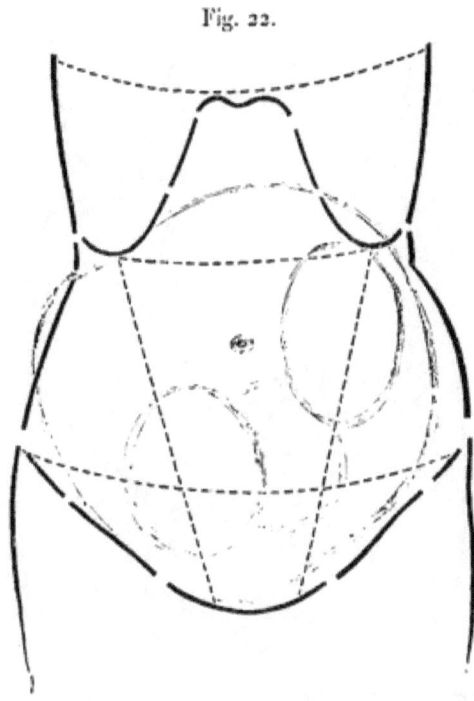

Fig. 22.

Fig. 22. Sketch, drawn upon a stencilled outline, to illustrate the indications derived chiefly by the touch, in a case of compound ovarian cyst.

Sometimes the sense of fluctuation is very indistinct or very partial, and various parts of the tumour yield it in different degrees. At other times, the fluctuation is even more evident than in the most extreme cases of ascites; and sometimes, as the patient lies on the back, a thin layer of fluid is discoverable, external to the great distending tumour, so that when the points of the fingers, placed on the surface, are moved forwards with a jerk, they are evidently resisted, after pressing aside a little fluid, by the surface of the tumour within. Sometimes this layer of fluid extends over a wide space, and the fluctuation it yields by percussion may be plainly

Fig. 23.

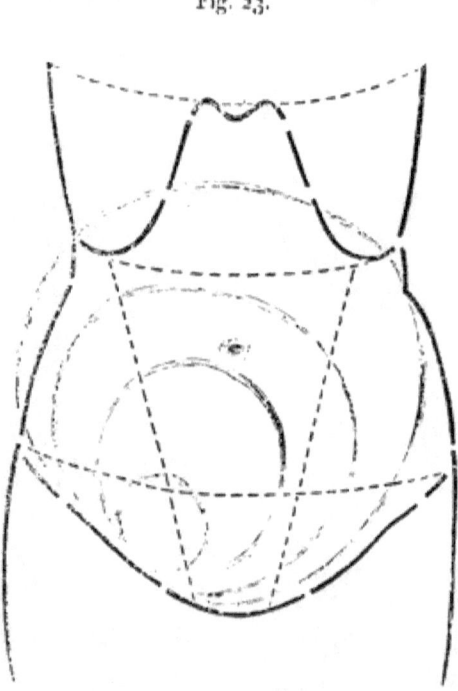

Fig. 23. Diagram, showing the gradual enlargement of a tumour of the right ovary, till at length it fills a large portion of the abdominal cavity, forcing the intestines into the lumbar regions, where they may be recognised by percussion.

felt, or even seen as a wave passing over a large portion of the abdomen.

The use of percussion is likewise very important in these cases, not only as detecting the existence, precise situation, and extent of fluctuation, but as eliciting sounds, hollow or otherwise, in the various parts of the abdomen. These will, of course, vary as the disease advances, pushing before it the hollow viscera; and in this consists one of the remarkable differences between ascites and ovarian disease. In ascites, as long as the peritoneum has undergone no serious change, the hollow viscera float upon the surface of the fluid, and rise to the highest part, whatever position almost the body assumes; but the ovarian disease displaces these viscera, and retains its relative position under all circumstances; so that instead of discovering the clear sound yielded by percussion in the umbilical region, or at the scrobiculus cordis, or in the lumbar spaces, according as the patient lies upon her back, stands erect, or reclines to the right or to the left side, we find the chief sound of the hollow viscera always on the side opposite to the tumour, till by its encroachment it has driven the intestines entirely into the outskirts of the abdominal cavity (Fig. 23); and to this the exceptions are very rare, unless it be in those cases where communications have taken place between the cyst and the intestines, and thus air has been admitted.

Having ascertained the existence of a tumour or cyst, it will still further be right to examine carefully the state of the subcutaneous cellular membrane, to detect any traces of the existence of scirrhous or other tubercles deposited in it. And lastly, by applying the palm of the hand pretty firmly on the integuments covering the tumour, we should endeavour to ascertain whether, by its motion, we can discover any such crepitation or rubbing sensation as would lead us to infer the probability that adhesive effusion or adhesions existed between the tumour and the peritoneum lining the parietes of the abdominal cavity.

When by all these indications and, if any doubt have arisen, by an examination per vaginam, the extent, the nature, and the circumstances of the tumour, and the existence of a fluid have been ascertained, then, if the various functions have suffered so much interruption that prudence will allow of no further delay, the fluid is drawn off by the trochar; ten, twenty, or thirty pints of the contents of the cyst are discharged, varying in quality, but generally less clear in its colour and more mucous in its consistence than the serum of ascites.

The operation is attended with very little pain, and followed by very little constitutional disturbance, but affords the most marked relief; and, for a few days, the comfort of being freed from such a burden is most gratifying to the patient. Still, however, she is not unfrequently disappointed that the size of the abdomen is not more completely reduced, and the large masses and nodules, which were but indistinctly felt or discovered by the dullness yielded locally by percussion, are now not only easily grasped by the hand, but present large and obvious elevations and irregularities in the contour of the flaccid abdomen (Fig. 22). Not many days elapse, before the regular and spontaneous tightening of the bandage with which the body has been swathed, and which percussion shows to depend on no accidental evolution of flatus, gives warning of the speed with which fresh accumulation is taking place, and there is too often reason to believe that the rapidity of the effusion is increased by the withdrawal of the fluid. The nodular masses again become indistinct; in the course of a few weeks the abdomen has arrived almost at its former size, and perhaps before two or three months have elapsed the operation must again be performed. It may be that the patient still retains a fair state of general health; but if the accumulation be rapid, the system soon begins to suffer, the body to emaciate, the countenance to fade, and if pain be added, as is not unfrequently the case, when the disease assumes its more active or virulent forms, the suffering of the patient greatly reduces her strength. The interval between the operations become less, and at length, after the lapse of an uncertain number of months or years, she dies worn out. Or, on the other hand, if the suffering continues comparatively little, and operation after operation be borne without a visible decrease of bodily power or mental energy, yet, at length, some inflammatory process, apparently accidental, or some state of unexpected collapse for which no reason can be ascribed takes place, and the patient sinks. To assign any precise or specific time to the course of this disease, from its first appearance till its fatal termination, is impossible, the difference in this respect being great; but, from what I have myself observed, I should be inclined to state, that cases which continue above four years from the first necessity for the operation of paracentesis, bear a small proportion to those which prove fatal before that time.

Such is the more general course of this disease, but there are cases in which the latter part of the history is considerably varied; as, for instance, we find some in which from various circumstances no attempt has been made to relieve the distension by operation, and then death usually follows, by the slow exhaustion of the powers of life, through irritation, or through the obstruction which the pressure of the tumour occasions, interfering with the various essential functions, and sometimes by compressing the lacteals, positively cutting off some of the avenues by which nutriment is conveyed to the system. Other cases there are where nature performing the work which is more usually attempted by art, adhesions take place, and the fluid is evacuated through the intestines—the orifice remaining open, or being easily renewed, and a gradual decline of powers leads to the fatal termination. In some cases the cyst, through accident, or through a process of ulceration commenced in the inner lining, bursts into the peritoneal cavity, and then death sometimes speedily follows, either by the effects of the shock, or by inflammation and its results; or, occasionally, recovery seems most unexpectedly to follow. Too often, however, the improvement is but for a time, and the disease returns under still less favorable circumstances than before the rupture. In some cases, after the performance of paracentesis, the wound refuses to close, or bursts out afresh, and sometimes, for months or years, a discharge continues; and this event may not be peculiarly prejudicial, but rather serve to prolong the patient's life. Such then, with various modifications, is a short history of the disease of which I shall now proceed to give a few cases, and in the following details I intend to illustrate many of the circumstances I have stated, and to bring into view the nature and extent of the structural changes by which the disease is marked; commencing by saying a very few words on those cases of ovarian tumour which are probably devoid of a malignant character.

The cases to which I am able to refer with certainty, as those where the simple serous cyst has occurred, are all of them instances in which it has attained a very small size, and has not been discovered during life. The patients have been of various ages, and in various conditions; and all the circumstances of their cases have appeared so little connected with the existence of the cyst, that it is quite unnecessary to detail them. I shall simply mention two: one, on account of the tender age of the subject; and another, from its connexion with other evidences of irritation in the uterine appendages.

Case 1.—I was, during the last year, called upon to attend an infant of five months of age; in whom, from the symptoms, scarcely a doubt existed that the obstructed condition of the bowels depended on some mechanical cause, and this we believed to be intus-susception. The child died on the following day; no relief having been obtained to the obstinate constipation under which it laboured. After death our conclusions were verified to the fullest extent; for we found the whole cæcum and the arch of the colon, and a portion of the ileum, swallowed up by the descending colon.

All the other organs were in perfect health; but from the appendages of the uterus on the left side we discovered a cyst of the size of a pea, hanging by a footstalk half an inch in length.

Case 2.—A young woman, about eighteen years of age, died worn out with chorea.

"The uterus was rather large, and its cavity was extensive; in the left corner was a deposit of as much clear transparent mucus as would cover a sixpenny-piece. The ovary of the right side contained a cyst of the size of a small hazel-nut, full of a tenacious, dull-red substance, of just sufficient consistence to allow of being cut. The Fallopian tube on the same side was quite pervious, admitting of the passage of air from the blowpipe; but it presented a remarkable appearance, having the points of the fimbriated extremities tipped with deposits of semi-transparent bone, looking like large grains of sand of irregular and rather botryoidal form; and a deposit of the same kind was found on the outside of the broad ligament. The ovary on the opposite side was more healthy, but had in it a few vesicular bodies. The Fallopian tube on that side had none of the bony deposits. Attached to the ligaments of the uterus, on each side, was a small vesicle of the size of a pea, hanging by a peduncle, along which vessels were seen to pass from the peritoneum."

Having mentioned these two cases, I may simply refer to what I have said in page 59; where, likewise, will be found a few observations on another form of simple cyst when it is sessile or developed, apparently beneath the peritoneal covering of the broad ligament and the Fallopian tube; as, likewise, some reference to the cysts which are formed by the dilatation of the Fallopian tube itself.

With regard to the simply distended Graafian vesicle, without malignant tendency, the cases which have occurred to my observation scarcely go further than to throw an air of probability on the occasional existence of such diseases. There is nothing like a convincing anatomical demonstration of the point; and, in the very next case I shall relate, what I consider, partly from the analysis of the fluid contained, and partly from the structure, to be an early specimen of the malignant disease; though the cyst appeared, when viewed externally, so completely to arise in the situation of the Graafian vesicle, to be so simple in its structure, and to be connected with so healthy an appearance of the ovary, that I at first considered it a simple non-malignant ovarian cyst. It is, therefore, my intention not to separate such doubtful cases; but rather to introduce them in the following collection, with such remarks as will show the reasons I may have for supposing it probable that they were of one character or the other.

CASE 3.—*Incipient ovarian dropsy, probably of a malignant character.*—S. P—, æt. 37, was admitted, under my care, into the Clinical Ward, November 1, 1837, labouring under ascites and anasarca. In the preceding August she had been delivered of a female child; and immediately afterwards profuse flooding followed, which was suppressed with difficulty; and about one week after she rose from her bed her legs began to swell; and in less than a month her abdomen also swelled; since that she had suffered from palpitation of the heart on exertion, and from prolapsus uteri. The fluctuation was very distinct in the abdomen at the time of her admission. The urine was not coagulable, and varied from one pint to two and a half.

After being in the hospital nearly three weeks she was suddenly seized with hemiplegia, and entirely lost all power over the right arm and leg, and was unable to articulate a word.

About six weeks after the hemiplegic seizure, when the ascites had almost disappeared, but the paralysis remained nearly unaltered; she was discovered one morning to be insensible, her eyes fixed and turned upwards, with her breathing somewhat difficult; and in two hours after she died.

Sectio cadaveris.—Some serum under the arachnoid. The whole anterior lobe of the left hemisphere of the brain was reduced to the consistence of a custard; so that it was only kept in its situation by the membranes, and the cineritious substance, which was of a yellow colour. This softening included exactly the corpus striatum and the anterior lobe. In the posterior part of the corpus striatum the most material mischief seemed to have taken place; and there was a small yellow stain, as if from a slight effusion of blood some weeks previously. The heart was small and weak, and perfectly adherent to the whole pericardium. There was fluid in both cavities of the chest, of which some was evidently of long standing. The uterus was healthy.

Fig. 24.

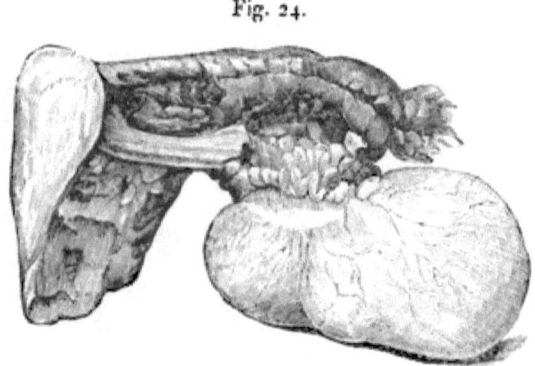

Fig. 24 represents a portion of the uterus, with the Fallopian tube and one of the ovaries, beneath the peritoneal coat of which a cyst of the size of an egg was developed; apparently, the early stage of a true malignant ovarian tumour.

One of the ovaries presented a beautiful specimen of the incipient stage of ovarian dropsy. A small semi-lobulated cyst seemed to proceed from the ovary; being completely covered by the tunic of the ovary, so as to form, apparently, a continuous portion of that organ. Its size was about that of a small hen's egg; and vessels proceeded from the ovary over its surface. (Fig. 24.) The investing tunic of the ovary could be traced to some distance over the cyst; and then became lost in its parietes. These parietes were about as thick as two or three folds of writing-paper; and when the cyst was opened, the external lobulated appearance was found to depend, not on the existence of separate cysts, but to be the results of bands or folds which formed one or two imperfect septa. A few vessels were seen in the inside of the cyst likewise; but whether these belonged to the inner surface, or were seen through from without, was not quite decided (Fig. 25). When

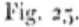

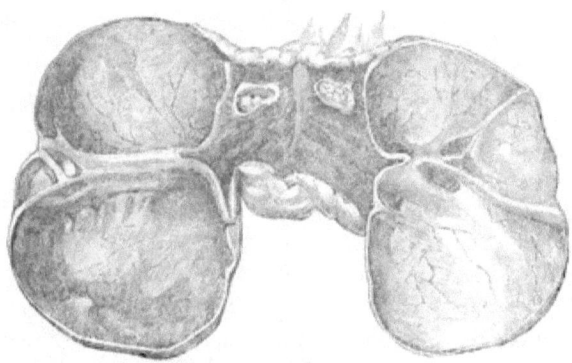

Fig. 25. A section of the ovary and cyst, represented in Fig. 24, showing its partial division by septa. It was filled with a glairy fluid, of which the analysis is given above; but whether it originated in the cellular tissue of the ovary, or in one of the Graafian vesicles, is uncertain; the peritoneal coat of the ovary may be traced a short way over its surface, before it becomes lost in the cyst itself. One of the Graafian vesicles is seen in a diseased state; and the same was observed in the ovary of the opposite side.

opened, the fluid it contained, which was clear, limpid, and slightly mucilaginous, was carefully collected; and Dr. Rees undertook the analysis; which will be found to correspond very closely with other analyses in this paper, of fluids taken from malignant ovarian tumours.

"Guildford Street, Jan. 11th, 1838.

"My dear Sir,—I enclose the account of the fluid from the cyst developed in the ovary. It is very different from serum of blood, containing no extractive soluble in alcohol, and no alkaline phosphate.

"P.S.—I experimented on 400 grains, and have given the result in 1000 parts.

"Yours very sincerely,
"G. O. REES."

ANALYSIS OF A FLUID FROM A SMALL CYST IN AN OVARY.

Water	. . . . .	940·10
Albumen	with traces of fatty matter of the blood, and phosphate of lime . .	47·75
Albumen, existing in solution as albuminate of soda		6·69
Chloride of sodium	. . . .	3·76
Carbonate of soda, with traces of sulphate	. .	1·70
		1000·00

This fluid was alkaline, producing a permanent effect on reddened litmus. Its specific gravity was 1018·2. Water being 1000.

There was the distinct appearance of a diseased and thickened Graafian vesicle in the same ovary; while in that of the opposite side four or five similar bodies were seen.

From the circumstance of this cyst being developed so completely beneath the peritoneal tunic of the ovary, and from other Graafian vesicles being enlarged both in this and in the opposite ovary, I was at first inclined to consider this a case in which a collection of serum had taken place in a Graafian vesicle, in contradistinction to the more ordinary form of ovarian disease; but the analysis of the fluid leads me to a contrary conclusion; and the structure of the cyst, though simple, bears very much the appearance which is occasionally presented in certain portions of the complicated cysts; so that this case somewhat adds to the doubt I have already expressed, of having met with any very distinct case of dropsical accumulation in the Graafian vesicles, as distinguished from the disease which runs into the malignant ovarian tumour. Considering this, then, to be, as I believe it is, an example of a very early stage of the malignant ovarian dropsy, I introduce it here; and may just notice, that in the case of M— (Case 17), an instance of a still more early and partial development of the disease will be found associated with extensive and well-marked disease in the ovary of the other side. And, as I conceive this to be the incipient state of the disease in its mildest character, I shall follow it by a case somewhat more advanced, and differing in some respects, which well illustrates the connexion between the class of diseases which we are considering, and the truly malignant action going on in the system. The following case I have taken from the register of Guy's Museum; and in Fig. 26 will be found a reduced sketch of the ovary and uterus, as they are still preserved.

Fig. 26.

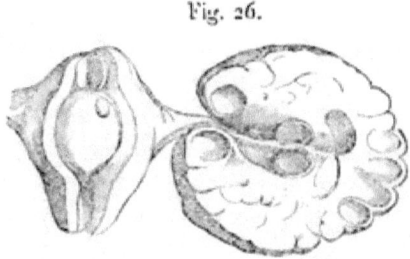

Fig. 26. The uterus and ovary, from a patient who laboured under scirrhous mamma, and in whom other organs were similarly diseased. The ovary appears to show the early stage of the malignant ovarian disease; and several cysts are already formed. The uterus is also affected, having a fibrous tubercle in the parietes of its fundus; and another obtruding on the cavity, which it distends. (Case 4.) This preparation is preserved in Guy's Museum; and the length of the diseased ovary is about three inches and a half.

CASE 4.—*Diseased ovary, with cysts, in a case of extensive malignant disease of other organs.*—Anne —, æt. 48, admitted 30th August, 1830, into Dorcas's Ward, under Mr. C. A. Key, for scirrhous mamma. Her health was not then much disordered; but the existence of several hard subcutaneous tumours, of various sizes, about the abdomen, and the discovery of similar disorganization in the liver, marked the extensive nature of the disease. Her principal and almost only cause of complaint was, of pain in the right side. She sunk gradually on the 13th, having exhibited no remarkable symptoms.

Sectio cadaveris.—The body had undergone much cadaveric change; it was not emaciated. A hard scirrhous mass occupied the situation of the left mamma; the right was slightly affected in the same manner. The tumours beneath the skin had the appearance of diseased absorbent glands; sections of them showed, in all, the same scirrhous structure. The chest contained about two pints of serum, rather turbid, and much tinged with blood; probably the result of cadaveric transudation. The fluid in the pericardium was about two ounces in quantity, and also very much tinged. That in the abdomen was small in quantity, and of a reddish-brown colour. Well-developed tubera, of scirrhous character, from the size of a walnut downwards, were found in great numbers in the liver. The smallest and latest formed of these had the appearance of round, flat, circumscribed opaque marks on the surface of the viscus; the larger ones were flat externally, or depressed in the centre. Small bodies, of a scirrhous character, were thickly dispersed throughout the omentum and mesentery, and other parts of the peritoneum; but none of a large size. Both ovaries, the right in particular, were much enlarged and indurated, their surfaces being very irregular; the Fallopian tubes, however, seemed free from disease. The body of the uterus contained a tumour the size of an egg; but the surface of the organ was sound, as were also the os tincæ and vagina. No unnatural appearance of the peritoneum had taken place in any of these situations. The pleuræ were partially connected by old adhesions. A few marks were found on the surface of the heart and of the spleen, resembling the commencement of disease as described in the liver. On the lungs these were more numerous; and in some few had acquired a consistence resembling cartilage. The substance of the pancreas and spleen, the kidneys, with their tunics, and the brain and its membranes, were healthy. No fibrin or coagulum was found in the heart or in the large vessels; these last were stained of a red colour. All the tissues had undergone much softening. The right ovary was about three inches and a half in its largest diameter; it was much corrugated, and raised into irregular elevations on its surface; and when cut into, showed a most diseased structure throughout; the section laying open five or six vesicles, each approaching the surface, and about the size of a large hazel-nut, filled with fluid. These appeared to be Graafian vesicles; but the whole structure of the ovary was a mass of hard, malignant disease. (Fig. 26.)

This case serves to show the connexion between the cystiform enlargement of the ovary and malignant disease, which developed itself in various parts of the body in the form of scirrhus, and in the uterus, probably, as the fibrous tubercle.

CASE 5.—*Ovarian dropsy of eleven years' standing.—Death probably from inflammatory changes going on in the interior of the cyst.*— Esther W——, a woman of light, sandy complexion, was first admitted under my care September 8, 1824, when her age is set down at 27, and she stated she had then been ill for a period of nine years. Her general appearance was that of a woman some years more advanced in life than this statement would point out; but if correct, she must have begun to feel her present disease at the age of eighteen. It is certain, that nearly two years before her admission, that is, in May, 1822, the operation of paracentesis had been performed, and a quantity of fluid, amounting to two pailsful and a half, or about five gallons, had then been drawn off. Nearly an equal quantity had been taken away in June, 1823; the same quantity in December of that year, and in February and June of 1834.

At the time of admission, her abdomen was generally and greatly distended; and, on even a superficial examination with the hand, three or four large masses were to be felt, which, from the situation they occupied, were considered by some to be probably enlarged viscera, as the spleen and liver. However, a more attentive examination, together with the history of the case, easily explained their nature and situation; for there could be no doubt that this was a case of ovarian tumour, and that these were subordinate cysts growing into the cavity from the parietes of the larger cyst. Her general health was suffering somewhat, from the pain she occasionally experienced in the abdomen; I therefore ordered her to be tapped; and sixteen quarts of thick, opaque fluid were taken away, with great relief; and when the abdomen was examined, the hard masses were felt even more distinctly than before. After a short time she left the hospital, but returned in February, 1835, on the 18th of which month twenty quarts of fluid were taken away; on the 9th of April, twenty-six quarts were drawn off; on the 5th of July, sixteen quarts; and on the 8th of November, sixteen quarts and a half; at the next operation seventeen quarts and a half; and at the next, twenty-one quarts were removed, on July the 10th, 1836. Again, in October, 1836, twenty-two quarts were taken; and in the end of January, 1837, an equal quantity. The last two or three operations had been attended with more inconvenience than the former, and the fluid had become more puriform in its appearance; and a sense of sinking and lowness, with tenderness and abdominal pain, bespoke mischief, probably of a low, inflammatory character, going on. All these symptoms became aggravated after the operation in the end of January; and on the 8th of the following month she gradually sank.

Thus, during a period of between four and five years, this patient had been tapped fourteen times; and in that space had lost sixty-eight gallons of the thick, glutinous fluid characteristic of this disease.

Sectio cadaveris, February 9th, 1837.—The general aspect greatly emaciated; no œdema in any part; the abdomen very large, but not distended, appearing quite flaccid. On opening the abdomen to the left of the umbilicus, nearly a bucket-full of turbid yellow fluid resembling pus in appearance, and just like that which had come away by tapping, was removed. On making an opening at the scrobiculus cordis, in the direction of the linea alba, another cavity showed itself also, containing a fluid not very different, though somewhat less turbid and thick than that in the chief cavity. About two full wash-hand-basins of fluid were taken from this cavity.

On further examination, it appeared that the first cavity opened was the chief cavity, and that from which the fluid had always been drawn by tapping. It was a completely encysted cavity; whereas the other portion of fluid was contained in the cavity of the peritoneum itself. With respect to the encysted cavity, it appeared, on minute examination, that it was a large cyst, arising from the situation of the left ovary, and having the Fallopian tube of that side greatly elongated (not less than eight inches in length), attached along its outside; the fimbriated extremity being plainly seen at the end.

This cyst was attached most firmly and generally to the anterior parietes of the abdomen, so as to require careful dissection to detach it. It was thicker and stronger towards the left side, and in front; but was rather thin towards the right side and in the iliac region. It had formed no attachments to the viscera, except that at the upper part it was glued to the omentum; it quite filled the cavity of the right ileum; and the intestines were very much pushed aside by it towards the left side.

Internally, the cyst was very vascular, and was covered, in patches, with a deposit of puriform lymph of a yellowish-green colour; while in many parts it was rough, as if ulcerated. In other parts, tuberculated masses of different sizes were seen: of these, two were more remarkable; the one occupying a situation a little below the spleen, and the other a little below the liver, between the right iliac and lumbar regions; and as these were, in parts of the cyst, closely attached to the parietes of the abdomen, they had been perfectly discoverable by the touch for the last two years, and did not change their position in the least at the time the fluid was drawn off. Besides these two large masses, there were four or five others, smaller in dimensions, attached to the different parts of the cyst; one, which had been always felt about an inch above the umbilicus.

The smaller masses were like small, thick cysts; and one of the smallest being opened, it was found filled with a straw-coloured substance, semi-transparent, of a glutinous character, which separated with some difficulty from the sides of the cavity, and then disclosed another cyst of a more rounded form, semi-transparent, and beautifully vascular. (Fig. 27.) This appeared to be the more early stage of each mass—these internal cysts sprouting up from the bottom, and bursting the external cysts; and then the surface, so opened, becoming a secreting surface of that semi-gelatinous matter, which, in its more diluted form, seemed to compose the fluid which had been so frequently drawn off by tapping.

Fig. 27.

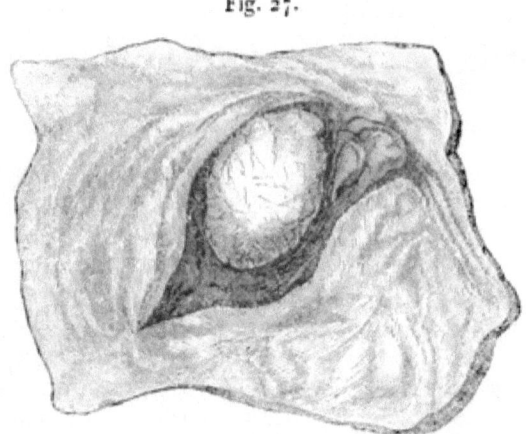

Fig. 27. The incipient stage of a tumour analogous to that represented in Fig. 28, and taken from the same ovarian cyst. In this case, the inner lamina had been divided by the scalpel. A tenacious mucus distended the cavity; but when this was removed, a transparent vascular cyst was seen projecting from the bottom.

On examining one of the larger masses, the cyst, out of which the tubercular-looking growth had proceeded, was seen opened, forming a margin round about two thirds of the mass; the other third became lost in the tubercular cysts; the internal lining of this was in the highest degree vascular. These cysts rose almost like a cauliflower-head, quite opaque and vascular; and one mass, which was more advanced, showed, on the surface, an appearance of irregularly deposited lymph. (Fig. 28.) Each of the masses, on examination, showed the same structure, with some variation; in some, the cysts were full of fluid or semifluid matter; while in others they were hard, and presented various approaches to the true malignant character.

Fig. 28.

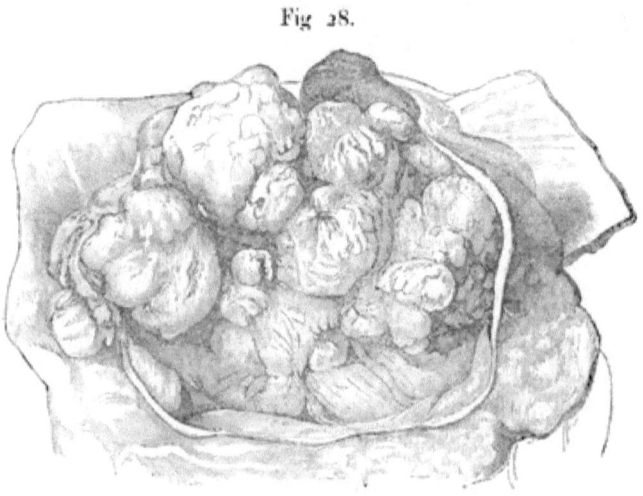

Fig. 28 represents one of the diseased masses which are frequently found connected with the parietes of the large cysts of ovarian dropsy. It projects from the inner surface of the cyst, originating between its laminæ; and a process of sloughing having taken place in the lamina by which it was retained, a crescentic margin is seen formed around it, with a clean, firm edge. The diseased mass was itself a fungoid growth, probably formed originally of more transparent cysts filled with glairy mucus, now become opaque and cerebriform.

The uterus, the right ovary, and the Fallopian tubes, were perfectly healthy.

The liver was pushed up to the diaphragm; and, having formed strong adhesions, remained in that situation when all the other abdominal contents had been removed; its lower surface apparently occupying nearly the natural position of the diaphragm itself. It was much enlarged, of a yellow colour throughout, and firm consistence, approaching to the udder liver. The gall-bladder was filled with a full-coloured and apparently healthy bile.

Spleen quite healthy. Stomach quite healthy, internally and externally, but containing a quantity of dark matter. Intestines throughout healthy externally; but through a considerable portion of the ileum, some feet in extent, the solitary glands were enlarged, and their orifices tinged with yellow, so as to give the appearance of pretty thickly disseminated yellow specks; this appearance diminished as you approached the jejunum. Colon healthy. Kidneys pallid in colour; and the tubuli uriniferi appeared blocked up with little concretions or sandy deposits. Heart rather feeble. Lungs most perfectly healthy throughout, without the least adhesion.

This case may be considered as presenting a well-marked example of the complicated ovarian tumour, which had proceeded through many years in the successive changes of its growth; and I give it as a fair specimen of a large class of such cases.

CASE 6.—*Ovarian dropsy, anasarca, and ascites. Death from peritonitis, after the fluid was partially drawn from the cyst.*— Anne M—, æt. 34, was admitted, under my care, into Guy's Hospital, March 25th, 1829, affected with ovarian dropsy, anasarca, and ascites. Her abdomen was more distended than I ever before witnessed; so that it hung over the thighs, chafing the groins; and the umbilicus was scarcely to be seen; it measured, on its most prominent parts, four feet ten inches in circumference; the cutaneous veins were very much distended, and fluctuation very distinct in the upper part of the tumour; but below the umbilicus the whole was hard, lobulated, and unyielding. Her general health was represented as pretty good, but she had lost flesh within the last two months; her countenance was placid; tongue clean, but purplish; and the respiration much impeded when in the recumbent posture. Pulse, 120, rather weak; urine scanty, of a dark colour, tinged with bile, and having a light-reddish sediment, not coagulable by heat.

Eighteen months ago, she lay-in, having been extremely large during her pregnancy, and after her confinement never diminished to her usual size. A month afterwards she was tapped in the usual place, rather below the umbilicus, but not more than a quart of yellow, gelatinous matter came away. The catamenial discharge occurred quite regularly till three months ago, since which it has ceased; and it is only for the last two months that her urine has been scanty and high-coloured.

She took medicines, gently to regulate her bowels, and to act on her kidneys, till the 15th of April; when having had a consultation with other medical officers upon the subject, and perceiving that the abdomen increased, and the breathing had become so impeded that she was constantly obliged to sit erect in her bed, I recommended paracentesis. As there was no fluctuation to be felt below the umbilicus, it was judged right to make the opening some inches above it; and fearing the effects of the large depletion, the canula was withdrawn when eleven pints of coffee-coloured fluid had been extracted.

16th.—She was quite comfortable, and free from all pain; and she remained so well till the 22d, that we were already beginning to consider at what time the remainder of the fluid might be drawn off; but her nights now became restless, though she denied all pain; her breathing became shorter; and she felt generally worse.

24th.—Pulse, feeble, 140; respiration 40; hands clammy; no tenderness on pressure of the abdomen, unless it be very heavy just below the scrobiculus cordis. She vomited once in the night. The abdomen was covered with a large mustard poultice, and simple injections were administered. The next day she seemed relieved, but gradually sank; the tongue becoming dark; and she denying, to the time of her death, that she suffered any pain.

Sectio cadaveris, April 26th, 1829.—The distension of the abdomen was very great, and the recti muscles were spread like a panniculus carnosus over the abdomen. A puncture being made, above two pailsful of green fluid were drawn off, turbid, and containing some shreds of recent coagulable matter; the parietes were then laid open, and were found to be adherent in some parts by tolerably firm adhesions to a large sac, which now appeared to occupy the whole abdomen. The viscera were all thrust by this so far upwards, as to lie within a line drawn across from one false rib to another. The colon was seen of a black colour, projecting at the top, greatly distended with flatus, and looking like another large cyst. The whole of the cyst was covered with shreds of lymph, showing recent inflammatory action; and the colon was glued to the cyst, to the liver, and to the stomach. When these adventitious unions were broken down, the whole of the small intestines were found closely compacted together below the inferior part of the colon, and the cysts united to each other by a dark gray or black fibrinous deposit. The cyst was separated with tolerable ease from its attachments; and was held only by the round ligament of the uterus. Its coats were a quarter of an inch thick, and it contained several pints of grumous, brown fluid; and around the sides was deposited a light-brown, fibrous matter, like the fibrin separated from the blood; masses of which came away from cells connected with the larger cyst, and opening into it by well-defined crescent-like openings, of which the edges were entire. Some of these cells were capacious enough within to hold a quarter of a pint of such soft fibrinous matter; and when it was emptied out, several globular, transparent cysts came into view. On the lower part of the tumour, turned towards the pubes, was situated the chief mass of globular cysts. These were situated completely between what appeared to be the laminæ of the membrane composing the large cyst; and were freely supplied with vessels from it. When this was cut through by one clean incision (Fig. 29), several tumours were divided, and found

Fig. 29.

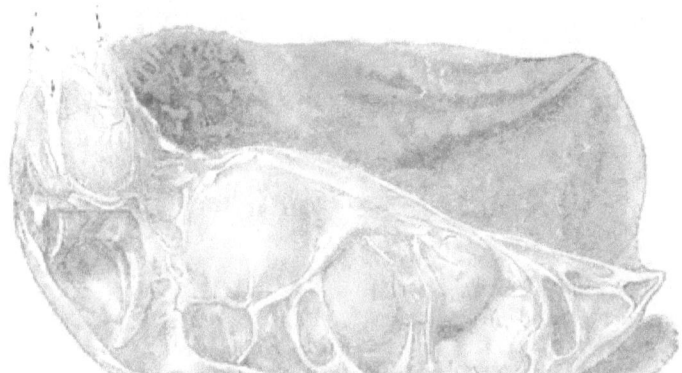

Fig. 29 represents a mass of cysts included between the layers of a large ovarian cyst, apparently owing their peculiar form and arrangement, in some degree, to the cellular structure connecting the layers. Some of the cysts are complete, without any opening; but many communicate freely one with the other by openings only partially closed by folds, some of which form bands and imperfect septa through the mass.

to be full of a yellow, glairy fluid, something like oil, while others remained perfect; and some crescentic margins or bands were seen, which had half divided the cysts, laid open. A few very small cysts were seen sprouting out of the parietes; and a very peculiar structure, like a network of fibres, from beneath which the cysts were in some parts seen sprouting, as if forcing open and distending the meshes. (Fig. 30.)

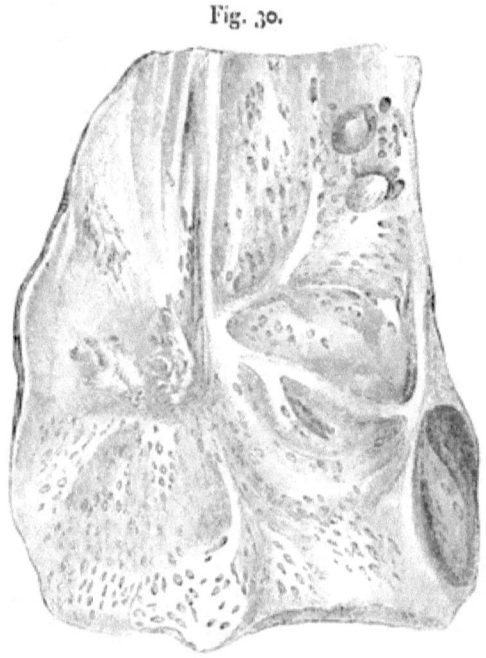

Fig. 30.

Fig. 30. A portion of the internal surface of a large malignant ovarian cyst, showing a peculiar but not unusual reticulated appearance, apparently the result of the thickening of cellular tissue; and between the meshes may be seen occasionally small cysts projecting.

The whole of this diseased mass was in the exact situation of the right ovary, and appeared to be formed by a gradual distension of the broad ligament at that part, in such a way that the Fallopian tube was bound round it; and the covering of the tumour was, to all appearance, a continuance of the covering of the ovary, very much thickened; the ovary itself being quite lost in the mass.

In this case, the whole bore the appearance of having been the result of a disease in the ovary itself; the cells of which had been distended by an enormous secretion within them; and the reticulated parts seemed to be little other than the cellular membrane of the part thickened into cartilaginous bands.

The immediate cause of death was the extensive peritoneal inflammation, which, in all probability, was chiefly owing to the fluid not having been more completely emptied out of the cyst, and some of it consequently escaping into the peritoneal cavity.

CASE 7.—*Ovarian dropsy of many years' duration, showing several cysts in different conditions; with the analysis of the fluids they contained.*—Maria N—, æt. 35, was admitted, under my care, into Guy's Hospital, December 3d, 1834, apparently the subject of a very large ovarian tumour; she had been married above eight years, and had borne three living children within that period. It seems to have been about the time of her marriage that she first experienced some pain and swelling at the left side of the abdomen, in the inguinal region; and the swelling gradually increased so much, that about five years and a half ago, it was necessary to draw off the fluid it contained, with the trochar; it then very slowly increased, and it was not till after three years and a half that a second operation was performed. The increase was then more rapid, for she was again tapped after a year and a half, which was in June last; so that less than six months have passed, and now she is nearly as large as she ever was. The abdomen is very greatly distended, and the fluctuation is very distinct in every part, even in the lumbar spaces; the body is emaciated. On the 8th, four gallons of fluid were drawn off, of a dingy colour, and containing numerous small, shining flakes of what appeared to be cholesterine; and which Dr. Rees, who collected a considerable quantity of this matter, and examined it more minutely, at my request, decided to be so. On the fifth day after the operation a brisk purge of rhubarb and calomel brought away much hardened fæces; and the abdomen being then flaccid, I examined it carefully, and plainly discovered three or four hardened bodies appended to the parietes of the cyst. The urine was sufficient in quantity, light-coloured, and not coagulable. Within a fortnight the fluid had obviously accumulated considerably; but her feelings being very comfortable, she wished to return home about three weeks after the operation.

August 12th, 1835.—She was again admitted, under my care, being as large as before the last operation, but suffering less from sickness, dyspepsia, and general symptoms of oppression, than has usually been the case. On the 14th, four gallons and a half of fluid, moderately coagulable by heat, were drawn off; after which she suffered some pain and tenderness, with a quickened pulse, requiring leeches, and calomel and opium, for a few days, till the gums were very slightly affected.

The two most obvious hardened masses were to be felt; one, low down on the right side; the other, above the umbilicus, to the left. (Fig. 22.) She remained in the house till the 14th of September, when, although the fluid was again accumulating, she preferred going home to her family.

March 9th, 1836.—She was again admitted, and on the 15th, twenty-five quarts of fluid were drawn off; after which, the two tumours, which had been before felt, were very distinctly found. In about three weeks she left the house, but the fluid was again accumulating.

August 3d.—Again admitted; and the following day, five gallons and a quart were again drawn off; which she bore without any unpleasant symptoms, and returned home in about a fortnight.

November 15th.—She was again admitted; on the 25th, twenty-four quarts of fluid were drawn off: it was of a darkish colour, with some ropy sediment, and tinged with some red particles. On the 12th of December she returned to her family.

March 22d, 1837.—She was again admitted, and again about the same quantity of fluid was drawn off, on the 30th. On the 5th of April shivering took place, accompanied by swelling, apparently glandular, in the pelvic and inguinal regions, which required a good deal of attention and treatment; however, on the 15th of May she left the hospital, in her usual state of health.

Maria N— (now called Price, having lately married again) was admitted, under my care, July 26th, 1837, with the abdomen again distended to the utmost, and complaining of sickness, for which I gave the hydrocyanic acid.

On the 31st of July, when the sickness had subsided, and the bowels were opened, twenty-three quarts of serum were drawn away, of a muddy colour, slightly oleaginous, and moderately coagulable by heat; after this, considerable inflammation took place, which was subdued by calomel and opium; but it was three weeks before she was able to return home.

In this case, we observe a disease which, in all probability, depends upon a structural change in the ovary, very similar to that which was discovered in Waite, proceeding, as yet, in a comparatively mild course. That the tumour consists of a large sac, in the parietes of which hardened enlargements are developed, scarcely admits of a doubt; but though the secretion seems to proceed with an accelerated progress, we have reason to believe, from the character it bears, that the surface of the cyst has not yet undergone these changes from the bursting of the smaller cysts, which are apt to produce the still more irritating or less mild character in the discharge. It is, however, but too obvious, that the disease is now making inroads upon her constitution, and that the symptoms which have attended the two last operations have been more alarming than on former occasions. Up to that time, she suffered scarcely any pain from the disease, or any unpleasant results from the operation; indeed, the increasing bulk of the tumour has been almost the only source of inconvenience; and no less than nine years and a half have now elapsed since the swelling was so large as to require the first operation, but the disease has certainly existed between eleven and twelve years. The form of this tumour is highly characteristic of an encysted accumulation of fluid; so that I have had it engraved (Fig. 31) as an example of that form, from a sketch which was taken

Fig. 31.

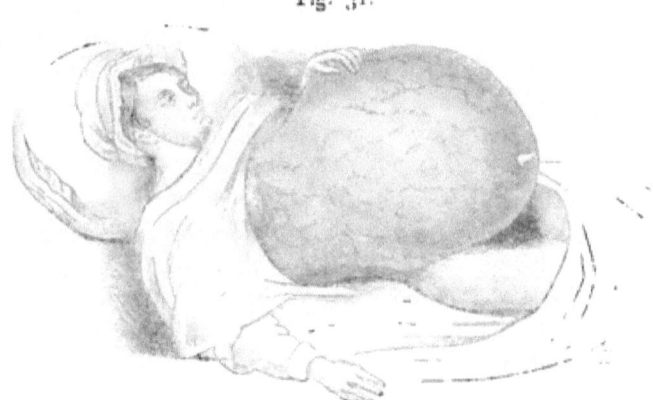

Fig. 31 represents the abdomen distended by an ovarian cyst, which, notwithstanding its enormous size, interfered little with the posture assumed by the patient in bed. The surface was covered by a network of distended veins, in consequence of the pressure of the tumour on the veins internally. They conveyed the blood from the iliac to the intercostal veins chiefly; and as the cava is generally simply compressed in these cases, and not obliterated, the circulation is partially restored to its natural course, when the fluid is withdrawn and the pressure removed.

two or three years ago; and the patient is still able to lie recumbent on her back, as here represented, without suffering from dyspnœa even when the accumulation is at its utmost. The only alteration I have had made in the sketch is, strengthening the appearance of the superficial veins, which remain nearly the same in distribution, but are more distended.

Thus far I had written this case, and prepared it for publication, when, on the 13th of December, 1837, the subject of these observations again applied for admission under my care; but her appearance was dreadfully changed. She was greatly emaciated; her voice was feeble; her eyes sunk; her pulse was extremely weak; her bowels were in a state of constant irritation; and her stomach was unable to retain the least food. The form of the tumour, however, was nearly unaltered, but a little more pendulous in the lower part as she lay on her back; and the veins on the surface, though almost exactly the same in distribution as had been marked in the sketch, were become larger and more obvious; and in some parts, owing to the thinness of the skin, from which every particle of adipose matter had been absorbed, they seemed to have communicated a stain around them by transudation, producing a kind of ecchymosis. The tumour was about the size which it had reached before the former operations, and the fluctuation was remarkably distinct in every part; nor did any part yield a clear sound on percussion, though a small space in the left lumbar region was rather more resonant than the rest. I learnt that the operation of paracentesis had been performed at her own house in the end of October, just five weeks before; and that three pailfuls, certainly amounting to four or five gallons, had then been drawn off; but she had never left her bed till the day she came to Guy's Hospital, and had, for the last three weeks, been subject to constant diarrhœa. By means of gently astringent injections, the bowels became less irritable, and her stomach was enabled to retain some small quantities of nutriment; so that for a day or two she left her bed, and sat by the fireside. She strongly objected to having the operation performed, nor could I, in her present emaciated and enfeebled state, press it upon her; though I had no doubt that, if she bore the operation, she would derive much temporary relief. The amelioration of her symptoms was but of very short duration. The diarrhœa returned, and with it increased irritability of stomach. She suffered considerable pain, particularly in the right side, where tenderness was experienced. Such palliative means as appeared admissible were assiduously administered; but she sunk on the night of the 7th of January.

Sectio cadaveris.—The integuments were reduced to their utmost tenuity, and were in many parts so closely adherent to the sac of the tumour, that the thickened peritoneum seemed to split into two layers, in the attempt to remove them. When the tumour came into view, it appeared to occupy the whole space of the abdomen, forcing the ribs up, so as to give the chest a bell-like form. (Fig. 32.) The adhesion of the cyst was chiefly confined to its anterior part; and a slight evidence of recent peritonitis was found in the right lumbar space. When the tumour was removed, it was found to be appended to one ovary alone, which was considered the right; though from the twisted position of the uterus, I was not quite convinced that it was. The other ovary was small and dwindled. The tumour

Fig. 32.

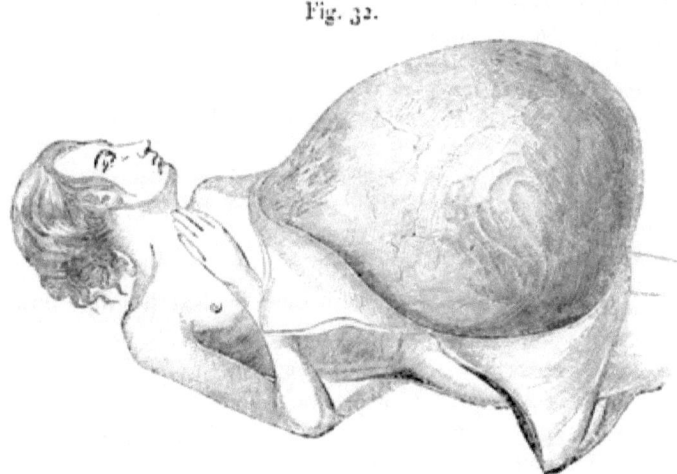

Fig. 32 represents the ovarian tumour when the integuments had been removed.

did not adhere to any of the viscera, except partially to the omentum; which came into sight on opening the integuments, spread over a small extent of the upper part of the tumour.

The liver lay closely driven up into the hollow of the diaphragm, encroaching on the chest as high as the fourth rib; and being slightly adherent, did not come into view, even after the tumour was removed. (Fig. 33.) The stomach, and the whole of the intes-

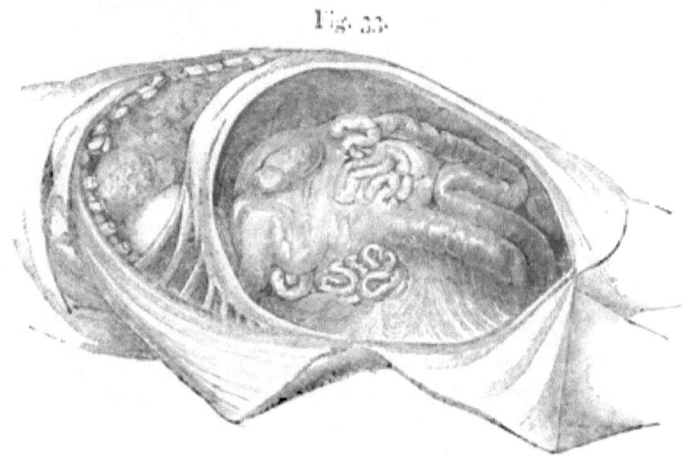

Fig. 33.

Fig. 33 shows the situation which the abdominal viscera had occupied, in consequence of the pressure of the ovarian tumour during a period of several years. When this sketch was taken, nothing had been done beyond the careful removal of the tumour, that no disturbance might be given to the viscera as they lay. The liver was seen pushing the diaphragm as high as the third rib. The stomach and intestines, greatly reduced in size, occupied the posterior and upper part of the abdomen, where they afforded hollow sound, on percussion; and where alone the movements of the intestines were felt by the patient.

tines, except the descending colon, were pushed likewise into the hollow of the diaphragm, and were exceedingly contracted; so that altogether they seemed to bear no proportion to the enormously increased dimension of the abdominal cavity. The stomach was contracted to one fourth its natural size; and the colon, as well as the small intestine, had very nearly the same relative dimensions. The descending colon was seen running down, closely bound to the parietes of the right lumbar space, and terminating in a very strongly-marked sigmoid flexure. None of the intestines bore marks of peritoneal inflammation, either old or recent; and no remarkable disease was discernible in the mucous membrane of the stomach, or any part of the canal. The structure of the liver was tolerably healthy, as was that of the spleen. The kidneys were partially absorbed, owing to the obstruction which the ureter had suffered; and this was particularly the case on the left side, where the ureter was not only dilated, but much thickened; and the enlarged infundibula contained a puriform fluid. The bladder was contracted.

The lungs adhered to the ribs, and were extremely small, from the encroachment of the tumour, but were not otherwise diseased. The heart presented a remarkable specimen of atrophy; and the aorta, through its whole extent, corresponded well with the heart.

The ascending cava lay quite flat and empty, and small upon the spine: it contained neither blood nor coagula, but did not appear diseased, nor was there any approach to obliteration.

The iliac and connected veins contained firm coagula of recent red blood.

The tumour itself consisted of one large cyst, which contained a bucketful of rather tenacious, straw-coloured fluid, which towards the bottom became opaque and puriform. In its parietes, towards the left side, was a large mass, like a placenta, consisting of several semi-transparent cysts, which yielded a very transparent, gelatinous fluid, containing portions more opaque; and within the large cyst arose two smaller ones, each containing above a pint of fluid; one of a limpid straw colour; the other a more turbid fluid, loaded with little shining particles of cholesterine, corresponding precisely with the fluid which had been drawn off, to the extent of four gallons, on the first admission of the patient, just three years ago, in December, 1834.

The cyst which contained this fluid was somewhat thicker than the large cyst; and it had undergone changes which seemed to bespeak that, in all probability, it had at one time been much larger than it at present was; for many plates of a cartilaginous hardness were found imbedded in its parietes. Its external surface looked diseased and rough, and puriform matter was attached to it; while its internal surface was smooth and polished, presenting a shining membranous appearance.

One of the masses which occupied the parietes of the larger cyst had begun to sprout out, and become opaque, yielding puriform matter, quite analogous to the change which I have described, and endeavoured to represent by an engraving, in the case of W—— (Fig. 28).

Thus the fatal result and consequent examination confirmed the similarity of this case to that of W——; proving the same changes, but rather in a more advanced degree, had taken place in the large cyst; and the puriform matter which had been drawn from W—— would have been exactly imitated in this case, had the operation been performed; that fluid being probably yielded, in part, by the fungoid mass growing from the surface, and, in part, by the lining membrane of the cyst, in which a process of superficial ulceration had taken place.

It was a matter of considerable interest, both with myself and Dr. Rees—who had examined the fluid, drawn at the first operation, performed under my care just three years ago—to ascertain whether any of the cysts contained cholesterine in the state we then discovered; for we had conjectured, from the total absence of that substance in the fluid drawn on a subsequent occasion, that the same cyst could never have been again opened, as it appeared very improbable that the fluid should have been so completely removed and never have formed again; and this proved to be the case; for after I had obtained specimens of the fluid from each cyst in succession, we at length (but not till the fourth cyst was opened, and I had begun to despair of finding cholesterine) came to the cyst which contained that substance. I immediately put all the four specimens into Dr. Rees's hands, whom I knew to be sufficiently interested in the case to undertake these analyses; and of this I was the more desirous, in the hope that we might be able to derive some guide in our diagnosis between encysted dropsies and ascites, from the actual chemical properties, as we do already, to a certain degree, from the obvious and physical character of the fluids. How far this hope has been realised, must be gathered from the following analyses and observations.

Examination of four fluids drawn from secondary cysts of an Ovarian Tumour, and of one (No. 5), probably from an Ovarian Cyst, by Dr. Rees.

	No. 1. (Clear, light straw-coloured, alkaline, sp. gr. 1017.)	No. 2. (Dark-coloured, muddy, neutral, sp. gr. 1017.)	No. 3. (Approaching in character to white of egg, alkaline.)	No. 4. (Clear, straw-coloured, containing flakes of a pearly scaly-looking substance.)	No. 5. (Sp. Gr. 1026, alkaline, very tenacious, see Case 8.)	Analysis of serum of blood, for comparison.
Water	190·9	190·70	195·2	187·7	195·32	181·2
Albumen, with traces of fatty matter	4·1	4·25	1·8	7·6	0·54	16·5
Albumen, existing in solution, as albuminate of soda	3·7	3·62	1·1	......	*2·22	0·4
Alkaline chloride† and sulphate, with carbonate of soda, from decomposed albuminate	0·8	0·78	1·2	4·0	‡1·08	1·6 ⎫
Extractive, soluble in water, and alcohol	0·4	0·45	0·5	0·5	0·54	0·3 ⎬
Chloride of sodium with carbonate, from decomposed lactate of alcoholic extract	0·1	0·20	0·2	0·2	0·30	...... ⎭
Totals	200	200	200	200	200	200

* This albumen existed only in part as albuminate of soda.
† In very small proportion, being in great part separated with the alcoholic extract.
‡ This was from decomposed lactate, with traces of phosphate.
§ The whole of the alkaline salts are estimated together in the analysis of serum as indicated by the line.

It will be seen, on comparing these analyses with that of the serum of blood, that in every specimen there is a considerable excess of water and extractives, and a deficiency of albumen. As all these fluids were of that mucoid, tenacious character so well known to those who are in the habit of examining the cysts of ovarian dropsies, I am inclined to conclude that this peculiarity in appearance is attributable to the presence of a large proportion of extractives, particularly the albumen combined with soda (aqueous extractive insoluble in alcohol); which opinion is confirmed by the experiments of Dr. Babington, who has succeeded in forming a mucoid fluid by the addition of alkalies to albuminous secretions.[1] If we regard the salts present in proportion to the quantity of solid matter, we shall find that Nos. 1 and 2 contain an excess of salts; for the solid matter in 200 grains of serum is equal to about 18·8 grs., and the proportion of alkaline salts 1·6; while the solid matters of Nos. 1 and 2 are 9·1 and 9·3 in 200 grains, and the proportion of salts 0·9 and 0·98; whereas their corresponding proportions would be about 0·77 and 0·79; for $9·1 \times 1·6 \div 18·8 = 0·77$; and $9·3 \times 1·6 \div 18·8 = 0·79$. My reason for regarding the salts in relation to the solid matter, is that the peculiar mucous character of the liquors is owing to the *nature* of the solid ingredients; and quite independent of any particular proportion of water, as might at first be supposed. If No. 3 be compared, we observe a very great excess of salts in proportion to the solid contents, which are very small. No. 4 gives likewise an excess of extractives and salts taken together: the proportion of salts alone was not ascertained in this specimen, as a loss was experienced while determining their weight. The fat contained in these fluids (which was estimated with the albumen, and existed as a mere trace) consisted of the ordinary fatty matter of the blood in Nos. 1 and 2. Nos. 3 and 4 contained cholesterine, as the fat.

The flocculi of pearly, scaly matter were separated from No. 4 previous to analysis by diluting the portion of liquor containing them with a large quantity of water, and allowing it to drain through a fine linen cloth; the residue on the filter being well washed with cold distilled water. Of this substance, 5·3 grains were obtained:[2] on examination, it was found to be composed of

Cholesterine . . . . 3·4
Albumino-cerous matter,[3] with traces of albumen . . 1·9

The alkaline salts obtained from the ovarian liquids differ from those of the

---

[1] Vide 'Guy's Hospital Reports,' vol. ii, p. 534.

[2] From eighteen ounces of the liquid.

[3] First noticed by Dr. Marcet, as existing in a diseased thyroid gland; afterwards by Dr. Bostock (who gave it the above-mentioned name), as found in tumours of muscular parts. More particularly described by Dr. Bostock, as found in a hydrocele of some years' standing.—Vide 'Med.-Chirurg. Transact.,' vols. ii, iv, and xv.

It may be well to mention, that this substance differs from albumen in not being soluble in a solution of potassa, and from cholesterine by its insolubility in boiling alcohol. It otherwise closely resembles cholesterine in its chemical properties.

blood in not containing any phosphate which can be recognised even as a trace in the quantity of solid matter obtained from 200 grains; experiments made on larger quantities, for the express purpose of detecting an alkaline phosphate, showed a trace only. I may observe that the albumen from these liquids yielded a scarcely perceptible portion of earthy matter on incineration; this, most probably, was phosphate of lime.[1]

The proportion of water and solid matter in No. 5 approaches very nearly to that of No. 3. It contains much less free albumen, however, and more albumen in combination. I have no doubt that many alkaline salts, as well as any free alkali present, have the power of retaining albumen in a soluble form after a heat of 212° has been applied to dry it; for the salts, from the aqueous extractive in this specimen, yielded less carbonate than did that of No. 3, notwithstanding the excessive proportion of combined albumen. I am inclined to attribute much of this solvent power to the lactates, which exist in greater proportion in this specimen than in any of the kind that I have yet examined.

CASE 8.—*Malignant tumour in abdomen, probably ovarian; discharging constantly from the wound made by paracentesis.*—E. D——, æt. 34, ill six years, of moderate stature, dark hair and eyes, single, and employed as governess in a family, was admitted into Guy's Hospital in February, 1838. Between her sixteenth and seventeenth year the catamenia first appeared, and have continued, at the proper times, till within the last four years, since which period they have appeared irregularly. She says, that she has not enjoyed good health for many years past, having had repeated attacks of inflammation of the bowels, head, and chest. About six years ago, one month after the last severe attack of inflammation of the bowels, she first perceived a general swelling over the anterior half of the abdomen, apparently commencing rather above and to the left of the umbilicus. This gradually increased in size downwards; and after two years had elapsed paracentesis was performed, and six and a half gallons of glutinous fluid, of the colour of mustard-whey, were drawn off. Two months after the abdomen again enlarged; and about one pailful was discharged through the former opening, which gathered, and burst of its own accord. A few months after an abscess formed at the opening, which burst, and discharged to the amount of a wash-hand basin; since which, although there has been a constant discharge, the abdomen has enlarged, the superficial veins are distended, and the umbilicus is entirely obliterated.

[1] The analysis of specimen No. 5 was performed after these observations were written.

The parietes of the abdomen are not at present (March, 1838) greatly distended, but the skin feels flaccid under the hand; the chief prominence is around the umbilical region; but the tumour may be traced into the left iliac fossa, and into the pelvis on that side; no fluctuation, or very little, is to be felt. The tumour is hard to the feel, and irregular on its surface, and appears glued to the parietes. In the situation of the puncture made by the trochar, a vascular excrescence arises, of the size of a small bean; from beneath which a fluid distils, so as to keep the napkin constantly moist; it is clear and slightly mucilaginous, and, according to the analysis of Dr. Rees, to whom I gave some, which she collected for me in a phial, it agrees very closely with the fluid contained in the ovarian cysts. (See Table, No. 5, p. 93.) She says that the tumour has decidedly diminished latterly; and her health is tolerably good, with the exception of occasional vomiting. Tongue clean; pulse feeble; appetite good; but she has emaciated lately, and complains now and then of pain in her loins.

The whole history of this case seems to bespeak a malignant ovarian cyst, which has formed adhesions to the parietes, followed by a fistulous opening externally; and, judging from her present condition, her capability of walking about, her general manner, and aspect of tolerable, though weak health, there seems little reason to doubt that this circumstance has conduced both to her comfort and to the prolongation of her life.

CASE 9.—*Compound ovarian cyst. Death from exhaustion.*— Susan W—, æt. 25, was admitted into Charity Ward, July 14th, 1830, the subject of ovarian dropsy, for which she had already been twice tapped. Her abdomen was very large, and she had a red, sandy complexion; and, although not under my care, she struck me immediately, from her strong resemblance to my former patient W— (Case 5); and when I examined her abdomen the similarity was still more striking, for in different parts of the large fluctuating tumour other small, irregular, hard tumours were distinctly felt. Her health appeared good, except so far as the size of the abdomen interfered with it. She was three times tapped when in the house, and bore the operation well; a large quantity of thick, glutinous fluid was drawn off each time. The last operation took place on the 9th of November; she seemed very well for a day or two; but about ten days after, without any very obvious cause, became exceedingly exhausted, and died on the 23d of the same month.

Sectio cadaveris.—November 24th, 1830.—On opening the abdomen, the cyst, which had been tapped, occupied the lower part, pushing the intestines to the left side; while a large growth from the tumour appeared like an independent body in the right side, pushing the liver upwards. This upper portion of the tumour was divided into several lobules; and a few serous cysts were hanging from it.

On carefully examining the attachment of this diseased mass, it was found to arise entirely from the situation of the left ovary. The Fallopian tube on that side was stretched over it to a considerable length, and the uterus was a little drawn from its place. No adhesion had taken place to the parietes, and only a few slight filamentous attachments to the omentum.

When the large cyst was laid open, three or four pints of fluid escaped, which was like thin water-gruel in consistence, but a little more mucilaginous; and in two or three parts, when the fluid was completely removed, subordinate tumours were seen rising from the lower part of the cyst. In several parts the lining membrane was evidently undergoing a process of softening, or a kind of sloughing, so as to allow of the protrusion of small cysts through orifices which were then surrounded by marginated bands circular or crescentic, the central softened portions of such parts of the cyst being yellow and friable; and when removed, a quantity of thick mucus, like birdlime, issued from the orifice.

There was not more than half a pint of fluid in the abdominal cavity, and no evidence of recent inflammation. The absorbent glands along the course of the left iliac vein, near its exit, were enlarged; which seemed to account for a considerable swelling during life in the leg and thigh of that side.

This case, which is one of well-marked malignant disease of the ovary, proceeded rapidly, so that paracentesis was required no less than three times in the space of four months. It is chiefly valuable, as showing one of the circumstances which occasionally occurs, perhaps as the result of operations (but even that is uncertain), where an almost sudden and unexpected state of exhaustion or collapse takes place, and death ensues without any obvious sign of inflammation being observed afterwards, except that which may be supposed to have been taking place in the interior of the cyst itself.

The appearance of the interior of the large cyst illustrated very strikingly the same process in the development of the small cysts, through openings taking place in the membrane, and leaving crescentic margins, as in the case of W— (Case 5, fig. 28); or in that of M— (Case 6, fig. 30); an appearance which possibly results from the original cellular structure of that part.

CASE 10.—*Compound ovarian cyst; the fluid never removed. Slow exhaustion and death; adhesions of the tumour to the parietes discerned during life.*—The following case has been already published in a paper treating on the subject of peritoneal adhesions, in the 'Transactions' of the Royal Medical and Chirurgical Society; but as the case involves the history and termination of ovarian dropsy when no operation has been performed, and as the illustration it affords of the means of diagnosis in cases of adherent peritoneum is necessary for the completion of the present subject, I think it well worth introducing in this place.

Sophia Y—, æt. 30, was admitted, under my care, into Guy's Hospital, February 24th, 1830, with a large swelling of the abdomen. She had borne five children; and since August the catamenia had not appeared till three weeks ago, when there was a slight appearance; and at the time of her admission she laboured under menorrhagia. The tumour occupied the whole abdomen, and was of a very irregular form. She stated, that it had at first shown itself at the lower part of the abdomen, on the left side; but now the most prominent part was on the right side, not far from the head of the colon, where a hard, round projection was both seen and felt. Several other round, hard masses might be plainly ascertained by the touch; one nearly in the situation of the liver, and another to the left of the umbilicus, and one below. There was, besides, a distinct general fluctuation; and in several parts, on making the parietes move gently, a peculiar feel, like a slight crepitus, or like the crackling feel of new leather, was to be distinguished.

I considered this to be either an ovarian tumour, or a collection of hydatids; and that the peculiar sensation communicated to the hand arose from adhesions between the tumour and the parietes of the abdomen. I thought it by far more probable that the tumour was ovarian, from the history, from the fluctuation, and from the hardness of some portions of the tumour. As the tumour was large, and from its size exceedingly inconvenient, I spoke about tapping, in her hearing, but found she most resolutely refused to consent to an operation. My treatment, therefore, was confined to the application of leeches, to relieve local pain (from which she suffered much), and the regulation of the bowels, together with a few other internal remedies, which suggested themselves as likely to retard the increase of the morbid growth and effusion.

On the 7th of July she left the hospital, decidedly increased in size, but still retaining a tolerably healthy appearance in other respects.

When she had returned home, she continued to increase in bulk —her legs swelled, becoming œdematous, and then inflamed. She gradually sank, and died on the 31st of December, 1830.

Sectio cadaveris.—The upper part of the body greatly emaciated; the legs œdematous, with desquamation of both shins. The abdomen was of the most inordinate size, and very irregular in its form; numerous veins ran over the tumour, and were seen forming large plexuses on the chest.

Fig. 34.

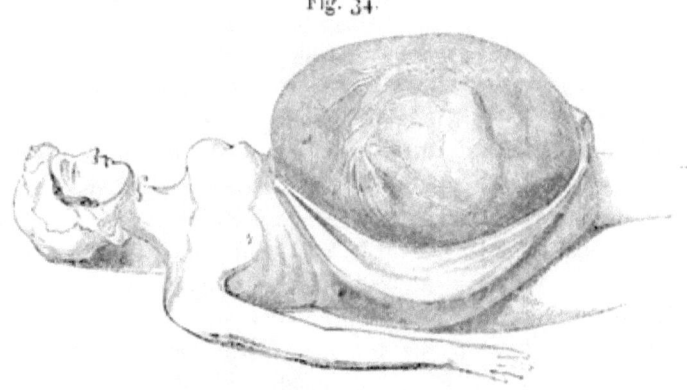

Fig. 34 represents the appearance of an ovarian tumour, when the integuments had been carefully removed; and is chiefly given to illustrate the difference of the form which the abdomen assumed, and its irregular shape; and also as an instance of the rapid growth which sometimes takes place in the ovarian tumours; for the disease in this case had not attracted notice above two years, at the utmost. On one portion of the right side of the tumour, crepitation had disclosed the existence of adhesions; and the cellular membrane forming them is marked in the sketch.

The parietes of the abdomen were found to adhere very generally, but chiefly about the central part, from side to side, to the tumour within; and there was only about a quart of limpid, straw-coloured serum in the cavity of the abdomen. When the integuments and the attenuated muscles had been pretty well detached from the contents of the abdomen, a tumour, exactly resembling the external form of the abdomen, was fully brought to view—the only difference being, that the projections on its surface were rather more marked. (Fig. 34.) It was now quite obvious to the feel, that the whole was one large cyst, with several hard, flattened bodies, almost like the placenta, formed in its parietes. The intestines were forced back, out of view, to the left side, and the liver was quite pushed under the ribs, so that nothing was to be seen but the large ovarian tumour. An opening being made into the cyst, nearly six gallons of a tenacious, dingy-coloured fluid, of the consistence of thick gruel or very thick linseed-tea, were drawn off; and the cyst being laid open, a tolerably healthy surface was exposed, with a few uneven parts, where smaller cysts seemed to be pushing forwards into the cavity. The greater part of the thick, cake-like masses, which occupied at least two thirds of the whole parietes of the tumour, were developed in the substance of the parietes, and projected outwards rather than inwards. Cutting into these masses, they afforded an appearance of cells filled with thick mucus, not unlike, in some parts, an enormous honeycomb filled with its contents (resembling Fig. 29); and in one part, near the iliac region, a large, rounded mass projected, as an external appendage to the great tumour. On examination, it appeared that this was a cluster of cysts, more or less globular, which projected into a kind of chamber connected with the large cyst; the opening being formed by two or three crescentic margins, some parts of which were serrated with very fine spicula of bone. This mass of disease was attached entirely to the left broad ligament of the uterus; the ovary itself, however, could not be traced. The uterus and the right ovary were perfectly healthy; but the uterus was drawn round by the weight of the tumour, which, though it arose in the left side, lay very much to the right of the abdomen.

The viscera of the abdomen were in general healthy, as was the peritoneum of the intestines, which in no part adhered to the tumour, though the parietes adhered so generally. The liver was healthy. The kidneys were flaccid, and pale.

The chest was diminished in size by the tumour, which rose almost to the third rib. The lungs were healthy in structure, but gorged with blood.

In this case it was not possible, from the want of observation by the patient, to say at what exact period the tumour first appeared; but it had not attracted her notice till August, 1829, when the irregularity of the catamenia roused attention. The whole course, however, of the disease, from the time it was discovered till it proved fatal, did not exceed a year and a half.

Dr. G. H. Barlow has kindly furnished me with the following case, illustrative of the fatal result of the ovarian tumour, when left entirely to pursue its course; and I shall give it in his own words.

Case 11.—*Compound ovarian cyst; the fluid never removed. Death from irritation and exhaustion.*—Mrs. N—, æt. 35, had been delivered of three stillborn children, and had menstruated regularly till January, 1837, at the end of which month the catamenia appeared for the last time. She soon after observed her abdomen gradually enlargeing; and in the middle of June she made application to an accoucher to arrange for her confinement, which she said she expected would take place towards the end of October. At the time of her application, she was, I am informed, about the size of a woman in the fifth month of pregnancy, and she said that she felt the motion of the child. She appears to have had no misgivings till within a few weeks of the time of her expected confinement, when she said she felt as she had never done during any former pregnancy; her bowels were then exceedingly irregular, and she had occasional vomiting. The tumour, I am told, then felt rather lobulated. She continued to enlarge, and suffer increasing inconvenience, till January, 1838, at the end of which month I saw her for the first time. She had a dingy sallowness of complexion, and was then unable to lie down, owing to the pressure of the distended abdomen; which was of a size far exceeding the greatest enlargement of pregnancy, and was marked by a number of veins of great size. The abdomen felt rather lobulated, and there was rather indistinct fluctuation at the upper part; but inferiorly there was none; and at this part the abdomen felt as if it contained a large, hard mass. There was no resonance upon percussion about the epigastrium;

but there was some in the right iliac fossa. Her urine was very scanty. Paracentesis was suggested, but to this the friends would not consent. I saw her a few days afterwards; when her legs were much swollen, and had given way in several parts. The abdomen then felt exceedingly tense; but the sickness had been less distressing. She continued for about five days to undergo no change, except that of increasing debility, and a return of the vomiting; at the end of which time she sank exhausted.

Sectio cadaveris.—The abdomen only was examined. It contained a large tumour, which was nearly free from adhesions, so that it could be removed entire. It appeared to have originated in the left ovary, which was adherent to or rather seemed to form part of it. The small intestines were nearly all collected in the right iliac fossa; and portions of them, as well of the jejunum as of the ileum, were of a deep-brownish red, both externally and internally, as if from excessive congestion. At these parts, grumous-looking blood could be squeezed from the mucous membrane. The tumour, when removed, was seen to be nearly spherical, and measured just two feet in diameter. That part of it which was situated superiorly, consisted of three or four large cysts, which contained a thin, glairy fluid. The inferior portion was of a much more complicated structure; it consisted of cysts of every size, from that of a large orange to that of a pin's head, the larger cysts being lined by smaller ones. In the lowest part of the tumour, all regularity of structure seemed merged in that of a cellular substance, containing here and there a cavity of the size of a large pea. The contents of these cysts varied from the clear, glairy fluid, mentioned as having been found in the larger cysts, to an opaque substance of the colour of pus, and having the consistency and tenacity of the muco-purulent expectoration sometimes voided by bronchitic patients. The kidneys were healthy.

In this case we have another instance of death from the simple effects of the enormously enlarged ovarian tumour; and scarcely more than a year had elapsed since the first discovery of the disease. The cyst afforded a very excellent example of one form of the complicated tumour; but although this and the last case ran their course so rapidly, when unaided by art, there is reason to suppose that a great many cases would be much slower in their progress to a fatal termination.

Case 12.—*Ovarian dropsy, fatal from peritonitis after the partial abstraction of the fluid.*—A. B—was admitted into the hospital on the 8th of April, with a large, fluctuating tumour, of a globular form, occupying the whole abdomen. After being in the house a few days a portion of the fluid was drawn off, and proved to be of a dark coffee-ground appearance. She became very low, with a dry and brown tongue. Pulse faltering; abdomen very tender; and in this state she remained till the 10th, when she died.

Sectio cadaveris.—Signs of inflammation displayed themselves very extensively on the peritoneum, which contained two quarts of dark-coloured serum. One large cyst occupied the greater part of the abdomen, the parietes of which were about a quarter of an inch in thickness; and within might be felt other cysts, rendering the parietes more hard and unyielding. It was removed from the abdomen entire; and was found to be behind the right Fallopian tube, which was extended across it to the length of at least a foot, and was not amalgamated into its substance. The fimbriated extremity was free, but the orifice appeared obliterated. The tumour arose distinctly from the situation of the right ovary; and the ligament was seen gradually dilating to cover the sac, affording a radiated, vascular appearance. No remnant of the natural ovary could be discovered; and in all probability its whole structure formed the basis of the tumour.

The cyst was injected; and, when laid open, was found to contain five or six quarts of brown, opaque fluid. The wall of the cyst was about a quarter of an inch in thickness, somewhat laminated in its structure, and having vessels in its substance, the cut ends of which were seen when a section was made, giving an appearance not unlike a section of the uterus. There were also some cysts formed in a mass between the layers of the chief cyst, and nearer the external than the internal surface. This mass was formed of forty or fifty flattened, semi-transparent cysts; some of the size of an egg, but many of them not larger than a marble. On the inside of the large cyst arose two brown, fungous masses, apparently breaking down; and in one part a portion of the internal lining of the cyst was detached, forming a kind of blister large enough to contain a pint of fluid. There was also a small cluster of three or four pellucid cysts, which seemed to have been contained within the cavity of another which had sloughed away. On the outside of the main cyst were one or two fungous masses, not discoloured or sloughy.

When the parietes of certain parts were taken between the fingers, they were obviously much thicker than the rest of the cysts, and were elastic; and on being cut into, found to be separated, as splittings of the lamellæ of the cyst filled with grumous fluid; and within this was a deposit like the fibrin of blood coagulated and brown, but not having any cyst-like arrangement. The left ovary was quite natural, and the Fallopian tube on that side perfect.

This case furnishes an example of the compound ovarian cyst, involving, distinctly, the whole right ovary; and while its general structure was quite analogous to that which has been already described, it presented some peculiarities in the unusual vascularity of the chief cyst, and the circumstance of its dividing into lamellæ, between which grumous fluid had collected.

This case also affords another example of peritonitis, following shortly after the partial abstraction of the ovarian fluid.

CASE 13.—*Cyst, probably a diseased Graafian vesicle, communicating by ulceration with the colon. Death from irritation of the mucous membrane of the large intestine.*—Mary Ann J—, æt. 22, of a sallow complexion, was admitted, under my care, November 2d, 1835, with an indistinct tumour in the lower parts of her abdomen, and suffering great and constant pain. It appeared that about twelve months before she first felt a tumour in the left iliac region, which had gone on increasing till about three months ago, when diarrhœa came on, and with it the tumour decreased; so that it was now very much diminished; and was rather a diffused hardness than a defined tumour, extending from the crest of the ilium to the pubes, two or three inches in width. The motions were frequently very copious, and of an unhealthy, muddy appearance, but not obviously containing pus. The tumour seemed to vary in size in some degree, according to the extent of the fæculent discharges. She suffered much pain and griping; the tongue was glossy and dry. Anodynes and the gentlest laxatives, as manna and castor-oil, injections of gruel and poppy fomentations, formed the chief remedies; and by taking them with the mildest diet she continued fluctuating, and occasionally affording some apparent hope of recovery; but at length she sank under great mucous irritation, after being in the hospital nearly four months.

Sectio cadaveris.—On opening the abdomen, the omentum, somewhat loaded with fat, came into view, covering the whole intestines and glued down to the pelvis, passing over a tumour which arose over the pubes, nearly in the centre, but rather to the right side. There were no signs of recent peritonitis. On examination, it appeared that this tumour had probably been developed in the right ovary; but it had passed behind the uterus to which it was attached, and it had likewise become slightly glued in the sigmoid flexure; but the chief adhesion was to the cæcum, or commencement of the colon; and here ulceration had taken place, and an opening was formed; and when the cyst was squeezed, bubbles of air escaped through an opening into the cæcum. The fluid it contained was of a dirty dull-red colour. The cyst was firm, and nearly half an inch in thickness; its internal lining presented a very curious appearance, which I ascribed entirely to the contraction which had taken place since the evacuation of the fluid; it had an appearance of corrugation or mammillation, being thrown into folds of irregular polygonal forms, with deep fissures between them. The colour of this membrane was a dark olive-green. (Fig. 35.) The ascending colon and the arch were full of dark-coloured fluid, resembling that found in the tumour; but as the whole surface of these viscera had evidently been recently irritated, so as to present many small points of blood, it was difficult to say whence the fluid

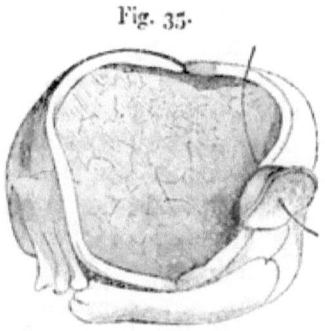

Fig. 35.

Fig. 35. The internal view of a cyst, believed to be ovarian, which had emptied its contents into the colon, at the point where the bristle is introduced. Its surface was curiously corrugated, apparently from the contraction which had taken place in the cyst since its contents had found an egress. This cyst which is preserved in the Museum of Guy's Hospital, is about six inches in diameter.

had come. The descending colon was more healthy, and, at its sigmoid flexure, was slightly attached to the tumour.

The uterus was large and flaccid.

In this case we have an example of the mode in which life is generally terminated, when a cyst communicates by ulceration with the intestines; the irritation of the mucous membrane usually, sooner or later, exhausting the powers of the patient. In this instance, I think it likely that the cyst was of a less malignant character than is most common, and probably had its origin in a disease of the Graafian vesicle; of this, however, there is no proof.

CASE 14.—*Ovarian cyst, probably a diseased Graafian vesicle; fluid partially removed; inflammation of cyst and peritoneum.*—H—, æt. —, died on the 20th of April, 1837. She was not under my own care, and I only saw her once or twice during life. In this case it was intended to try how far the ovarian cyst might be gradually contracted by drawing off small quantities of the fluid by successive operations; however, considerable inflammation succeeded the first attempt, and she had suffered a great deal from pain and tenderness of the abdomen ever since; an abscess had formed in the parietes, extending downwards towards the pubes. For some days before death constant sickness, and frequent wandering and delirium, had marked the progress of the disease.

Sectio cadaveris.—On opening the abdomen, it was found that the parietes adhered closely over the whole lower part of the abdomen to the omentum, which was spread out over the cyst. The adhesion was so strong, that it was necessary to tear it away in every part; and the omentum and the peritoneal lining of the abdominal parietes were deeply stained with that carbonaceous deposit, which is the result of an alteration taking place in blood effused during or subsequent to inflammation.

The cyst occupied so large a share of the abdomen that its upper portion rose to the situation of the stomach, and the intestines and liver were pushed up under the concavity of the diaphragm and ribs; and as the adhesions by which it was connected with the parietes were torn through, the cyst gave way in two or three parts, and puriform fluid escaped.

The cyst, when opened, proved to consist of one large cavity, which was filled with puriform serum; the whole internal surface being irregularly but thickly coated with layers of yellow, coagulable matter; and a process of ulceration was going on in those parts of the cyst which had given way when the parietes were being detached.

The fluid in the cysts differed entirely from that which had been drawn off two months before, which was a coffee-coloured, somewhat grumous fluid, sparingly coagulable by heat; and there is no doubt that the purulent character which it now bore was the result of the inflammatory action set up in the cyst. The dark, carbonaceous colour exhibited by the omentum and peritoneum had, in all probability, taken place subsequently to the tapping, as the abdomen had previously appeared quite free from inflammation; and there is little doubt that it depended either on the escape of a small portion of the fluid from the cyst, or on some slight sanguineous oozing from the wounded vessels of the omentum.

The perfectly simple character of the cyst in this case inclined me to consider it as probably an example of one of the non-malignant forms of ovarian cysts; though I own it was a point admitting of great doubt.

Case 15.—*Ovarian dropsy; paracentesis. Death from peritoneal inflammation.*— —, at. 44, was admitted into Guy's Hospital, June, 1831, affected with a large ovarian dropsy. She dated the commencement of her complaints to the day of Queen Caroline's funeral, when she caught cold by exposure to wet, and was confined for four weeks with inflammation of the lower part of the abdomen; and, although she then appeared perfectly well, yet in a very short time she perceived a swelling in the left side of the abdomen, towards the bottom; and from time to time was subject to indisposition, generally affecting the abdomen. Although the swelling continued, she was married about six months before her admission, and since that time the swelling had increased more rapidly; but it did not interfere much with her proceedings; she could walk from Peckham to London and back, and she was fond of dancing.

June 18th, 1831.—She was tapped in the middle line, about an inch below the umbilicus; a few drachms only of fluid came away; when a little cyst protruded, almost like an hydatid; but it was attached within, and was returned; a small quantity of blood escaped. Within an hour or two of the operation she began to experience collapse, and died within twenty-four hours.

Sectio cadaveris.—From external examination it was concluded that there was one large sac occupying the greater part of the abdomen so generally, that it did not appear to belong to one side more than to the other; but on the slope of the tumour, to the right side, in the iliac region, was distinctly to be felt a part harder than the rest; and here a projection could be perceived by the eye. The fluctuation in the great tumour was decided, but far from remarkable. When the parietes were removed, one large sac came into view; and a few drachms of puriform fluid escaped from between this and the parietes. The omentum was thin, and stretched over the right side of the sac. It was exceedingly vascular; and attached to a second tumour, of the size of a large fist flattened, which had formed the projection in the right iliac region. This tumour was lobulated in appearance, and of a dark gray colour. Across the large tumour, and running in a diagonal direction from the lower part of the right iliac region upwards to the left, passing within half an inch of the umbilicus, was a fleshy band, rounded at its upper margin, and becoming thin below. In this was perceived the slight scar of the incision which had been made to evacuate the fluid. Just below this belt, which ran below the umbilicus, and was about an inch in width, were two or three transparent vesicular bodies, hanging on peduncles.

On further strict examination, it was found that the large cyst arose from the appendages of the uterus on the right side, and that the fleshy band which crossed it was composed, in its upper part, of a large vein; and in its lower of the Fallopian tube, connected, and formed into a mass by the thickened ligaments of that side of the uterus. The smaller tumour was appended to the larger, and hanging upon it. On opening the larger sac it was found to be very thin, and contained a large pailful of brown, glairy, mucous fluid. The inside of the tumour was, for the most part, pretty smooth and even, but in one or two parts presented the projections of secondary cysts. At the lower part of the tumour was found some gelatinous matter, which appeared to have subsided from the fluid contained in the cyst. The tumour in the right iliac region was filled with a peculiar mass, of the consistence of natural fæces, and brown in colour, with large flakes of white matter, which resembled adipocere; and when this was completely evacuated, some small portions of bone and a little hair were found attached to one side of the parietes. The uterus was healthy, except that the neck was elongated by being drawn out by the tumour.

The intestines all showed distinct marks of recent inflammation on their peritoneal coat, which was vascular, particularly in two stripes where each came in contact with the neighbouring convolution.

This case is very interesting, as it shows the great caution which is necessary in the performance of paracentesis in this disease, and, indeed, the impossibility, in some cases, of avoiding parts which may be displaced. The unnatural elongation of the Fallopian tubes, and of the appendages, is by no means uncommon amongst the displacements which occur in tumours of this kind. The tendency to inflammation of the peritoneum, where the parts are greatly distended, and the sudden prostration arising from it, is also very worthy of observation.

CASE 16.—*Cyst in the broad ligament of the uterus; ruptured. Death sudden.*—Jane R—, æt. 42, a married woman, was admitted into Guy's Hospital, June 30th, 1830. It appeared, from her account, that she had been in the hospital rather more than a year before, the subject of an abdominal tumour, with œdema of both her legs, which was supposed to arise from venous obstruction. From the central position of the tumour, pregnancy was at first suspected, but this idea was abandoned. She was at that time rather stout, and left the hospital free from anasarca, though the abdomen remained unchanged.

She was somewhat emaciated in appearance. The lower part of the abdomen tumid and hard, with scarcely any perceptible fluctuation. The lower extremities œdematous; the superficial veins of the abdomen much distended. She stated that she had passed no urine for some days, except a little which came away in certain positions of the body. The catheter was passed with much difficulty, owing to the orifice of the urethra being drawn back. The urine was slightly turbid. Twenty leeches were applied over the abdomen, followed by fomentations and poultices, and soothing injections were administered.

On the seventh day after her admission, having been sitting up a few hours before, and speaking of no new symptom, except a sensation, at one time, as if her bowels turned over, she died quite suddenly.

Sectio cadaveris.—The appearance of circumscribed swelling had entirely subsided. The abdomen, though swollen, was flaccid, like a half-filled bladder; and the idea immediately presented itself that the rupture of the cyst had taken place; which, on laying open the abdomen, was found to be the fact; for a quantity of discoloured, ropy fluid escaped, which was found to have proceeded from a large cyst which entirely occupied the lower part of the abdomen. The parietes of the cyst were extremely unequal, in some parts thick and fleshy, in others thin and tender; and it was in one of these thin parts that the cyst had given way, allowing the escape of its contents. Considerable evidence presented itself of peritoneal inflammation, particularly about the spleen, where adhesions had taken place.

The cyst had evidently originated in the broad ligament, near the uterus; and had insinuated itself even under the peritoneal covering of the uterus.

CASE 17.—*Ovarian tumour, partly fluid, partly fungoid; paracentesis rendered necessary, from the great pain experienced. Death, after several operations, from peritoneal inflammation.*— Mary M——, æt. 53, was admitted into Guy's Hospital, under my care, October 17th, 1832, the subject of ovarian tumour, from which she suffered extreme pain. She had been the mother of eleven children, of whom the youngest was twelve years old. It appeared that about twelve months since she had been apparently in perfect health; but about eleven months ago, she was supposed to be labouring under a liver-complaint. Six months since, she passed what were considered several small biliary calculi; and about that time she first felt a swelling at the bottom of the abdomen, towards the right side. This gradually increased, from the size of a potato till it occupied a large portion of the abdomen, and was attended with most violent pain. Having suffered this pain for about a month, it became almost insupportable; and two months and two days ago she was tapped, when eight pints of dark, thick fluid were drawn off, with the greatest immediate relief to the pain, and increased freedom of passing urine; and she left the hospital in ten days, at which time the accumulation was already taking place, and it had continued to increase till it was now arrived at its original size, and had latterly produced great pain, particularly at the time of passing fæces. Urine scanty, but general health good.

A dose of castor-oil was ordered; and on the 20th, three quarters of a pailful of greenish straw-coloured fluid, mucilaginous in appearance, with much yellow, flaky matter, were drawn off; and when the cyst was emptied, two other tumours were plainly to be felt. The next day, the pain she had experienced was quite gone, but a little tenderness remained on the right side of the abdomen. I ordered the ointment of the hydriodate of potash to be rubbed in on the abdomen; but she was so well, that, although the fluid had begun to accumulate again, she left the hospital on the 6th of November.

December 12th.—Was again admitted, under Dr. Back; the tumour having arrived at even a larger size than before. A purgative was administered, and in two days she was tapped. The fluid drawn off was described as being very thick, almost like jelly; and after the puncture had been bandaged up, it broke out again, and flowed in large quantities into the bed.

17th.—She appears very well; the hard masses, which are evidently cysts in the parietes of the large cysts, are very evident.

22d.—For a full week after the operation the fluid continued to drain off; it has now, however, quite stopped, and considerable accumulation has again taken place.

26th.—She was sitting up, eating her dinner with other patients; and she shortly afterwards left the hospital.

January 30th.—She was again admitted, suffering great pain, with a tumour occupying the whole centre of the abdomen, fluctuating, and very tender, particularly on its upper part.

February 2d.—Suffered most acutely from pain in the back, and round the abdomen, during the night. Mr. Callaway made a puncture with a lancet, an inch and a half below the umbilicus, and introduced a canula. Four quarts of ropy, greenish fluid, containing some white flakes, were drawn off. At one time the canula was obstructed by a portion of fine membrane, which was drawn out and cut off, having a small cyst attached. A bandage was applied, with moderate pressure. The abdomen diminished about four inches in circumference, and a hard, transverse tumour could be felt on the left side, extending from below the umbilicus towards the loin. The most prominent hardness was on the right side. In the evening she was sick, and dyspnœa came on.

4th.—Abdomen very tender; and the cyst has filled so much that she measures within one inch and a half of her size previous to the tapping. The tumour in the lower part is hard, and very distinct fluctuation is felt in the upper.

7th.—All tenderness is gone.

13th.—Some shooting pain in the right side, extending into the iliac fossa; and that part is very tender to the touch.

March 2d.—Nearly as large in measurement as at the time of admission.

14th.—Has suffered much pain in the loins, and round the upper part of the abdomen, and cannot cough or take a deep breath without pain. Paracentesis was performed, as before; at first, some serum escaped, which was supposed to be from the peritoneal cavity; and then some ropy matter, which, towards the termination, was of less consistency, and changed from a dirty white to a light-greenish hue. Several portions of opaque membrane of some strength, and one of them in the form of a cyst, escaped at the orifice, and required to be detached by scissors. The quantity drawn was about two quarts; she felt afterwards rather exhausted, but the breathing was better than before the operation.

16th.—Passed a tolerable night, and appears quite cheerful. Sickness has subsided; pulse 100, soft; some healthy dejections passed, with less pain than before tapping.

18th.—Was very comfortable yesterday; but on getting out of bed this morning, and coughing, the puncture reopened, and some fluid has been oozing. Passed a pint and a quarter of urine. The fluid being inclined to flow, about three pints of a yellow, turbid fluid, slightly unctuous to the feel, were drawn off.

19th.—More fluid, to the amount of one or two pints, escaped from the orifice; feels weaker; pulse feeble; tongue clean; not much abdominal tenderness; no stool; more urine.

20th.—Vomited last night, and continued to retch all night; has vomited this morning; and at present there is coldness at the extremities. Pulse 104, very small.

21st.—Has been getting much worse since half-past two this morning, not having spoken. At present she is almost in a comatose state, giving no answers to questions put to her. Vomited last night; bowels not open; extremities warm; but her pulse flutters, and is scarcely perceptible; occasional subsultus and picking of the bedclothes.

Sectio cadaveris.—March 23d.—Much emaciation; the superficial veins, both on the hands and legs, very strongly marked. Opening the parietes of the abdomen, they were found very closely attached, particularly at the upper part, to an ovarian tumour. This tumour was composed of two parts, very different in their appearance; and seemed to fill every portion of the abdomen when it was first opened. The upper part passed quite under the ribs, on both sides, and in the middle, and was exceedingly thin, so that the fluctuation could be seen plainly through the integument of the abdomen. The lower part of the tumour, which was the size of a half-quartern loaf, was apparently solid; and, externally, somewhat botryoidal, and very vascular. The thin part of the tumour was also somewhat vascular, and had upon it some very peculiar white marks, terminating abruptly in the vascular parts.

The thin tumour contained several pints of very tenacious matter, which flowed out precisely like the white of egg, falling to the ground, from the table, without the least noise, or making any splash; exactly as the white of an egg falls into a basin; it was of a dingy, brownish colour. The inside of the cyst had but little appearance of vascularity; was in some parts quite smooth, like membrane, and in other parts botryoidal, from other cysts pushing forward; some, small as peas; others, particularly in the neighbourhood of the hard tumours, a good deal larger, and opening spontaneously, to let out some more fluid still more tenacious, like glue or birdlime, which separated from the cavities in which it was contained, leaving them quite dry, but showing fresh botryoidal masses shooting up.

The hard tumour, when cut completely through, showed a section which exactly resembled a somewhat magnified fungoid testicle; in which every shade of colour, and every variety assumed by the fungoid disease, occupied the various cysts of which it was composed; some were still like white of egg, but others were bloody; and some of the colour of the cheesy matter of scrofula.

The whole of the tumour arose from the right broad ligament; and it appeared to be the ovary itself. The Fallopian tube, still quite pervious, and about six inches in length, lay extended over the tumour. The left ovary was shrunk and small; but at its lower part there was a vesicle of the size of a bean, which seemed to be formed within the tunic of the ovary, and was filled with a pellucid fluid, bearing very much the character of that represented in Figs. 23 and 24, and in all probability, the incipient stage of the same disease as that which occupied the other ovary.

The uterus was healthy, with some white mottling, probably the result of frequent childbearing. The peritoneum was extensively inflamed; and besides containing some of the ropy fluid which had escaped from the cyst, had poured out a good deal of puriform lymph.

Almost the whole of the natural contents of the abdomen were pushed into the two lumbar regions; and the tumour appeared to have made such pressure on the lacteals carrying the chyle from the small intestines that they were enormously distended, and a most extensive extravasation of chyle had taken place into the mesentery, about midway along the small intestines; and, at the same time, many small collections of chyle were seen immediately beneath the mucous membrane of the intestines, between that and the muscular fibres.

The liver was rather soft and yellowish, and was pushed upwards by the tumour, so as to be lodged under the third and fourth rib. Spleen, pancreas, and kidney, healthy.

In this case, we see very plainly marked the transition from the less malignant form of the ovarian cyst to the most complicated varieties of fungoid disease; for though the large cyst was filled with the usual mucilaginous matter found in the cells of ovarian disease, yet the harder part, which formed no small portion of the whole, presented all the various modifications of the cerebriform and hæmatoid fungus.

The progress of this disease had been rapid; for not above eleven months had elapsed since it first made its appearance. In about four months from its being first discovered, it was necessary to draw off the fluid, which was again so far accumulated, as to be most inconvenient and painful within two months afterwards. After that time, it was again necessary to have recourse to the operation; then in six weeks; and again in a still shorter time. Nor did she long survive this fifth operation; but a small quantity of the fluid having been effused into the peritoneal sac, inflammation came on, and she died. But while inflammation appeared to be the immediate cause of death, the rapid emaciation plainly showed that there were other causes in operation; and the remarkable instance this case affords of the effect of pressure, in cutting off the supply of nutrition, and actually preventing the lacteals from absorbing the chyle, sufficiently explains the source of emaciation.

The urgency of the symptoms, the pain, and the white flaky matter which was mingled with the fluid drawn away, may all be considered to have indicated the peculiar character of the disease.

CASE 18.—*Ovarian dropsy; possibly enlarged Graafian vesicle; rupture of the cyst internally. Death from inflammation of the cyst and neighbouring parts; the cyst tympanitic.*—Jane ——, a married woman, æt. 37, was admitted, under my care, into Dorcas Ward, September 2d, 1835. She had a light complexion, and was by no means emaciated. When she presented herself in the room for admission, she stated that she had observed a swelling of the abdomen for two years, but that for the last six weeks only had she suffered from it; since which time the pain had been great and constant. As she sat, the abdomen was evidently much enlarged at the lower part, and yielded an indistinct sense of fluctuation. I considered it ovarian, from her history. On questioning her more particularly, when removed to the ward, I found that she had been married for many years; the catamenia had always been regular, but she had borne no children. About two years before, she had first perceived, or at least had her attention particularly drawn to, a swelling in the lower part of the abdomen; it was accompanied by a stoppage in the urine, which rendered it necessary to have a catheter passed. She seems at that time to have been ill for a considerable period; but ultimately the swelling subsided completely. It, however, again made its appearance, and a second time subsided; so that for a time, as she stated, the abdomen was as flat as ever it was. Six weeks before admission, she again perceived the enlargement, and from that time she had suffered great and constant pain. On careful examination, I could discover no distinct tumour, no marginated enlargement, no lobulated or hardened knots; there was indistinct fluctuation, and the abdomen was tender on pressure, without acute pain. Pulse 120, sharp; tongue slightly furred and dry; and she altogether appeared greatly prostrated.

The conclusion to which this examination led me was, that there could, at all events be no hard or malignant disease of the ovary; that there was probably chronic inflammation of the peritoneum, excited by the previous disease; and that the membrane had become thickened and altered, so as to prevent that distinct fluctuation, which otherwise, from the considerable size the abdomen had obtained, might have been expected. I thought it right to have the catheter passed; but no material quantity of urine was found in the bladder. Twenty leeches were applied to the abdomen, followed by a poultice; and a pill, composed of a grain of opium and calomel, and one fourth of a grain of tartarized antimony, was given three times a day. The following day the tenderness was somewhat diminished, and the bowels had been twice relieved—the motions loose, but well supplied with bile. A small quantity of blood was taken from the arm, and again leeches applied to the abdomen; but the irritation of the bowels increased, and it was necessary to have recourse to starch injections with opium, and gently to give support; however, the tenderness of the abdomen increased; it became tympanitic; a large tympanitic ridge, corresponding to the arch of the colon, passed over the abdomen, above the umbilicus; while the lower part was also tympanitic; but fluctuation could still be discovered in its lower part, as she lay on her back. On the 11th of the month, that is, ten days after admission, she sank.

Sectio cadaveris.—No obvious change had taken place in the appearance of the abdomen since death; it still presented two remarkable elevations—the one crossing the epigastric region, the other occupying the hypogastric and umbilical; and both were decidedly tympanitic on percussion; but fluctuation was still ascertained in the inferior and posterior part of the lower tumour. When the parietes were divided, a spherical tumour came into sight, completely occupying the lower part of the abdomen; while, nearer to the diaphragm, the colon, greatly distended, filled all the remainder of the cavity which was brought into view. They were both evidently distended with gas, yielding a tympanitic sound on percussion; and it was at once obvious, that the lower tumour was attached to the uterine appendages, as the left Fallopian tube was seen drawn over its exterior surface. When pierced by a scalpel at its upper part, nothing escaped but a large quantity of fetid gas; and attempting to turn aside the arch of the colon from the tumour, it was found to adhere firmly; and many pints of a fetid, grumous fluid flowed from the sac, through the rent made in its walls by this attempt to detach it. Examining more carefully, it was found that a similar attachment had taken place to the head of the colon, and that the sac was, moreover, closely glued to the small intestines; and that a collection of ill-conditioned pus had formed in the folds of the mesentery, at that part. On laying open the tumour, it was found to consist of one sac, about the sixth of an inch in thickness, apparently quite simple in its structure. Its internal surface was somewhat flocculent throughout; but in the parts where the adhesion had taken place, both near the head of the colon and at the mesentery, the internal membrane of the sac was softened, ulcerated, and cerebriform, so as to allow of communication with the adventitious abscesses, which had been formed externally by layers of coagulable lymph and folds of the mesentery.

From the simple structure of the cyst, and from the condition of the right ovary, in which more than one of the vesicles of De Graaf were diseased (one forming a cyst representing in miniature the large one, and the other filled with yellow matter), there was reason to believe that this tumour might have arisen from one of these vesicles in the left ovary.

All the peritoneum showed marks of recent inflammation going on in many parts, to the formation of tender bands of adhesion between the different portions of the mesentery and the intestines. The internal membrane of the last few feet of the ileum, and that part of the colon near the valve about which adhesion had taken place, presented most extensive evidence of old ulceration; but whether any actual communication existed between the intestine and the large cyst, was not completely made out, though the appearance greatly favoured the idea. The mucous membrane of the stomach was unusually mammillated, but colourless. The kidneys and bladder were healthy; indeed, except some concretion in the gall-bladder, and some old adhesions of the pleura, all other parts appeared healthy.

Reviewing the history of this case, and comparing it with the appearances after death, the conclusion to which I come is, that this was probably a non-malignant disease of a Graafian vesicle; that the cyst had twice burst, and emptied itself into the cavity of the abdomen; but that, though no fatal result had immediately followed, the consequence was such a change, from the inflammatory action excited, as to lead ultimately to the extensive formation of abscesses in the lymph deposited between the folds of the peritoneum; and hence arose the lesion of the intestines, and the inflammation of the sac, which formed the chief part of the disease under which she sank. From the situation which the cyst occupied with relation to the

Fallopian tube, it is evident that it had been developed in the appendages of the uterus; and it was equally evident, that neither its structure, nor the fluid which it contained, nor the effects of the inflammation excited, bore any resemblance to those which mark the malignant or specific forms of ovarian disease. The inflammation which had left its traces in the peritoneum was evidently of old standing; and, supposing the adhesion of the cyst to have taken place on the first occasion of the disappearance of the tumour, we perceive a sufficient reason why the more satisfactory result, which probably sometimes follows such occurrences, did not take place in this case.

The circumstance of gas having collected in the cavity of the tumour, and thus affording a tympanitic sound, was one which seldom occurs; but where it does, it will be very apt to mislead us in our diagnosis, as the absence of the tympanitic sound on the upper part of the tumour generally distinguishes the ovarian from the ascitic tumour. Perhaps, could we trace with certainty the result of those cases which are reported as recoveries from ovarian dropsy by rupture, many would be found to correspond very exactly with that of R——; or, to give evidence of a still nearer approach to the malignant form of disease, being scarcely more retarded in its progress by the internal rupture than it would have been by the operation of paracentesis. Thus, for example, in the case recorded in the first number of the 'Guy's Hospital Reports,' although the relief experienced after the rupture was so great, yet scarcely had two years elapsed before the patient returned to the hospital with the abdomen enlarged nearly as much as before the occurrence; and in a short time her death afforded an opportunity of examining the condition of the abdomen, and discovering that the ovarian disease had been of the specific character, and that an extensive rupture, several inches in length, had suffered the fluid to escape. I will subjoin the examination, in the words stated in the book of Guy's Hospital Museum.

CASE 19.—*Malignant ovarian cyst ruptured internally; subsidence of the tumour. Death in about two years, from increase of the disease.* —Ann ——, æt. 47, was readmitted into Guy's Hospital, July 19th, 1836, under Dr. Addison, and died on the 19th of the following month. Her case will be found in page 41, vol. i, of 'Guy's Hospital Reports,' where it appears that she was admitted in March,

1834, on account of the rupture of an ovarian tumour which had been observed for a period of five years. After having been in the hospital about six weeks, she left it, returned to her duties as a servant, and is reported in the December of the following year to have experienced no return of the dropsical effusion, though a small tumour was still perceptible.

"*Sectio cadaveris.*—The body was much emaciated. The chest presented little that was unhealthy, besides one or two sub-pleural tubercles of a vascular and firm medullary matter, thin and flat, and rather less than a sixpence. The middle of the anterior face of the right ventricle presented a patch of simply thickened pericardium, as large as a shilling. There was a little serous effusion in the peritoneum, with much thickening and adhesion, especially about a cyst which was at once brought to view; the remaining serous surfaces were somewhat scabrous. The liver was nearly twice as large as usual, from the development throughout its substance of malignant tubera, differing in size from that of a pea to that of a walnut. These were globular, medullary, vascular, soft, and reticular, and containing coarse grains of strumous deposit, partly inclined to soften down. Few of these tubera were flattened at the surface of the liver, or they were less so than usual, being rather prominent. The hepatic substance was much injected, coarse and firm; some parts had the character, slightly, of fibrous medullary degeneration. The surface of the liver was pretty generally concealed by adhesions, and its edges rounded by the development of great tubera. The bile was dark, watery, and in moderate quantity. The spleen was of a full size, much enveloped in adhesions; and one fifth of its tunic was thickened, cartilaginous, and yellowish; its substance lacerable, softening, yet fibrous. The kidneys were large, vascular, somewhat mottled and firm, not easily parting with their tunics. The ureters were thick; the omentum a good deal contracted, and sprinkled with firm, palish, medullary tubera. The pancreas was firm and close, and much enveloped in morbid thickening and malignant deposit.

"The cyst occupied the true and false pelvis. It was globular, and separated with difficulty. Its serous surface was thickened and irregular; in parts smooth; and in parts adherent by bridles, and a dense cellular membrane to adjoining surfaces. Between this and the pubes the bladder was compressed, but pretty natural in appearance. The walls of the cyst varied in thickness about one third of an inch; some firm, pale, medullary tubera were found about it; and the absorbent glands were much affected with a similar degeneration. The contents of the cavity were nearly two quarts, of a puriform and rather pasty fluid, darkish, as if discoloured by admixture of a little decomposed blood; the smell was not remarkably offensive. The lining of the cavity consisted mostly of a rough, thickish, and pretty firm layer of unorganized and, as it were, strumous matter. A puriform cell was found at one point on the walls. Across the front of the tumour the wall of the cyst presented a band formed by its reduplication—a thickened portion of three layers, firmly and closely glued together, and each a little wasted, evidently produced by the former shrinking of the cavity. Posteriorly, it was quite evident that a rupture had occurred, perhaps eight inches in length. The inferior lip of the rupture projected into the cavity in the form of an elliptical layer, of about six inches square; of which one margin was free, like a recently clean-cut surface; and the other simply continuous with the proper walls; whilst what had originally formed the outer surface, though bathed in the contents of the cavity, was still a clear, dense, peritoneum, and the face correspondent to the lining of the cyst resembled it (the lining) in all respects.

" The rectum wound over the hinder face of the sac; and beneath the promontory of the sacrum was loosely enveloped in tubercular disease. The uterus was nearly twice as large as is natural, in consequence, as it seemed, of a kind of fibro-scirrhous degeneration, uniform throughout its texture. The right ovary was pretty natural, but enclosed in adhesions; the Fallopian tube dilated, tortuous, and sealed towards the morsus; the left broad ligament not traceable. The os uteri tumid; and its inner lip afforded a short footstalk, a third of an inch thick, to a tumour the size of a chesnut, soft, vascular, and full of large mucous cells."

There is, I think, in this case, reason to suppose that the extensive rupture of the ovarian cyst, by diffusing the malignant matter in the peritoneal cavity, facilitated greatly its absorption into the system; as shown by the occurrence of the disease, not only in the parts to which it was immediately applied, but in parts, as the substance of the liver and the pleura, where no such contact could have taken place; for we certainly find, in a great majority of cases where this malignant disease occurs in the ovary, that it confines itself very much to that organ, being almost insulated by the cyst in which it is contained; and that when it becomes more general, it is often after inflammation has been excited by paracentesis.

The case which I shall now shortly relate, from the report of my friend, Mr. Beaumont, of Gravesend, was followed likewise by a fatal termination within three years of the accident; and, except that the sac appears never to have filled again, bears much resemblance to the case I have just mentioned, and was, in all probability, brought to an end by the development of the disease in some internal organ.

CASE 20.—*Ovarian cyst ruptured internally. Death after three years, with emaciation.*—" My dear Sir,—The case you refer to was that of a woman who was a second housekeeper at Cobham Hall; she had laboured under ovarian dropsy many years, but had never been tapped; she was very large, and I had thought of performing the operation. However, she fell from some high steps in brushing the ceiling of a very lofty room, and burst the sac. The immediate effect was fainting, from which she soon recovered by the administration of some stimulants. About two days after I was desired to visit her, and found her without pain, but feeble; and my attention was directed to the quantity of urine she had passed; at the same time her attendant produced three large chamber-pots full of urine, which had passed in twenty-four hours, and which increased quantity continued for four or five days afterwards. I ordered her to be supported; and a bandage to be applied to the abdomen, the pressure being increased as it became slack. In a week or ten days she resumed her duty. About six or seven months after this I lost sight of her; but to-day have learned that she became a monthly nurse; and that she never filled again, but, on the contrary, became very thin and emaciated, and died in London about two years afterwards.—Gravesend; Jan. 19th, 1838."

CASE 21.—*Compound ovarian cyst, ruptured internally; followed by death from peritonitis.*—S. G——, æt. 44, who had been affected with ovarian tumour for five years, was already dead when brought to Guy's Hospital on the 22d of December, 1832; and we were informed that it was believed the cyst had burst internally.

Sectio cadaveris.—December 22d, 1832.—Great emaciation; slight yellowness on some parts of the skin, more particularly on a blistered surface at the scrobiculus cordis. The veins of the legs, particularly the right leg and thigh, dilated and turgid. On examining carefully, a massive, irregular tumour was felt, occupying the central part of the abdomen, capable of being pushed upwards above the umbilicus, but by no means to the scrobiculus cordis; it might be pushed downwards to the pubes. Fluctuation was to be felt all over the abdomen, even to the scrobiculus cordis and in the lumbar regions; but the abdomen was far from being tense; it was flaccid; and in the lumbar spaces, particularly the right, there was no difficulty in perceiving that there was a cyst externally, to which fluid was effused.

Fig. 36.

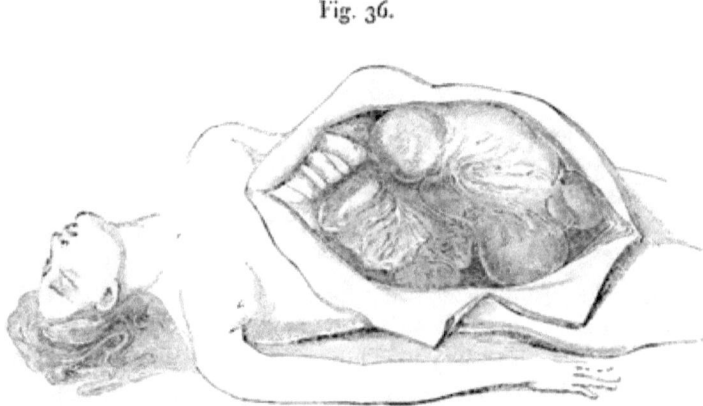

Fig. 36 shows the appearance of the abdomen in a case where an ovarian cyst had been ruptured by ulceration of the inner membrane, during life. The intestines had been forced by the tumour, when fully distended, into the upper and posterior part of the abdomen; and had not recovered their natural situation, the cavity having been filled by the fluid which escaped from the ruptured cyst.

When the parietes were opened, a quantity of brown-red fluid, of a thin, serous consistence, immediately flowed out from the general peritoneal cavity; and, as the opening was enlarged, the surface of an irregular lobulated cyst came into view, on which was deposited a thin coating of coagulable lymph, the product of inflammation, stained brown by a grumous deposit. (Fig. 36.) The same deposit was found upon the convolutions of the intestines which came into view above the cyst; but in the upper part, and more particularly over the surface of the liver and the diaphragm, this soft, brown deposit, which was evidently a combination of the lymph effused by inflammation and some foreign matter deposited, was much more abundant; and the liver was bound to the diaphragm by several adhesive fibres of half an inch in length, but pretty easily torn away.

The convolutions of the intestines were glued together, but separated with moderate ease. A part of the small intestines, the arch of the colon, the stomach, and the omentum, lay all very confusedly glued together between the tumour and the liver. The substance of the small intestines was somewhat peculiar in appearance, being more massive and opaque than natural, and seemed to have been thickened by the irritation and pressure of the tumour on the large intestines; they were not, however, distended; and the mucous membrane was healthy. The sigmoid flexure of the colon was exceedingly contracted, with a few small pieces of fæces in it, not larger than peas; and the caput cæcum was compressed and pushed completely into the space above the right ileum.

The kidneys were very small, and of a pale-yellow colour. The liver was remarkably friable; so that in squeezing it between the finger and thumb, the finger immediately broke through the peritoneal covering, and lacerated the substance.

The lobulated tumour at once showed itself to be a compound ovarian growth, a larger cyst of which had burst towards the upper part of the mass, where an orifice, not larger than a small quill, allowed a fluid precisely of the same character as that effused into the general cavity to escape; showing at once the nature of the circumstances which had been going on previous to death. On opening this cyst more freely, a considerable quantity of brown, grumous matter, almost like the soft curd strained from treacle posset, was found deposited about the internal parietes. In the substance of the parietes, and shooting up in it, were many of the subordinate cysts clustering together, one within the other. They contained fluids and substances more various in character than we often find. In none, however, was there the ropy, gelatinous matter, which is most frequent; in some a yellow, transparent fluid—in some that fluid tinged with blood—in some small ones almost entire blood; and in one large mass all the cells were filled with a fungoid matter, almost cerebriform, with some cavities containing blood, giving the whole greatly the aspect of the fungus hæmatodes.

The whole mass was attached to a single broad ligament, which was somewhat twisted on itself. There was no other attachment, but a very recent bridle of adhesion towards the right side of the tumour.

The uterus was more bulky, round, and white-coloured, than natural. The other ovary was not implicated.

CASE 22.—*Malignant disease of the ovary; fibrous tubera in the uterus; paracentesis; subcutaneous tubera on the abdomen. Death from extensive scirrhous disease.*—June 7th, 1829.—I was requested to see, in consultation, an unmarried lady, considerably past the meridian of life, who had been under treatment fourteen months for ovarian dropsy. For several months before that time it had been observed that she grew large; but it was not looked upon as disease till fourteen or fifteen months ago; for the last three months the tumour had been rapidly increasing. It was in consequence of the absence from town for several weeks of the physician who had previously been consulted, that I was called; and the points to be decided were, whether it would be right to draw off the fluid; and, likewise, whether it would be advisable to extirpate the whole tumour; for she had heard so much of the success of the last mode of cure, that she was quite prepared to submit to it, if recommended, and, indeed, unwilling to submit to any less decisive remedy. During the last week the oppression and the general suffering had so much increased, as to lead to a feeling, that without some relief she could not long survive. I found the abdomen greatly swollen, and the ovarian tumour was plainly felt, extending within a few inches of the scrobiculus cordis, consisting of one large cyst, and of a mass of lobulated substance, which appeared to be a number of other cysts, situated towards the left side and on the inferior part, extending as high as the umbilicus.

It was likewise quite obvious, that a quantity of serum was effused into the cavity of the abdomen lying partly between the cyst and the abdominal parietes, where it could be felt covering the upper part of the tumour over some space, and forming a thin layer of fluid on the side of the tumour; the fluid could also be discovered filling the lumbar spaces. She was much emaciated, and very feeble; the legs greatly swollen; more particularly the left, which was inflamed, and going into a state of ulceration; the right was less advanced in the same form of disease; this inflammation of the legs having taken place within the last week. The tongue was aphthous and naked. Pulse 124, weak. She suffered from very frequent hiccough, particularly excited by swallowing anything.

It was our opinion, in consultation, that to attempt extirpation would be certainly fatal; and that possibly paracentesis would be so likewise, by the subsequent inflammation either of the cyst or of the peritoneum; but as it was likewise certain that she must die speedily by the inflammation of the legs and the suffering of the distended abdomen, we judged it right to draw off the fluid by paracentesis.

A large trochar was introduced three inches below the umbilicus; and a pailful of dark-coloured fluid, like black tea or weak coffee, was taken away; and towards the end of the operation many shreds and masses of lymph and puriform matter blocked up the canula, but came away by the use of a probe; at length, all that could be obtained was drawn off; and she bore the operation well. A large flannel bandage was applied, and an opiate given. She passed an easy day; and a tranquil, though sleepless, night.

June 8th.—The hiccough better; the legs much reduced; but as the pulse was quick and rather sharp, we feared inflammation, and ordered her to take two grains of calomel, with half a grain of opium, every sixth hour.

9th.—A tranquil night; no pain; bowels well opened; hiccough much better; legs diminished; inflammation subsided; but the abdomen evidently again filling.

From this time I did not see this patient again till after her death, which occurred on the 1st of July. I understood that no alarming symptoms of inflammation ever showed themselves, but that the abdomen continued to fill, and that she grew gradually weaker.

Sectio cadaveris.—Great emaciation, legs œdematous, abdomen greatly distended, as in the full period of pregnancy. The integuments for six inches round the umbilicus were thickly beset with small, hard, flat tubercles, about the size of a split horse-bean, or smaller; the skin was generally not discoloured upon these tumours, though a few of them appeared slightly vascular; these were precisely the subcutaneous tubercles observed in cases of scirrhous mamma, when the constitution is completely infected with the most malignant form of the disease; they were placed, like little glands, in the cellular tissue, immediately under the skin, were almost of cartilaginous hardness, when cut into; of a dead-white colour, and very slightly transparent. On inquiry, it appeared that these tumours had first made their appearance, like slight rings of ecchymosis, a few days after my last visit to the patient, and had since become hard and elevated. The discovery of these at once forced upon us the belief that the ovarian tumour would be found to be of a truly carcinomatous character.

Above five quarts of clear serum, not unlike high-coloured urine, were drawn from the cavity of the abdomen; and about half that quantity, of a darker colour than we had obtained by tapping, flowed from the cyst. This was a good deal tinged with blood, and was accompanied by a large mass of brown, coagulable matter, which, from its peculiar membranous and reticulated appearance, suggested the idea, as it pushed its way out of the orifice, of its being a portion of omentum.

When the parietes of the upper half of the abdomen were laid open, the colon came in sight, greatly distended with flatus; the omentum, rolled up and attached along the upper surface of the colon, of a dark-gray colour, and studded with hard, white tubercles, from the size of a small shot to that of a pea rather flattened; the edge of the liver was also seen, and about an inch in circumference of the large curvature of the stomach. The fundus of the ovarian tumour, now collapsed by the abstraction of the fluid, was also seen suspended by firm attachments to the anterior part of the abdomen about the umbilicus. On further examination, it appeared that these attachments of the cyst to the parietes were very firm, and formed by the deposit of an irregular layer of the same scirrhous matter which formed the external tubercles; and each attachment corresponded in its centre with the space occupied by one of the tubercles. It extended, however, considerably further on both sides; the sides and the lower part, as well as the fundus of the cyst, were free from attachments, and must have admitted the serum from the cavity of the abdomen to lie between them and their parietes, as was easily detected in the first examination. Having torn the adhesions asunder, the lower portion of the abdominal parietes was laid open; and we then found that the cyst arose by a broad basis, not less than three or four inches in circumference, from the broad ligament of the uterus, which dilated, as it were, into the cyst. The Fallopian tube, nearly as large as the little finger, and elongated considerably beyond its natural length, lay firmly attached to the back of the tumour; it was hard, and its fimbriated extremity could scarcely be recognised; it was thick, red, and warty in appearance, plainly partaking of the general disease.

The external surface of the cyst exhibited on its left side, where we had felt the lobulated mass, the appearance of a true scirrhous disease—vascular, lobulated, and of a cartilaginous hardness, and a large network of veins ran over part of the surface; but the most striking appearance was seen near the attachment, and towards its right side, from which a pendent cluster of vesicles hung into the pelvis, mingled with a gelatinous fluid, which filled the cavity of the pelvis where it was not occupied by disease. This cluster of vesicles corresponded with what Dr. Hodgkin has described as the essential formation of many adventitious structures, and particularly scirrhus; it was quite obvious that it arose from the bottom of a cyst which had burst or dilated, so that it now formed a crescentic margin, or rather a circular fold round the basis of the pendent vesicles, which all seemed to rise by comparatively small bases nearly from the same point—they were highly and beautifully vascular. The internal surface of the cyst was hard and scabrous throughout; it contained gelatinous matter, fibrin, and a clot of above two ounces of pure coagulated blood; some of the contents seemed to be glued to the parietes by soft, carcinomatous, and fatty-looking deposits, but I did not observe any subordinate cysts opening into the large cyst.

The uterus was also involved in the disease. From its fundus arose a large, oval, hard, and elastic tuber, of the size of a pigeon's egg; and in the substance of the uterus another was imbedded.

The right ovary was large, appearing somewhat, though slightly, affected with the same disease. The whole peritoneum of the pelvis was rendered rough by confluent flat tubercles of the same carcinomatous deposit, and the same might be said of the peritoneum lining the parietes of the lower part of the abdomen. The other parts of the abdominal peritoneum were thinly studded with similar deposits, as were the lower surface of the diaphragm and the ligaments of the liver. I did not perceive any of these tubera upon the peritoneum covering the intestines, but some portions of the small intestines had a thin, gray deposit upon them, which felt quite scabrous to the touch.

The bladder was greatly distended and vascular, and in one part slightly scabrous. The kidneys not obviously diseased. The liver was tolerably healthy, with no tubera in its substance. The gallbladder empty. The stomach was pushed upwards and backwards, and was so small that it would scarcely have held six ounces of fluid. The heart and pericardium perfectly healthy.

In the chest great disease had been going on in the right side; it contained about four pints of serum; the upper part was clear yellow, but below was deposited grumous, bloody fluid, and yellow, gelatinous matter, not unlike what we found in the pelvis, and the whole pleura costalis was thickly covered by small, scirrhous deposit, rendering it completely rough and hard; the lung was contracted to one sixth of its natural size, but the upper lobe contained air, and was rather emphysematous. On the surface of the liver, below the pleura, were some small, flat deposits of carcinomatous matter. The left side of the chest contained a very small quantity of fluid; the pleura costalis was scarcely affected with the scirrhous disease; the surface of the lung, in two or three places, had clusters of small yellow or white carcinomatous deposits.

The foregoing case presents an illustrative example of one of the more malignant forms of ovarian tumour, approaching to the true scirrhus; and shows, in a strong light, the morbid tendency which often pervades the whole system when this destructive disease has once displayed itself. In this case, we likewise see some of those modifications of the disease which take place when it develops itself in different structures. The uterus, the ovaries, and the various reflections of the serous membranes, were the parts chiefly affected. In the solid, fleshy substance of the uterus, the disease had shown itself in the form of hard, fibrous, elastic tumours; in the serous membranes it was seen as flat, circular patches, of various sizes; in the integuments it formed small, rounded bodies, like enlarged glands; in the loose texture of the ovary it expanded into cysts; and probably, in each of these different parts, the disposition of the cellular tissue had the chief influence in directing the course of the morbid matter, the tendency of which is always, as it would appear, to deposit itself in that structure; and it seems that, wherever inflammation is excited, when such a decided tendency prevails, the disease springs up. At what period of the complaint the peritoneum and pleura had taken on this morbid action cannot be decided; but that a very short time is necessary for effecting such changes as they exhibited, is plainly proved by the deposit of malignant tubercles in the cellular membrane of the abdomen, within a few days after the irritation of passing the trochar.

The length of time in which this disease ran its course is not distinctly ascertained; but although the size of the body had evidently increased for some months previously, it does not appear that medical advice had been sought above fifteen months; and judging from the rapid progress made after this time, it is not unlikely that less than two years would include the commencement of the morbid growth; and it is even probable that the extension of the mischief beyond the ovary itself only dates from the time of the paracentesis being performed, when some of the fluid may have escaped into the peritoneum and cellular tissue.

It is but too well known, that a case of this kind admits scarcely of palliation, much less of cure; and it is well that this should be impressed on our minds, seeing how much misery and mischief may be added to the necessary grievances of disease by the rash interference of our art. Whether there had ever, in this case, been a serious thought of attempting the extirpation of the malady by the knife, I could scarcely take upon me to say; but certainly so much had passed, as rendered the patient herself anxious that something of the kind should be tried; and what the result of such a trial would have been no one can doubt—useless agony to the patient, and deep mortification to the operator.

CASE 23.—*Ovaries affected with a modification of the malignant disease; the peritoneum extensively involved in similar affection.*—August 25th, 1820.—I was present at the examination of a patient who had died worn out under a malignant form of ovarian disease. We found both the ovaries equally involved; and together they almost occupied the whole cavity of the abdomen, pushing the viscera completely aside. The appearance of the ovaries, when cut into, was as if they were filled with a gelatinous matter, intersected by a multiplicity of vascular membranes, forming cysts. These held the mucilaginous matter, which resembled calf's-foot jelly imperfectly cooled, so closely, that it was with great difficulty drawn out, but it appeared as if the general cyst or covering of the ovary, enormously distended, formed the general covering of all these minor cysts. In this case, most of the other viscera were tolerably

9

healthy; but the malignant disease showed itself very extensively on the peritoneum; for on first opening the abdomen, the omentum came into view as a flap of mucous or fatty, semi-transparent matter, granular in its texture, and slightly but universally adhering to the peritoneal lining of the muscles of the abdomen. This same granular growth sprung up as an irregular covering to the whole lower surface of the diaphragm and the peritoneum, extending along the sides of the abdomen to the pelvis. It covered the colon also, and formed a strong union between it and some portions of the small intestines.

Of the history of this case I have no record; but the disease of the peritoneum presented a modification somewhat different, yet nearly allied to that which occurred in the last case.

There is another modification which malignant disease occasionally assumes on the peritoneum, when the surface of that membrane, instead of being covered with flattened, opaque tubera, or with semi-transparent granulations, is beset more or less closely with pendulous bodies, varying somewhat in the firmness or fluidity of the matter they contain. As an example of this variety of malignant disease connected with ovarian dropsy, I shall here introduce another case, which I received from Mr. Beaumont, in the same letter as the case I have lately cited.

CASE 24.—*Ovarian tumour, with extensive growth of pendulous malignant tumours from the peritoneum.*—" Mrs. — had for many years laboured under ovarian dropsy. I was requested to see her with the gentleman who had been in attendance upon her, and we drew off thirteen pints of a fluid resembling thick water-gruel. She soon got about, but, within four months, filled again. In the mean time I had seen my friend Dr. Blundell, and mentioned the case to him, when he requested that she might be sent to Guy's Hospital. She went, and was examined by the doctor, and by one of the surgeons. The opinion was, that when she became so large as to require the operation it should be repeated, and she should then be sent back to the hospital, that she might again be carefully examined. This was done, and the letter she brought back stated that it was considered an unfavorable case for the operation of extirpation, on account of her general health, and a suspicion of adhesion having taken place with some of the viscera. She died, and, upon examination, we found that there were adhesions, but none which were not easily broken down by the finger. The tumour, or sac, was of an immense size, and nearly of an hour-glass form, attached by a neck about the diameter of a thumb.

"The most curious part of this case was, that there were innumerable pendulous tumours, like polypi, transparent; and filled with a watery fluid, attached to the various reflections of the peritoneum, some of the size of a small pear. They were not hydatids."

I may remark on this case, that though I have occasionally seen the pendulous form of malignant tuber in different states, and amongst these a few containing a fluid, yet I do not remember to have met with any in which the affection has been so extensive as here described by Mr. Beaumont, nor in any case do I remember it as connected with ovarian dropsy. This, however, goes to show how completely the ovarian disease identifies itself with all the varieties of malignant growth.

CASE 25.—*Malignant ovarian tumour, with ascites, communicating disease by contiguity to the sigmoid flexure and rectum.*—Mrs. B—, æt. —, had been in the Clinical Ward of Guy's Hospital during the winter of 1835; at first under the care of Dr. Cholmeley, and afterwards under mine.

At the time she came under my care, she was affected with a tumour lying obliquely in the lower part of the abdomen, very hard and lobulated in its feel, which continued to increase very gradually, while at the same time an accumulation of fluid took place slowly in the general cavity of the peritoneum, which was most distinctly to be felt fluctuating, as a thin layer over the tumour; but the circumstance which was peculiar, and most distressing, was the condition of the bowels, which were greatly constipated, rendering injections constantly necessary, and the pain she suffered in passing her stools was so great as to require the frequent use of anodynes, and the dejections were composed chiefly of shreds of bloody mucus with a little fæces. She emaciated rapidly, and finding no improvement, but, on the contrary, a gradual loss of power, she left the hospital.

I more than once referred to this case in the clinical lectures; all the symptoms leading to the supposition, that there was a malignant ovarian tumour which made pressure on the sigmoid flexure and the rectum, and had probably communicated disease of the same character to the intestines themselves.

After leaving the hospital, she came under the care of Mr. Kingston, of Walworth; and the ascites having increased very much, and become very oppressive, he relieved her by drawing off serum to the amount of eleven quarts. But the operation afforded only temporary ease; the serum accumulated again rapidly, and she died, exhausted, about a month after, on the 21st of May.

Sectio cadaveris.—May 22d.—The abdomen greatly distended, and two or three small scirrhous subcutaneous tubercles were felt in the parietes. The intestines, distended with flatus, were distinctly seen, and recognised by percussion, floating on the serum. On opening the parietes, a great many quarts of yellow serum were found in the peritoneal cavity, and when this was drawn off, the edge of the liver, and part of the fundus of the gall-bladder, were seen at the upper part; beneath these the colon was much distended, and below this, several portions of the small intestines occupied, together, above half the abdomen, while an ovarian tumour was situated in the lower half.

The tumour was formed in the left ovary, drawing the uterus out of its place, while the Fallopian tube and the broad ligament were stretched over it. It was composed of several cysts; the largest, about the size of a large melon, contained fluid. The different parts of the tumour were in different states. Some parts bore the appearance of fat, while some were decidedly cerebriform, and on the outside of the tumour were several lumps of a truly scirrhous hardness. It was attached closely by adhesions to the sigmoid flexure, and at the lower part glued to the rectum, which was converted into a scirrhous mass; a state of things which I understood had latterly become cognizable by the touch.

The whole of the lumbar glands formed one scirrhous mass; the mesentery was studded with small, hard, round, scirrhous tubercles, and a few were distributed on the peritoneal covering of the intestines.

The stomach and its pylorus healthy; the liver healthy, but a little pale; the gall-gladder distended with bile; the pancreas rather hard, and of a yellow colour, but without distinct scirrhous disease; the kidneys healthy; the uterus, although pressed upon and displaced, also apparently healthy.

This case presents a well-marked instance of a very malignant form of disease, showing itself by its extension to the various parts with which it came in contact, particularly the glands of the loins, the peritoneum, and, above all, some portions of the large intestines. The cerebriform, the scirrhous, and the cystiform characters of the disease were all exemplified in this case; and the small subcutaneous tubercles presented an unerring proof of the peculiarly malignant nature of the affection.

Case. 26.—*Ovarian dropsy; cerebriform disease, communicating to contiguous organs.*—In the month of September, 1837, I was requested to see, in consultation, a lady, the mother of a family, who, about eighteen months before, had suffered from prolapsus uteri, which had been relieved at the end of seven months, at the same time that a tumour had appeared in the right side of the abdomen, and it was conjectured that the rising of the tumour out of the pelvis had drawn the uterus up with it. In the course of about three months fluctuation might be indistinctly felt upon the left side, and became gradually more and more distinct, occupying a larger portion of the abdomen. At my first visit, I found that she had been labouring for the last three weeks under severe irritation of the stomach and bowels, sometimes vomiting bile, bowels irregular, appetite bad and capricious, much griping, peculiar spasmodic pain brought on by motion or by coughing, tongue red at the tip and edges, lips parched, general emaciation to a great degree; she was quite unable to leave the sofa. The tumour appeared to be one complicated ovarian mass, having a large collection of cysts in the parietes of its left side, with two or three smaller masses, besides one large cyst very thin and full of fluid towards the left. It was to be feared that this case having advanced so rapidly, and the constitution failing so much, a fatal termination would take place at no very distant period; although, at that time, there were no symptoms of a near approaching fatal event.

October 10th.—She has, upon the whole, been considerably better in her general health and spirits; the gentlest means having been used. Two or three doses of three grains of compound ipecacuanha powder daily, and a small dose of castor oil occasionally to regulate the bowels, with very careful attention to the diet. Latterly, however, she has suffered a good deal from the tumour and its pressure, and on one occasion, about a month ago, she complained of much pain in the upper part of the left side for a day or two, which went off suddenly, with a feeling of something bursting or moving quickly from its place. It was therefore determined to draw off the fluid by paracentesis; and a trochar having been used in the left side, six pints of fluid were drawn off. It was as thick as pea-soup, and of a pink colour, looking very much like pus tinged with blood. She bore the operation well, and the relief afforded was of the most marked kind. The appetite, which had been almost gone, returned, even in excess. No unpleasant symptom took place, and in about a week she got upon a sofa, and in a few days more was in the drawing-room.

November 6th.—I found her walking about the drawing-room; tongue less red, pulse below 100, countenance decidedly improved, abdomen a good deal enlarged.

December 3d.—She was greatly emaciated, and particularly for the last fortnight had been suffering a return of all her pains and all her worst symptoms; and, at a consultation, it was determined to have recourse again to paracentesis as a means of affording temporary relief. About six pints of thick, pink-coloured fluid were taken away with some difficulty, owing to the frequent obstruction of the canula.

For two days after the operation there was a slight rally; but then the pulse became quick, pains came on in the abdomen, the hectic symptoms returned, the appetite failed, and sickness ensued. She emaciated rapidly, and on the night of the 12th of December she died.

Sectio cadaveris.—December 14th.—The greatest emaciation; the abdomen was distended almost to the utmost; the integuments, from both these causes, were excessively thin; and adhered very generally, but not firmly, to the outside of the sac. The sac was remarkably thin, and occupied the whole of that part of the abdomen which came in sight on first opening it. It was also attached very slightly to some of the small intestines in the left hypochondrium; and the omentum was stretched over the tumour, and closely attached to it. The tumour was still more closely attached to the right side of the arch of the colon; where, indeed, they were firmly glued together in a cerebriform mass, which had so far consumed the natural parietes of the cyst, that, on detaching it from the colon, no cyst was found, but only the diseased portion which adhered to the colon.

It was plain that the whole mass of the tumour was attached to the Fallopian tubes and the ligaments of the uterus on the right side; and the Fallopian tube of that side was drawn out and stretched over the tumour; and carried in this so high, that the fimbriated extremity was attached to the margin of the right lobe of the liver.

All that part of the tumour which had felt so hard was one mass of cerebriform matter, assuming a somewhat lobulated form externally, and completely broken down internally. This cerebriform mass extended quite to the liver and colon; and the edge of the liver was infected with it, in the form of a tuber of the size of a filbert. The colon, though firmly attached to the mass, did not itself appear diseased.

There were at least two gallons of fluid removed from this cyst. That which first came away was fluid like sanguineous serum; but in the lower part of the cyst we had a thick, gruel-like matter, like that which had been drawn off. But the circumstance which first appeared peculiar was, that lumps of fatty matter, not unlike masses of dripping, were found floating in it; the origin of these, however, was soon discovered; for in the upper part of the cyst, under the arch of the colon, was discovered a mass of hair and fat, evidently one of the masses which develop themselves in these structures. There was still a very curious tumour discovered in the right iliac region, occupying nearly the natural situation of the cæcum. It was about the size of the kidney, felt cellular, but with a kind of cracking feel under pressure; it was supplied with vessels which ran over the brim of the pelvis towards the iliac vessels, but otherwise did not seem connected with any organ; it was easily torn from its attachments; and was then found to be a mass of hair and bony matter, containing two or three teeth with the alveolar processes, and apparently divided, in part, into cells.

On the convex surface of the liver was one fungoid mass, like fungus hæmatodes, of the size of a marble. A firm coagulum was found in one of the veins on the left side of the pelvis.

Carefully examining the uterus, no portion of an ovary could be detected on the left side; but on the posterior part of the broad ligament, very near to the uterus, was an obvious discoloured scar, with a few grains of bony deposit. There was likewise a very peculiar appearance in the upper portion of the Fallopian tube, which presented a somewhat bulb-like form, and seemed as if it had been cut off by previous ulceration. The kidneys were healthy. The chest was not examined.

In the foregoing case is an example of what is, perhaps, the most malignant form of the ovarian tumour—the true cerebriform disease. Of the rapidity with which this modification of malignant action takes place, we have, occasionally, most striking examples in the internal organs, but more particularly in the liver; and in the case before us, the whole period, from the first detection of a tumour in the inguinal region to the day when death occurred, with all the extensive ravages we have seen, did not exceed fourteen months. The cerebriform disease is, as far as I have observed, more apt to extend from viscus to viscus by contact, and less by what appears a diffused action through the system, than the true scirrhus; and this might readily be expected, from the rapidity and disintegrating nature of its progress, which generally gives much less time than the true scirrhus for the system to become extensively involved.

In this case, it appears probable that at some former period disease had taken place in the left ovary; which had actually been separated, and had fallen over to the right iliac region, where it had become attached; and that latterly the very same morbid tendency had developed itself in the right ovary; but here it had given rise to the most malignant form of disease.

In the cases which have now been brought together, we trace the history of the ovarian tumour through a great portion of the varieties it presents; and we find examples of most of the more striking circumstances which occur in the progress of the disease, and of many of the events on which its fatal termination depends.

In the first place, we have instances referred to, in which simple cysts have been found attached to the ovaries and uterine appendages, which have presented no character of malignancy, nor any apparent tendency to rapid increase. Cases are likewise stated by authors, where tumours bearing an equal and smooth surface have existed for a very considerable length of time, even for many years, without interfering much with the healthy functions. Well authenticated cases are on record, where such tumours have apparently been ruptured internally by accidental blows, and the accumulation has never again taken place. There is reason to believe, in cases of this kind, and in some of those in which the tumour has been emptied by operation an almost indefinite number of times, without aggravation of the symptoms, that the disease has consisted of an accumulation of the fluid in a simple cyst, without any tendency to a specific or a malignant action; but whether these collections of fluid are to be considered as belonging to simple serous cysts, to non-malignant disease of the Graafian vesicles, or to dropsy of the Fallopian tube, remains doubtful; and it is even possible that a certain proportion of these cases, as well as of reported cures by other remedies, may be set down as instances of erroneous diagnosis; for there is no question that the diagnosis is not always obvious; and there is one class of cases more particularly liable to lead the unwary and inexperienced into error respecting the disappearance of an abdominal tumour; I mean, cases of hysterical distension of the bowels; for although the swelling in these cases is essentially tympanitic, yet occasionally, from the singular way in which the intestines are partially distended, and remain so for days and weeks at a time, they sometimes give completely the forms of tumours; and sometimes even indistinct fluctuation may arise from fluid fæces, or even from the coexistence of a distended bladder; and sometimes the large accumulation of hardened fæces has led to a belief of a more solid tumour. And to show that such a solution is not altogether hypothetical, I shall insert the following example.

CASE 26.—*Hysterical distension of the bowels, mistaken for ovarian tumour; operation to attempt its removal.*—Susannah J——, æt. 30, said to have been ill for two years, was admitted under my care, into Charity Ward, September 29th, 1824, complaining of abdominal pain and some hysteric symptoms. She had, in the middle line of the abdomen, about half way between the umbilicus and the symphysis pubis, an unhealed scar, of about three inches in length. The deeper part of the wound had united; and it was filling up by granulation, as was a portion of the external part, at each end of the scar. It was evidently an incised wound; and the account she gave was, that her abdomen being swollen, as it was at the time she had formerly been in the hospital, a surgeon proposed to her the excision of a tumour which produced this swelling; and that, with two assistants, he prepared to perform the operation, and made a free incision into the abdominal cavity; but finding that there was no tumour, brought the wound together; which now, after the lapse of several weeks, was as we saw it. The wound healed completely, under common treatment; but her health remained in a most unsatisfactory state, both from the frequent tendency to diarrhœa, and from the succession of pains, with occasional puffing-up of the abdomen, of which she was the subject; so that she remained in the hospital till the 28th of December.

During this long confinement, the pains in the right and left sides of the abdomen frequently led her to request the application of leeches and cupping to these parts. Blisters were also applied; but the chief remedies employed, and which always proved most useful, were such as her hysteric symptoms were constantly suggesting. The tumour of the abdomen varied a good deal; and was, on one or two occasions, reported to have subsided entirely.

I may mention further, that I had seen this young woman many years before, when she was in Guy's Hospital for a supposed abdominal tumour, under Dr. Marcet; who, however, soon discovered its hysteric character; though, certainly, the abdomen bore a very peculiar appearance, strongly resembling an encysted tumour; but there were connected with this supposed tumour so many other ailments, embracing fits of hysterics, epilepsy, paralysis, abdominal and lumbar pains, so varied and so changing, that a little observation was sufficient to convince any experienced person of its real character.

By far the larger number of the cases in the foregoing series are, however, to be referred to diseases of a very different character, connected with a much more disastrous history. A tumour is observed arising from one side of the pelvis; and is perhaps scarcely noticed, till it has already ascended half way to the umbilicus. Its progress is moderately rapid; so that, in the course of the first year or eighteen months, it has risen above the umbilicus, has spread to the other side, or has perhaps apparently filled the abdomen, the surface of which presents a network of distended veins, owing to the pressure on the internal vessels. Fluctuation, which was at first indistinct, has become very obvious and general; so that in vain do we seek, by percussion, for the sounds of hollow viscera, till we pursue the examination quite into the lumbar region of the opposite side; and within six months more, the pressure occasioned on every side renders it almost indispensable that the fluid should be drawn off. This fluid is glairy, or mucilaginous, or dark, or turbid, or loaded with cholesterine. When the fluid is nearly withdrawn, floating, as it were, in the flaccid abdomen, one or perhaps two or three hard bodies are discovered; one round; another flat, and shaped like a placenta. The fluid now accumulates still more rapidly. In a few months it must again be drawn off. Its character is often changed; it is more gelatinous or more opaque, sometimes becoming puriform; or it is mingled with blood or cerebriform matter. Operation succeeds to operation, with diminished intervals; the constitution sympathises; and, after a limited number of months or years, the patient sinks exhausted by weakness, overcome by inflammation, or worn out by pain. Nothing can bespeak more plainly a disease differing widely in character from the simple cyst, or from any accidental collection of serous fluid.

From a consideration of the cases which have been now adduced, and others bearing on the point, we shall find that the diagnosis is not for the most part difficult, as regards the encysted character of the accumulation generally; but it is by no means easy, and is sometimes impossible to distinguish between the simple and the compound cyst; because the secondary nodules are often very small in comparison with some larger cyst; and are so situated as to be quite undiscovered till the fluid has been drawn off; and occasionally so small as not even to be felt when the cyst has been emptied.

The circumscribed extent of the tumour, and consequently of the fluctuation, distinguishes all ovarian cysts in the early stages from ascites. The fluctuation uninterrupted by the intestines in any part, distinguishes the disease in more advanced cases. The lateral situation of the tumour in the early stages distinguishes it from pregnancy in the normal state of the viscera. Its duration distinguishes it in the more advanced stages: the suppression of the catamenial discharge adds probability to the existence of pregnancy; but there is no certainty to be derived from this indication; as in ovarian disease, the catamenia are sometimes regular, sometimes irregular, sometimes wanting; alterations in the mammæ are likewise uncertain indications; and in doubtful cases nothing except examination by the vagina can give tolerable certainty; and then the shortened cervix, and the weighty feel of the uterus, would decide the question in favour of that organ. From the malignant disease of the fundus of the uterus the situation will in part distinguish it; the hardness of the tumour, and the peculiar abrupt nodules which the diseased uterus presents, contrast well with the soft and yielding feel which the subsidiary tumours of the compound ovarian cyst usually afford. The origin of these cysts from the pelvis generally distinguishes them from all tumours of the abdomen, except diseases of the uterus, or a thickened or distended bladder; and the central situation of both these viscera suffices, for the most part, to fix disease upon them when it exists.

When paracentesis has been performed, the obvious character of the fluid which is drawn off will generally, in doubtful cases, prove a guide (pp. 67, 73, 81-2, &c.); and it appears probable that the chemical composition of the fluid (see p. 82), may be further brought in aid of our diagnosis. Where the disease has assumed a very malignant character, we shall sometimes derive information of this fact from the hard subcutaneous knots which are developing themselves in the cellular membrane (pp. 75, 124, 132); and when it is of importance, with a view to the performance of an operation, to be made aware of adhesions between the tumour and the parietes, the peculiar feel derived from pressing the hand on the parts when the adhesion has taken place, will, in some cases, be instructive. (Case 10.)

There are occasional complications, which it is not easy to meet by any general rules, but which attentive investigation will greatly tend to unfold; as, for instance, diseases of the other viscera—as the kidney, or the spleen, or the liver—pushing the impregnating uterus to one side, and thus disguising the real cause of the increasing bulk of the abdomen, or impregnation taking place during the existence of an ovarian tumour, and obscuring the nature of both; or the combination of ascites with ovarian dropsy, more particularly should that ascites have assumed a chronic form, and be accompanied by thickened peritoneum; or even such chronic ascites uncombined may be easily confounded with the ovarian dropsy; or, lastly, such a condition of the cyst, that, owing to communication between it and the substance, gas is allowed to enter, or is generated in the cyst; in which case the tympanitic sound of the tumour would almost necessarily lead us into error as to its nature, were we not assisted by the history. (Case 18.)

Of such occasional complications I would willingly adduce instances, but, that the length to which this communication has already been protracted renders it impossible to add more details. I may, however, observe, that in Fig. 37, will be found a small sketch of an ovarian cyst, which, being complicated with a diseased condition of the peritoneum, from its thickness preventing the intestines from floating, served to disguise a case of ascites, and to lead to the belief that the accumulation was ovarian for a period of two or three years, during which the patient was tapped twelve or thirteen times; and it was not till her death afforded an opportunity of examining the general texture of the peritoneum, that its true nature was discovered. And I will likewise briefly mention, that a case occurred to me, of which I have the notes, where a woman was admitted with abdominal tumour of long standing, and having a completely ovarian history, but which she stated to have increased lately, and from finding that the breasts were now secreting milk, I was led to suspect the possibility of pregnancy; however, Dr. Ashwell examined by the vagina, and no alteration was discoverable in the neck of the uterus. The tumour went on increasing, on one side more particularly; and, in four months after, I again requested Dr. Ashwell to examine; and he then had no doubt that pregnancy was advancing; and shortly afterwards the motions of the child became very perceptible to the hand placed externally. In due time she was removed into another ward; had a natural and easy labour; but the ovarian tumour remained unaltered; and she was transferred back again under my care.

Fig. 37.

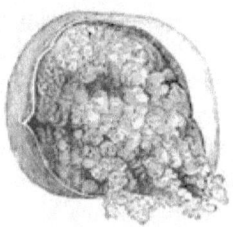

Fig. 37. A reduced sketch of a remarkably hard ovarian cyst, which occurred, in combination with ascites, in a case where the peritoneum was so much thickened as to give to the whole abdominal cavity the character of a cyst. The ovarian tumour, when opened, proved to be filled with a closely compacted growth, resembling a head of cauliflower, which sprung from one portion of the cyst more than from the rest; but the exact nature of this growth, though it appeared malignant, is not ascertained. The tumour, which is preserved in Guy's Museum, is nearly fourteen inches in its largest diameter.

With regard to our *prognosis*, the ultimate prospect is, certainly, most unfavorable. We find, in the cases above recorded, that the malignant ovarian tumour, left to itself, often destroys life in a short time, partly by irritation, but probably in a great degree by the mechanical pressure it exerts. (Cases 10 and 11.) That if paracentesis is performed, life may be prolonged; but that sometimes, from the inflammation excited by the circumstances attending the operation (Cases 6, 12, 14, 15, 17, &c.), and sometimes without any discernible inflammation (Case 9), death takes place. That in other cases the malignant disease seems to undermine the constitution, and gradually leads to a fatal result. (Cases 23, 24, 25, 26.) That, occasionally, the internal rupture of the cyst produces death. (Cases 16, 18, 19.) But still, with such a discouraging prognosis before us, we have every reason to feel that the interposition of our remedial means is productive of great alleviation, and is capable of prolonging life; and, although the duration of this disease is often limited to months, and still more frequently to a very few years, yet instances are not wanting, in which ten, twelve, or a still greater number of years have been passed in tolerable comfort; and, in giving our prognosis, we should suffer ourselves and our patients to have the full benefit of the hope which such cases are calculated to inspire.

I believe, as far as *cure* is concerned, the malignant ovarian dropsy admits of none, unless we may consider the excision of the tumour in that light; and this must ever be so doubtful an operation, surrounded by so much darkness, and attended with so much danger, that I can only look upon its happy event as the fortunate result of a bold and hazardous enterprise, which should not tempt us to adopt it as a rule of practice. When we consider the nature of the affection, we are at once prepared to find that all remedies specifically directed to its cure will prove useless. It is truly a malignant disease; and, though it usually assumes one, and that a milder modification, in preference to the rest, is not unfrequently found degenerating into the worst and most destructive forms of the fungous and cerebriform cancer; and it undergoes those changes by such insensible degrees, that it is impossible to draw the line, and deny a malignant character to one, while we grant it to the others. But, though we confess that we have no remedies to act directly upon the disease, a good deal may undoubtedly be done in regulating the various processes of the economy, so as to maintain the general health in a state unfavorable to the rapid development of the disease; and for this purpose we have to reinstate the natural secretions, to subdue excessive action, whether local or general, and to maintain the strength. It is not necessary, in this place, to enter into all the minutiæ of such treatment; it is enough to say that occasional local bleedings, blisterings, and counter-irritation, mild bitters and tonics, the taraxacum and the sarsaparilla, the alkalies, and a variety of other remedies, with conium, hyoscyamus, and different narcotics, afford the means, when varied according to circumstances, of preventing inflammatory action; of allaying the irritation, which is often discoverable by the pulse, and sometimes by the expressions of pain; and at the same time of assisting to maintain the powers of the system.

Iodine is one of the remedies which have been much recommended by some writers; but if administered, it must be done with all that precaution which naturally suggests itself, when employing a remedy capable of promoting the absorption of the natural structures, fully as much as it does of those tissues dependent upon malignant disease, and which sometimes leads to the most alarming state of nervous depression.

Dr. Barlow, of Bath, has published some cases, in which repeated bleedings from the arm, with leeching and cupping, seemed to have retarded the progress of the swelling, and almost anticipated that proof of the existence of the ovarian disease; but, I must confess, that however influential remedies may be in preventing the yet unformed disease, or in checking its progress, I am always inclined to look with doubt upon cases of supposed cure after the disease is once confirmed; as I think there is reason to suppose, that, from its very beginning, its character is often truly specific and malignant.

In the midst of our attempts to retard the progress of the disease, the question of paracentesis presents itself. There are, I believe, a few instances on record, where this operation has apparently been followed by complete cure; there are certainly cases in which the rupture of the cyst internally has been followed by no reaccumulation of the fluid; but whether, in these cases, the disease has been anything more than a simple serous cyst is doubtful. We have, however, at all events, great reason to believe, that, in some cases of a truly malignant character, an individual cyst has contracted after the fluid has been withdrawn, though other cysts in the same diseased mass have rapidly increased. (Case 7.) These considerations might lead to an expectation that paracentesis would prove more than a merely palliative remedy; but, unfortunately, this conclusion is not countenanced by experience; and although, by some rare combination of circumstances, the withdrawal of the fluid may be followed by a long respite, or even an apparent cure, yet we cannot look upon it, generally, in any other light than as a means of present relief. It is, however, an operation to which we must in many cases have recourse, if we would prolong the lives of our patients; and one or two important questions present themselves in connexion with it: first, as to the time, and then as to the manner of performing the operation. As to the time, it may be done early, while yet the tumour is small, and just rising from the pelvis; it may be done when the tumour is become large, occupying apparently the whole abdomen, but still attended by no great inconvenience, nor affording any apparent obstruction to the action of the viscera, or the abdominal circulation; or, thirdly, it may be deferred till the inconvenience is become very great, the stomach compressed, the intestines impeded, and the chest encroached upon. Of the first two of these I have very little experience; partly because cases of this kind are not generally brought under the notice of the physician in the early stages of their progress; and partly, because I always feel reluctant to recommend an operation, and the patient is unwilling to submit to one, when there is no obvious necessity, and when there is no imminent inconvenience to be removed. Besides this, our diagnosis is more certain as the disease becomes more advanced; and the operation is connected with less hazard at the time, and probably less danger from after-inflammation. Although, therefore, I have had but very little experience in early operation, yet, as I see no reason to suppose that by drawing off the fluid we shall change the malignant nature of the disease, but may probably accelerate its progress, I do not think it advisable to have early recourse to paracentesis. I have been much more in the habit of abstaining from operation, as long as the patient herself feels no urgent inconvenience; provided there is no direct evidence, in the interruption of functions, that the pressure is doing essential injury. The timidity of some patients, however, will render it necessary to interpose with strong advice; for there is no doubt that death will take place, and sometimes rapidly, from the effects of the pressure, and the irritation of the unrelieved tumour; as exemplified in Cases 10 and 11; and I conceive that the time for the operation is arrived when the tumour pretty fairly occupies a large portion of the abdomen, giving the appearance of pregnancy advanced to the last months, and before any material mischief seems to threaten either to the surrounding viscera, or to the parietes of the tumour itself; for there can be little doubt that the forcible distension of the sac continued beyond a certain limit will endanger its inner surface, and, perhaps, prove one cause for those ulcerative changes which often take place, and are the source of great constitutional irritation and of death, as seen in several of the foregoing dissections.

Supposing the period for performing the operation to be agreed upon, another question arises as to the part in which the puncture should be made. As the tumour is probably one of complicated structure, we must, by the hand and by percussion, ascertain as far as possible the part in which the parietes are yielding, and in which the fluid is chiefly accumulated, for I have known instances in which the operator has been foiled, and even obliged to make a second puncture, from having pushed the trochar into a solid mass; and even when distinct fluctuation has been ascertained, the thickness of the fluid has sometimes prevented its passing by the puncture; or, by opening into some secondary cyst, a few ounces only have been drawn off, to the great disappointment of the patient, who had made up her mind to the operation under the full expectation of being relieved of a large part of the burden with which she was oppressed. In one of the foregoing cases (Case 15), another source of disappointment has been seen, from the trochar passing into a firm band formed by the broad ligament and the Fallopian tube stretched over the tumour, and affording such resistance that the instrument pushed the parietes of the tumour before it; and when withdrawn, under the belief that it has gone deep into the cyst, no fluid escaped. Very attentive manual examination might possibly in general prevent such an accident, and there is scarcely any rule by which the operator can be directed, as these bands may cross the tumour in various directions, and in one of the cases mentioned in this paper (Case 26), it actually ran to be attached to the lobe of the liver.

It is right before operating to be quite sure that the bladder is empty; and, of course, enlarged veins must be carefully avoided, and in general it will be right to examine the state of the uterus per vaginam, more particularly if it be the first time that the operation has been performed. Should the sensation given by pressure on the abdomen lead to the belief that adhesions have taken place between any portion of the cyst and the parietes, it will be well to select this part for the operation, as we shall thus avoid one important source of danger—the escape of a portion of fluid into the abdominal cavity: and if in any case we might allow of a fistulous opening being established, this is it. (Case 8.)

Another very important point, is the quantity of fluid which should be drawn away; some there are who think that it is most advisable to take away but a small portion of the whole, just sufficient to relieve the urgent oppression; supposing that by this means the cyst is more likely to contract, and believing that the fluid does not re-accumulate so rapidly in this case as where the distending contents are at once withdrawn. On the whole, however, I generally recommend that as much of the fluid as possible should be removed, because I dread above every other danger that of a portion of the fluid escaping into the peritoneum, of which we run a great risk, if the wounded parietes of the tumour fall in upon a considerable quantity of fluid; and in order to avoid this still further, a regular gentle pressure should be maintained, as is usual during and after the operation in ascites; and for some days the most perfect tranquillity should be enjoined, the patient being treated like one who is recovering from labour.

There are other diseases to which the ovaries are subject; some of which produce manifest tumours, ascending from the pelvis, and are therefore by no means foreign to the subject of the present communication. Most of the enlargements of the ovaries would appear to be dependent on malignant disease; such, for instance, as the cellular enlargement, of which mention has been made in Case 4, and of which a sketch may be seen in Fig. 35; so likewise the deposit of bony matter in the ovary, which I have seen associated with the fibrous tubercle of the uterus. But in one rather remarkable specimen in Guy's Museum, both the ovaries are enlarged to the size of the kidneys, and are of a solid fleshy consistence. They had formed distinct tumours above the pubes; but whether they ought to be considered malignant or scrofulous, it is difficult to determine: certain it is, however, that their solid structure bears no analogy to anything we usually see associated with malignant disease in this organ. The short history which accompanied this preparation, in a letter addressed to the late Mr. Stocker, of Guy's Hospital, is worth preserving, and with it I will conclude my present communication on abdominal tumours.

"The woman had borne children, and when passed the menstrual "period of life, was seized with pains which were referred to the "uterus. These continued more or less acute for two months, when "a considerable indurated substance was perceptible in the regio "pubis, referable (as was considered) to a morbid state of the "uterus. After this time a difficulty in making water added "greatly to her sufferings; indeed it amounted to inability in the "erect position of the body, but the recumbent posture sensibly "removed the only impediment to its discharge. From anxiety, "which her intolerable pain induced, or from a combination of "circumstances, she became the most emaciated object I ever "witnessed. Jaundice supervened, attended with ascites; and in "this precarious situation, some one being consulted, took up the "idea of its being a scirrhous liver, and recommended a moderate "ptyalism to be raised and supported. The hardened substance "before mentioned was considered by him as a continuation of the "liver. Mercury, however, was only given in small quantity; and "soon after she began its use, death closed the scene.

"I solicited an examination of the body, and have sent you the "enlarged ovaries. (Fig. 38.) The liver was perfectly sound."

Fig. 38.

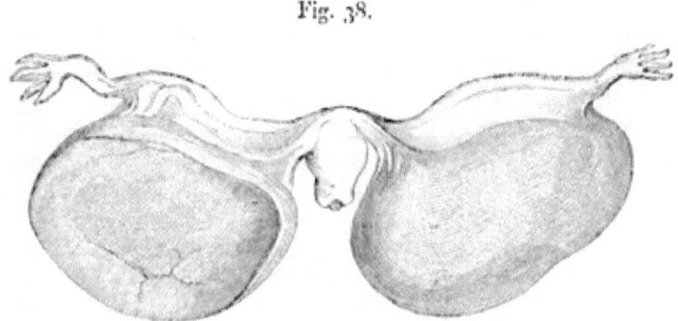

Fig. 38 represents the uterus, with the two ovaries greatly enlarged, independently of malignant disease; each ovary being nearly six inches in its longest diameter.

CHAPTER IV.

DISEASE OF THE SPLEEN.

The spleen is an organ which, both from the obscurity in which its natural functions are involved, and from the situation which it occupies in the body, presents, when diseased, some difficulties, in regard to diagnosis, which are not shared by many other organs. Moreover, its healthy condition probably admits of so much variety and so many changes, as to bulk and consistence, that, in a pathological point of view, it is not always easy to mark out the limit at which morbid change or degeneration of structure actually begins.

The situation occupied by the spleen is a portion of the left hypochondriac region: attached to the stomach and the pancreas, its lower angle touches the left kidney, while its convex surface fits into the concavity of the diaphragm. Thus, in its healthy condition, it is hidden from our view, and put beyond the reach of our usual modes of investigation; having the ribs and a portion of the diaphragm so placed as to prevent us from approaching it, on the one side, and the stomach and the colon on the other.

Its most usual appearance, after death, is an irregular flattened oblong body, varying in size, from that of half a lemon divided longitudinally, to four times that size; with a decided concavity towards the stomach, to which it is attached by vessels; and a decided convexity towards the diaphragm, against which it plays freely, without any attachment. Its colour is a purple, more or less dark in its shade, and of a somewhat silvery hue: its surface is sometimes smooth and polished; at others, corrugated: when smooth, the organ is firm and elastic to the feel: when corrugated, it is flaccid: when squeezed firmly between the fingers, the internal texture generally gives way, breaking down under strong pressure; while the tunic, with which it is invested, and the peritoneum, remain undivided.

With regard to the functions of the spleen, we have every reason to believe that it affords important assistance in preparing the blood; but whether chiefly as accessary to the process of digestion, or as having within itself the power of acting beneficially on the blood, I shall not now consider it necessary to inquire: it is an established fact, that it is provided with a structure which affords it peculiar elasticity, so that it can accommodate itself to great changes in the volume of the blood it contains.

That this power has reference to the varying quantity of blood with which it is supplied in the discharge of its duties, there can be no doubt; and the cellular, or, as I might almost say, the sponge-like arrangement of its parts, when coupled with its elasticity, plainly shows to what an extent its bulk may be expected to vary, under the ordinary circumstances which demand the filling or the emptying of its cells. From these considerations, it is obvious that, in the same individual, the healthy organ varies greatly in size: but besides this, the variety, as regards different individuals, is still more striking; and we have in the Museum of Guy's a specimen weighing only thirteen drachms and ten grains; while another apparently healthy spleen, in the same state, weighed nearly two pounds. Still, however, great as this variety is, and great as is the occasional increase of this organ, it perhaps never, in its healthy state, descends below the margin of the ribs, or becomes sensible to the touch in that part of the abdomen.

Like other organs, the spleen is subject to a variety of structural alterations, more or less permanent.

1. *Simple congestion.*—In this condition it would appear that the blood, having gained access to the cells, and over-distended them, the elastic power of the organ is too weak to send it forward, and the accumulation, consequently, goes on as far as the proper tunic and the peritoneum will permit. The spleen, in this case, retains its natural structure, and is, for a time at least, capable of being completely relieved. This condition of the spleen is probably often produced by repressed perspiration, and sudden or long-continued cold; it occurs in a more permanent way after some continuance of intermittent fever. (Figs. 41, 42, 43, pp. 160—162.)

2. *Congestion with enlargement, and probably partial organic change—the spleen still apparently able to discharge its function.*—In this state of disease, although the viscus is obviously and often greatly enlarged, yet, from the fact, that the constitution does not

materially suffer, that the countenance remains healthy, and that the spleen is subject to occasional fluctuations as to size, there is reason to believe that portions at least of the viscus, and most likely the whole, partially admits the usual passage of the blood. (Figs. 44, 45, pp. 168, 169.)

3. *Fleshy hardness.*—The organ is completely altered in its texture and characters; it becomes firm to the touch, cutting with as much resistance as an half-ripe apple, and the cut surface yielding the lustre of a firm damson-cheese; and sometimes the cut surface presents numerous opaque, whitish granules, apparently from thickened cellular membranes. It is probable that this condition is the result of chronic inflammation, or of frequent congestion; but as the spleen is often not materially enlarged, it happens that, in the present state of our knowledge, we have no means of ascertaining its induration during life.

4. *Fleshy hardness, with enlargement.*—In this state the spleen often attains to a prodigious size, filling up the whole left side of the abdomen. It produces very little constitutional irritation, and chiefly injures by its bulk, and its tendency to favour serous effusion. It is astonishing with what rapidity this enormous growth occasionally takes place; but in this respect we are liable to be deceived, for it is attended by so little pain, that, in many cases, the increase has been taking place gradually, long before some accidental circumstance leads to its discovery. In young children this form of disease is still more frequent than in adults, and with them it is more fatal. It often begins to show itself at two or three months of age, gradually increasing till it bears a very large proportion to the whole contents of the abdomen, and is to be traced quite into the pelvis, and extending far beyond the linea alba, towards the right side. In these cases it is often attended with the appearance of petechiae all over their cadaverous and pale bodies. Such children seldom live above a year, or two or three, and fall victims to emaciation, and often to mesenteric disease.

5. *Softening.*—This condition may exist in various degrees, and may depend on different causes. It is sometimes rather the result of rapid change after death than of disease. Where the colour of the organ is that of a deep venous blood, probably congestion and cadaveric change may be inferred; and where a lighter lilac colour, or a mottled red and lilac, is observed, it has been supposed to bespeak some form of inflammatory action.

6. *Inflammation.*—How much of the enlargement and the permanent hardening and softening, of which I have just spoken, may be the result of inflammation, and how much of congestion often repeated, may be matter of doubt; but that the spleen is subject to inflammation in its substance, like other organs, is certain; and although, from its peculiar character and colour, it is not easy to point out its appearance under recent inflammatory attacks, we have reason to suppose that certain alterations, with regard to its general vascularity and its consistence, must be so produced; and, perhaps, as I have said, the red and mottled lilac colour, accompanied with a degree of turgescence in the organ, indicates a state of inflammation.

7. *Suppuration.*—This proof of inflammatory action, though not very frequent, has come under my notice, in a distinct manner, two or three times. The spleen, under such circumstances, is apt to contract adhesions with neighbouring viscera, and either form a kind of shut sac by their assistance, or ulcerate through into some of the hollow viscera, as the colon or the stomach, and thus effect the discharge of the abscess without material injury to the peritoneum.

8. *Gangrene.*—This effect of inflammation is likewise occasionally found in the spleen.

9. *Tubercles.*—The substance of the spleen is occasionally sprinkled with genuine tubercles. They are often very regularly distributed through the whole substance, and, whether more or less frequent, seem to occupy every part equally. They are sometimes solid and hard, but very soon incline to soften at their centres, and early present the appearance of curdled matter contained in little cysts. The tubercles in the spleen are generally, but not always, accompanied by similar deposits in other organs, particularly the lungs and mesenteric glands; and the tubercular diathesis, in very young children, more frequently shows itself in the spleen than in persons of more advanced age, and seems to bear proportion rather to the disease of the glandular system, than of the lungs. (Figs. 47, 48, pp. 182 and 184.)

10. *Malignant disease.*—The true malignant tuber, both scirrhous and cerebriform, such as is found in the liver, is sometimes met with in the spleen, where, as in the liver, it probably occupies the cellular membrane, gradually insinuating itself extensively

through the substance of the organ, but having a tendency to the formation of rounded masses. (Fig. 50, p. 187.)

11. *Melanosis.*—The spleen, in common with almost all the organs of the body, is subject to this form of malignant disease. In the Military Museum of Fort Pitt, to which pathologists are every day more and more indebted, is a fine preparation illustrative of this fact.

12. There is another form of disease which appears to be of a malignant character, though it varies from the more usual forms of malignant disease; and which has been particularly pointed out by Dr. Hodgkin as connected with extensive disease of the absorbent glands, more particularly those which accompany the blood-vessels. The whole of these absorbent glands, or large masses of them, become large and firm, without any tendency to suppuration, as in ordinary scrofulous disease, or to soften, as in cerebriform disease: and, at the same time, the spleen becomes more or less completely infiltrated, throughout its whole substance, with a white matter of almost the appearance of suet. This matter insinuates itself into the cellular structure of the spleen; but it is no easy matter to point out what particular portion of the structure receives it. A section of the organ seems to show, from the irregular forms assumed, that it fills a cellular structure, and, in some degree, takes its shape from the cells into which it enters; having less tendency to assume the form of regular globular masses or tubera than other malignant disease. (Fig. 49, p. 186.)

13. *Fibrinous deposits, most probably from extravasated blood.*— In several cases it has been observed, in the examination of bodies, that the spleen has presented, when first brought into view, in the middle of its structure, a large mass, or sometimes two masses, of a yellow fibrinous matter, of uniform consistence. In some cases these have had all the appearance of being the remnants of blood thrown out, either like an apoplectic clot, or from the rupture or laceration of the spleen; they have sometimes presented, towards their edges, some appearance of an unconverted clot; they have not appeared to be in any state of active progress; they have generally been larger on the part seen externally, diminishing inwards, as might be expected if they had filled up a fissure or rent in the substance. In some cases the tunic of the spleen has not been distinctly to be traced; but in others the peritoneum, and perhaps the proper tunic, have seemed to pass uninjured over the yellow mass. (Figs. 51, 52, p. 194.)

14. *Bony deposits.*—It now and then happens that small rounded masses of bone are found in the very centre of the spleen; and in the only case I have recorded from my own experience, bony deposit was also found in some of the mesenteric glands;—a fact which is somewhat curious as connected with the facts I have already stated respecting the frequent coincidence of mesenteric scrofula with tuberculated spleen, and of a certain modification of malignant disease in the absorbent glands, with a corresponding disease in the spleen. (Fig. 39.)

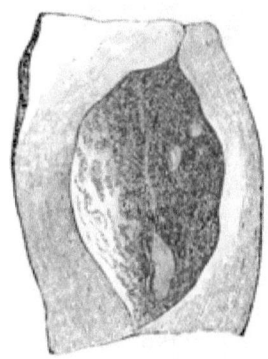

Fig. 39.

Fig. 39. Section of the spleen, showing two small deposits of bone in the substance of the organ.

15. *Cellular degeneration.*—There is an occasional appearance presented by the spleen, which I have also seen both in the liver and the kidney, where cells are developed, as if in the cellular membrane, filled with serous fluid. From these appearances, we should be inclined to suppose that they were of little importance, and only likely to interfere with the functions of the organ when they have occupied a much larger portion of it than I have ever witnessed. (Fig. 40.)

16. *Hydatids.*—The true acephalocyst hydatid is found occasionally involving, or arising from, the spleen; but by no means so frequently as from the liver. I have related, in a former number of these reports, a fatal case of an hydatid in the spleen bursting into the abdomen.

Fig. 40.

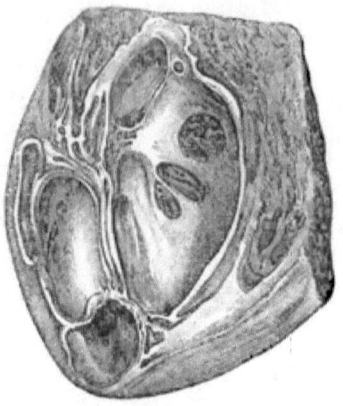

Fig. 40. Section of a small portion of the spleen, with cysts developed in the cellular membrane.

17. *Laceration.*—It happens, in cases of violent injury, not unfrequently, that the spleen is ruptured; and, in this case, haemorrhage may take place in the abdomen, and the patient die; this accident will be more likely to occur if the injury be inflicted when the spleen is in its turgid state. There are instances of laceration taking place without external injury; and the late Dr. Babington related to me a case where he had examined a patient after death, in whom the spleen had been completely detached, and was found loose in the pelvis. In that case, most violent sickness had taken place, and was believed to be the cause, not the consequence, of the spleen being torn from its attachment.

18. *Supernumerary spleens.*—It may be right to mention that it is by no means uncommon to find one, two, or three small spleens, from the size of a filbert to that of a walnut, quite separated from the large spleen. It is also said, but I cannot confirm it, that the spleen has been entirely wanting.

The peritoneal covering of the spleen is subject to all the usual alterations observed in other portions of that membrane. It may be vascular, from inflammation or congestion; it is subject to ecchymosis, adhesion, fibrinous deposit on its surface, cartilaginous deposit, and bony deposit. It may also be covered with tubercular matter, and with different forms of malignant growth.

1. The spleen does not, in general, show the *vascularity* of its surface so obviously as many other parts covered with peritoneum; and it is not common to find the membrane subject to marked vascular turgescence. Occasionally, however, that part of the peritoneum is most acutely inflamed, and the vessels sometimes distended.

2. *Ecchymosis.*—This condition is most frequently the result of accident, blows, and falls, accompanied by contusions or lacerations of the organ; but, besides this, it is sometimes seen as the result of disease; as when, in some cases of dropsy, the peritoneum has extensively put on the hæmorrhagic tendency; and this is more particularly favoured by organic changes in the spleen and liver.

3. *Adhesion.*—This result of inflammatory action is very frequently seen in the spleen, so that considerable force is necessary to draw it forward; and, in doing so, the peritoneum is often lacerated before the adhesion will give way.

4. *Fibrinous deposit.*—The surface of the spleen is often found covered with fibrinous deposit, when inflammation has existed in the peritoneum; for, owing to its dependent position, when the patient is lying on his back, it happens that the deposit has an opportunity of accumulating about it, and fixes itself permanently upon it.

5. *Cartilaginous deposit.*—The frequency of this occurrence is somewhat peculiar to the spleen; for there is no other organ so often found to be covered with a partial cartilaginous coating. The convex surface is the most frequent seat of this appearance. Sometimes the whole is covered with an even, shining coat of cartilage; at other times, it is distributed in masses of larger or smaller size, with intervening spaces; and sometimes it will be found nearly a quarter of an inch in thickness. This deposit seems to belong to the peritoneal coat, in the substance of which, or on its surface, it is probably formed; and it does not materially interfere with the elasticity of the proper tunic; so that I have seen a spleen covered with a coating of cartilage of extraordinary thickness, which had contracted, so as to bring the cartilaginous covering, which was incapable of contracting, into numerous folds. It is probably owing to the situation of the spleen favouring the accumulation of fibrin on its surface, and the peculiar and constant motion to which it is subject, in accordance with the motion of the stomach, and its own distension and contraction, that these cartilaginous patches are so frequent on its surface.

6. *Bony deposit.*—Occasionally, the change which takes place in the deposit goes one step further; and in portions of the cartilage, plates and spicula of bone are formed, or even a complete bony case.

7. *Cicatrices.*—It is not unusual to see appearances like scars, from healed lesions, upon the surface; and these sometimes penetrate quite into the substance. There is no reason to doubt that these are, then, results, either of accidental injuries, or of inflammatory, and, in some cases, perhaps, suppurative action.

8. *Tubercular deposit.*—When the tubercular diathesis is strong, and the serous membranes take on the action, or, as more frequently happens, when the newly-deposited products of inflammation receive the tubercular deposit, the spleen is often covered, either by a coating of such matter, or by innumerable miliary tubercles.

9. *Malignant deposit.*—The peritoneal coat of the spleen, and the cellular membrane beneath it, receive the different forms of malignant growth; sometimes the pendulous cysts and tubera, sometimes the creeping flat circular deposits, and sometimes the general even deposit of this kind.

Looking for the symptoms from which disease in the spleen is to be inferred, we find ourselves confined within very narrow limits. We know of no decided function which the spleen has to perform, of such a character as to direct us to the defect under which the system labours. We know of no secretion which it furnishes, nor of any excretion which it immediately influences; we therefore cannot be guided by any observations bearing upon these points. From experience, we know, that, not unfrequently, certain splenic diseases are concomitant with a peculiarly unhealthy, sallow, and anæmial character of countenance; we also know that, not unfrequently, an hæmorrhagic tendency is an accompaniment of such disorders; but neither of these are sufficiently defined; nor are they sufficiently limited to affections of the spleen, to furnish more than a clue in the investigation; and probably the local symptoms are those to which we shall turn with the greatest advantage. These local symptoms are pain, tenderness on pressure, and tumours. The pain is seldom acute, unless the peritoneal coat of the organ is inflamed; and then, owing to the proximity of so many other parts, as the heart, the lungs, the diaphragm, the stomach, the kidneys, the colon, it is very difficult to localize; although, by the method of abstracting one by one of the organs, in proof of the lesions, of which certain other symptoms are wanting, we may come to the conclusion that the pain belongs to the spleen. There is a dull and tensive pain sometimes complained of; but this, in general, does not occur till the tumour is already capable of being felt. The tenderness induced by pressure seldom leads us to the exact seat of disease, before the situation and circumstances of the tumour have already sufficiently explained its character. In most cases of splenic disease, there is neither pain nor tenderness; but when the organ is inflamed, it becomes intensely tender. The tumour is the most decisive indication; and in many cases it is scarcely to be mistaken: the character is, a smooth, oblong, solid tumour, felt immediately beneath the integuments, proceeding from under the ribs on the left side, a little behind the origin of the cartilages; often advancing to the mesial line in one direction, and descending to the crest of the ileum in the other; often filling the lumbar space, at its upper part. This tumour is very generally moveable; feels rounded at its posterior part; and presents an edge more or less sharp in front, where it is often notched and divided by fissures. If effusion takes place into the peritoneal cavity, a thin layer of fluid is early felt between the integuments and the tumour, but the intestines are not at any time found passing before the tumour.

The chief tumours which may be mistaken for an enlarged spleen, are, chronic abscess of the integuments, scirrhous thickening of the stomach, enlargement of the left lobe of the liver, diseased omentum, feculent accumulation in the colon, diseased kidney, ovarian dropsy, hydatids.

Chronic abscess beneath the integuments has sometimes shown itself so precisely in the situation below the cartilages of the ribs, which is occupied by the enlarged spleen, that difficulty has arisen in the diagnosis; but it will soon be perceived, that the swelling is too superficial, or too soft, to belong to an internal viscus, and more especially to one of the solid structure of the spleen.

Scirrhous thickening of the stomach sometimes gives rise to a tumour, which, from its being obviously deeper than the integuments, and descending from below the margin of the ribs, affords the subject of doubtful diagnosis; more particularly, as scirrhous attaching the substance of the stomach, and especially the left extremity, is often quite unattended by vomiting; while, at the same time, it is apt to be attended by a sallowness of complexion, not unlike that which bespeaks splenic disease. In this case, one of the best distinctive marks will be found in the sound elicited by percussion; which, when the stomach is so diseased, is usually clear and sonorous; while the substance is still harder than the enlarged spleen.

The left lobe of the liver is occasionally enlarged, either above, or out of proportion to the right lobe. In this case, the margin of the liver may be traced running towards the right side; while the bilious tinge of the skin and of the urine assist in the diagnosis.

The omentum is often the seat of disease; being either corrugated into a mass, or having scirrhous or scrofulous tubercles developed in its structure. In this case, the tumour much less obviously descends from beneath the ribs—cannot be traced backwards—extends across the abdomen—or is rough, knotted, hard, and uneven.

Feculent accumulation in the intestines is a very great source of difficulty in this diagnosis; for when it takes place in the descending colon and the left portion of the arch, it assumes nearly the situation of the enlarged spleen; and is scarcely to be distinguished, except by the history and by the result of medicine; nor must we, without the most persevering employment of purgatives, hastily conclude that the intestines have been emptied.

The kidney sometimes advances towards the left hypochondrium, and presents a tumour nearly in the situation of the enlarged spleen; but here we shall find, by tracing it backwards towards the loins, that its chief bulk is situated much further back, and that it is much more fixed; so that, if the patient be placed upon his hands and knees, it does not fall forwards with any freedom. On careful examination, by percussion at different times, we shall find that there is reason to conclude that the intestine lies between the tumour and the integuments of the anterior part of the abdomen when the kidney is enlarged, which is not the case with the spleen; besides all which, the history will most likely connect the tumour with some such peculiarities in the urinary secretion as will seem greatly to guide our diagnosis.

Ovarian tumours assume, as I have formerly said, the greatest variety of shape; and the hard masses which form in the parietes often mislead us, for a moment, into a belief that some other organs are implicated, and, amongst these, not unusually the spleen; but a knowledge of this fact, and of the general diagnosis of ovarian tumours, will soon correct this error

Of hydatids I have already spoken; their elastic feel and rounded form will generally distinguish them from enlarged spleen, even when the situation they hold would seem to lead us to a wrong conclusion. They are, however, sometimes attached to the spleen itself.

With a view of illustrating the foregoing statement of the pathological changes to which the spleen is subject, I shall now proceed to select a few such cases as appear to me most appropriate; and I shall commence by the simplest form of congestion, as presented during an attack of intermittent fever.

CASE 1.—*Simple enlargement of the spleen, connected with intermittent fever.*—Ellen C—, æt. 20, was admitted into the clinical ward, under my care, January 25th, 1832; a single woman, of florid complexion: she had been living for some time in the neighbourhood of Gravesend, in a low, marshy district. About one month before her admission, having been out in the rain, she was suddenly seized with cold chills, headache, and general pains; soon followed by heat, and afterwards by perspiration. These paroxysms returned regularly every other day, leaving her entirely during the interval. For the last three days, however, they had recurred daily, at nine in the morning, every alternate day; and in the evening at five, on the intervening day. She had no local pain; but general uneasiness continued, tongue moist and slightly furred, pulse 120 small, bowels regular, appetite gone.

She was ordered to take a little diaphoretic mixture; and nothing else, till a paroxysm should be coming on, when she was to have an emetic of ipecacuanha and tartarized antimony.

27th.—Yesterday afternoon, the cold fit having come on with great violence, twenty grains of the emetic powder were given, which produced vomiting of a quantity of yellowish fluid, and instantly brought on the hot stage; a slight perspiration then followed, and she slept pretty well through the night. She complained principally of pain in the head, which has left her this morning; bowels abundantly opened; motions feculent and healthy; pulse 80, and soft; tongue rather dry and brown; skin warm. The catamenia have not appeared since August.

Habeat Quinæ Sulphat., gr. ij, alternis horis.

28th.—Slept well, and feels tolerably well. There is a hard tumour in the left side, descending lower than the level of the umbilicus, which is evidently to be traced beneath the ribs, and is the spleen, slightly tender on pressure (Fig. 41); bowels not open this morning; pulse 100; skin cool; tongue moister.

    Applicentur cucurbitulæ cruentæ lateri sinistro, et detrahatur sanguis ad uncias decem.
    Habeat Pulv. Rhei c. Cal., gr. xv, statim.
    Rep. Quinæ Sulph.

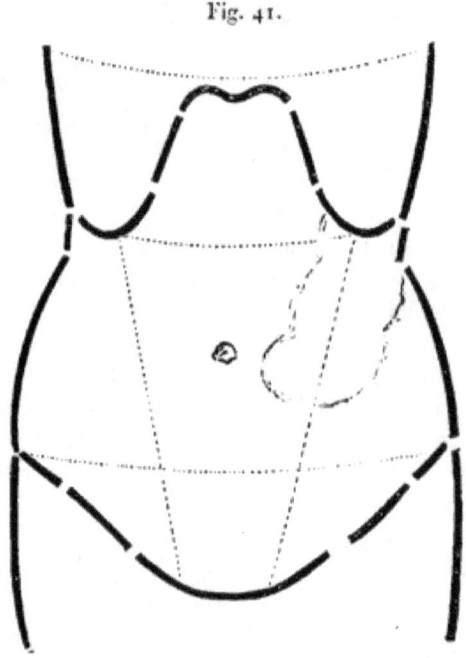

Fig. 41.

Figs. 41, 42, 43, present three diagrams, illustrating the gradual diminution of the spleen, in the case of Ellen C—, affected with intermittent fever. (Case 1.)

29th.—Slept but little during the night, from pain in the left hypochondrium; cupping gave relief, but the pain returned in the evening; no return of the paroxysm, and she is now perspiring profusely; bowels open; tongue dry and brownish; pulse 80, soft.

    Sumat Pulv. Rhei c. Cal., gr. xv, statim.
    Rep. Quinæ Sulph., gr. ij, ter die.

DISEASE OF THE SPLEEN. 161

30th.—No paroxysms; good night; the swelling is not so distinct, and there is no tenderness in the part; bowels freely open this morning; tongue moist.

> Applicentur cucurbitulæ cruentæ lateri sinistro, et detrahatur sanguis ad uncias decem.
> Rep. Quinæ Sulph. ut antea.

31st.—Good night; no paroxysm; spleen much softer, but nearly of same extent; no pain in the part; not above two ounces of blood could be obtained by cupping; pulse 64; skin cool; appetite improving; bowels open freely; tongue less dry.

Feb. 1st.—Tumour much softer and smaller (Fig. 42); tongue nearly clean.

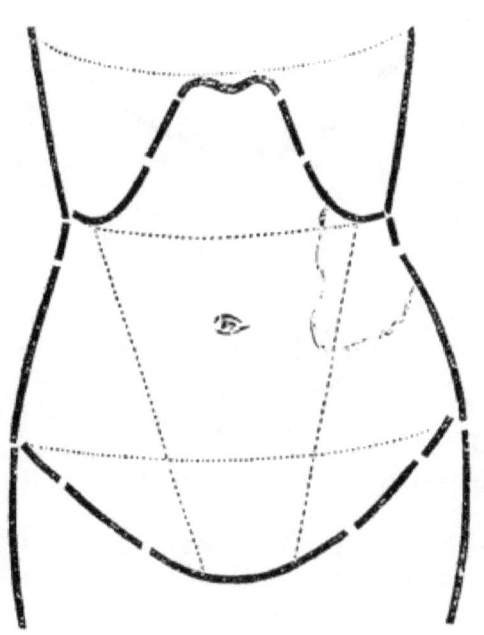

Fig. 42.

2d.—Improving daily; no return of paroxysm; swelling scarcely to be felt, and no pain in it. (Fig. 43.)

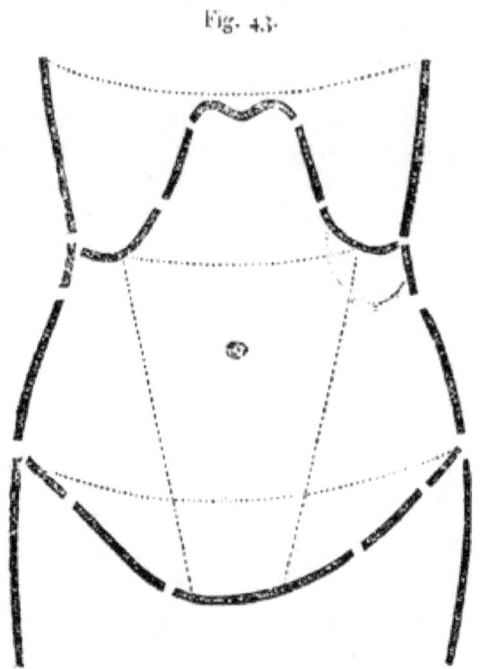

Fig. 43.

6th.—Tumour gone.

She remained a few days longer, on account of a slight diarrhœa; and left the hospital, cured.

In the following cases, the enlargement of the spleen has depended on congestion in the first place; but this has, in some instances, led to permanent change in the structure of the organ.

CASE 2.—*Enlarged spleen cured by tonics and purgatives.*— April 27th, 1835.—I was consulted by a gentleman of about 20 years of age, who had lately enjoyed good health, growing stout, and looking peculiarly ruddy. He was in the habit, whenever his bowels did not act for twenty-four hours, of taking a dose of colocynth and calomel, followed by a senna draught. On the 24th, he had first experienced a slight pain in his side, half way between the margin of the ribs and the crest of the ilium, and woke on the following morning with severe pain in that side, sickness, and bilious vomiting. There was no retraction of the testis, nor pain down the thigh; urine clear, but rather high coloured. On examining the abdomen, when standing erect, there was evidently a greater roundness on the upper part of the abdomen on the left side than on the right, and the ribs were somewhat forced out, giving an almost deformed appearance. Looking at the back, there was rather more hollow in the lumbar space than on the right. Laying him on his back, percussion yielded a dull sound below the ribs, in the usual situation of an enlarged spleen; but a very clear sound above, apparently in the situation of a portion of the stomach. Placing the hand on the left hypogastric region, a most distinct round tumour was felt just at the margin of the ribs; and placing the other hand on the lumbar space of the same side, a round tumour was also very perceptible; and when either hand was pressed, an impulse was given to the other by the motion of the tumour, which was evidently an oval mass, more or less long, egg-shaped, with its long diameter from before backward. When he was placed on the hands and knees, the tumour gravitated a little forward. There was slight tenderness, on pressure, on the back part of the tumour.

The exact nature of this tumour admitted fairly of some doubt. It might be the spleen, or the left lobe of the liver, the kidney, the renal capsules, or the colon. The tumour was rather more ovoid than the spleen usually is. It was not likely to be the liver, because it went so far back; and it could not be traced as having any connexion with the right lobe of the liver. The kidney would, by its enlargement, have produced a tumour extending, in all probability, further downwards; it would also have distended the left lumbar space—and perhaps have produced retraction of the testis, with pain down the thigh. The renal capsule has never, to my knowledge, been enlarged to such a size as this. A deposit of scrofulous matter under the tunic of the kidney, I have known to project more than this; but then it is more immovable. The colon might, by possibility, present a tumour like this. The left portion of the arch would occupy nearly this situation, if loaded with fæces; and the habitually costive state of the bowels would strengthen the suspicion.

The regular form of the tumour, and its general character, led me to express my full belief that it was the spleen; but I thought it right to give a fair trial to purgatives, and for this purpose ordered the compound scammony powder to be given, and followed by injections of infusion of senna and sulphate of magnesia. I also recommended frequent gentle friction on the tumour.

April 30th.—He has been very freely purged, but the tumour remains, and the bowels being emptied, the form of the spleen is more distinctly felt.

I ordered now twelve ounces of blood to be taken, by cupping, from the part, and, as soon as the wounds were healed, a large plaster of the Ammoniacum c. Hydrarg. to be applied, the compound scammony powder repeated occasionally, and two grains of sulphate of quinine to be taken twice a day.

May 10th.—The tumour somewhat softer. I desired him to go on as before, only using the combination of the compound extract of colocynth, the compound galbanum pill, and extract of hyoscyamus, instead of the scammony, as a purge.

June 15th.—He has continued the purging, the quinine, and the plaster; has had no return of pain, and feels generally better. The tumour is decidedly softer, and extends much less backwards into the lumbar region. It seems to have advanced a little towards the scrobiculus cordis. I desired him to persist carefully in the use of all his remedies.

July 3d.—I can no longer discover any tumour; and, on the most careful examination, is now to be perceived but a slight hardness under the angle formed by the ribs and spine, which is apparently the spleen. He has continued the quinine regularly, and has been obliged to increase the extract of colocynth. The weather having been very hot, he experienced great irritation from the Emplastrum Ammoniaci c. Hydrargyro, and has been obliged to leave it off for the last two days. I desired him to continue the treatment, but not to carry the purgatives to the extent of irritating his bowels, and, if necessary, to relinquish the plaster during the hot weather, resuming it as soon as he could.

May, 1836.—He called upon me to report that he had been perfectly well since he last saw me, a period of nine months.

Some months after, a relapse occurred in this case, but the same remedies again restored the spleen to its ordinary size; only, on this occasion, I had the cupping employed two or three times. This gentleman has since remained well.

I have at this time, under my occasional care, a case altogether analogous to the one just detailed, in as far as the very great and apparently sudden increase of the spleen is concerned, and its complete disappearance under the same plan of treatment; but in this case, unfortunately, the relapse which has occurred, has, for the present, bid defiance, not only to the same remedial means, but to the iodine and other powerful medicines. It was from this case that the diagrams in Figs. 44, 45, were taken; but they serve nearly as well to show the progressive decrease in the last case, except, that in that the tumour never descended so low towards the pelvis, but seemed more concentrated in the upper part, as if the spleen had enlarged rather in the hollow of the diaphragm, where it was possibly retained by some adhesions.

CASE 3.—*Enlarged spleen in a child.*—In December, 1837, I had occasion to examine a child aged two years and four months, who died, swollen to an enormous degree, with anasarca, and in whose abdomen was some serous effusion. This child had never flourished from its birth, and for the last year the spleen had been distinctly felt, occupying a large portion of the left side of the abdomen. Many petechial spots appeared on various parts of the body—whether the urine coagulated or not, I do not know. The spleen was found, as it had been felt during life, occupying the abdomen nearly to the pelvis, and extending almost to the mesial line. The liver was healthy; but all the glands of the mesentery were greatly enlarged, were hard, and of a red colour. The kidneys were remarkably hard and white.

I adduce this as an instance of the great size to which the spleen attains, during infancy. The case is a comparatively common one, and more marked cases, in younger subjects, will occur to my readers.

CASE 4.—*Remarkable distension of the spleen without disorganization. Death from the effects of diseased liver.*—George T—, æt. 23, a tailor, was in Cornelius Ward, in the autumn of 1832, under the care of Dr. Back. I saw him a few days after his admission, and was struck with his prominent abdomen, and the dark dingy tinge of icterus with which he was suffused. I found that the upper part of the abdomen about the umbilicus gave a most distinct hollow sound, on percussion, as he lay upon his back. In the lower parts, about the sides and over the pubes, fluctuation was equally evident. The veins of both sides of the abdomen were much enlarged; but this was most seen upon the left. There was an irregular tumour to be felt, descending from beneath the ribs on the left side nearly into the pelvis, and reaching, anteriorly, almost to the umbilicus. This I conceived to be the spleen; and a layer of fluid was spread between it and the integuments. At the same time, the liver was but very indistinctly to be felt, but what appeared to be the left lobe was just perceptible through the fluid. His tongue was furred, and of an ash colour; his stools light; urine deeply tinged with bile, and of a red tint; lips purple.

It appeared, from the history he gave, that about four years before, while sitting on his board, he had been greatly alarmed, and fell on the ground in a kind of fit; but though the blow was severe, he seemed to have derived no permanent ill from it; but a few months afterwards he found his clothes getting tight about his stomach, and this has continued ever since. About two years before his admission, he was in St. Thomas's Hospital, with slight jaundice, which had continued, occasionally, up to the time when I first saw him; but for the last month, his abdomen had been getting much larger. By the marks of cupping-glasses, it appeared as if the chief pain he experienced, at his first attack, had been in the region of the spleen, rather than the liver, as all the scars were on that side. Very little alteration took place in his condition, but the splenic tumour varied in size, as shown by some diagrams I made. His abdomen grew more distended, and his colour became more dark and dingy, assuming a green tint. About the 10th of January he expectorated a good deal of blood, which continued several days; petechial spots appeared on his shoulders and arms; and his legs became very painful, from the anasarceous distension; at length he died, on the 20th of January, 1833.

Sectio cadaveris, January 21st, 1833.—The body of a dingy light-green colour; the abdomen greatly distended, but flaccid, and the tumour on the right side was not to be felt.

The cavity of the thorax much encroached on by the fluid of the abdomen, which now pushed up the diaphragm, leaving the abdomen flaccid. The left lung adhered to the pleura, but was healthy, as was the right. The heart I did not see examined; it looked rather large, and was slightly tinged with bile.

On opening the abdomen, the small intestines were found only moderately distended, floating on the surface in the central part, and the colon some way above the umbilicus, with the omentum discoloured and rather puckered up. The liver lay quite in the hollow of the diaphragm, pushed upwards, and now presenting its edge only. It was small, contracted, hard, and lobulated, in a most extreme degree; the projections of the lobules of a dark olive-green colour; the rest of a silvery-white gray tint, owing to the thickened and diseased state of the peritoneum. On cutting into the liver, it was evident that the cause of its lobulated and misshapen form was the contraction of the cellular tissue. It cut almost as hard as gristle, and the bands of cellular substance appeared running through it, drawing the glandular texture up into nodules. Its colour was a deep olive-green throughout; a good deal of blood issued from the vessels in the substance of the liver when it was cut into, and many of the moderately sized biliary tubes contained bile of a thick consistence and rather mucous character.

The gall-bladder looked clear, as if filled with colourless fluid, or too opaque to show colour; it was distended, containing about three or four ounces of mucous fluid, and it was doubled over upon its duct, forming a kind of valve. The hepatic, cystic, and common ducts, were all much dilated, the cause of their obstruction being apparently several dark-coloured, hard, enlarged glands about Glisson's capsule.

The spleen was very large, and was plainly the viscus I had felt during life, but now it was flaccid, and evidently ungorged; besides which, the diaphragm being pushed upwards, it had subsided very much, falling back into the lumbar space, and hardly descending there below the level of the umbilicus. The weight of the spleen was three pounds ten ounces, and its structure was nearly natural.

The pancreas was hard, and appeared to have suffered the same contraction of the interstitial cellular tissue that had affected the liver, so that each little lobule seemed distinct and hard. The kidneys healthy; the colon tinged externally by bile, and the small intestines a little. A large quantity of very clear bilious serum in the cavity of the abdomen.

It is doubtful whether the accident, on which this patient laid much stress in his history, had any connexion with his subsequent illness; it is more probable that the whole depended on intemperate habits, which led to chronic inflammation of the liver and ascites. The important fact, as connected with our present inquiry, is the unusual size of the spleen, weighing, in its contracted state, no less than three pounds ten ounces, and still retaining somewhat of its healthy structure, which appears the more extraordinary, when we take into account the long continuance of the chronic hepatic disease. That the organ was capable of distending and contracting, appeared from the varying size denoted by the diagrams I made, which corresponded almost entirely with the two diagrams in Figs. 44, 45, of this communication. The occurrence of petechiæ might lead us to suppose that the spleen had been influential in the symptoms attending the fatal termination; but it is more probable that this was merely a manifestation of that general hæmorrhagic tendency, so conspicuously marked in many cases of long-continued jaundice.

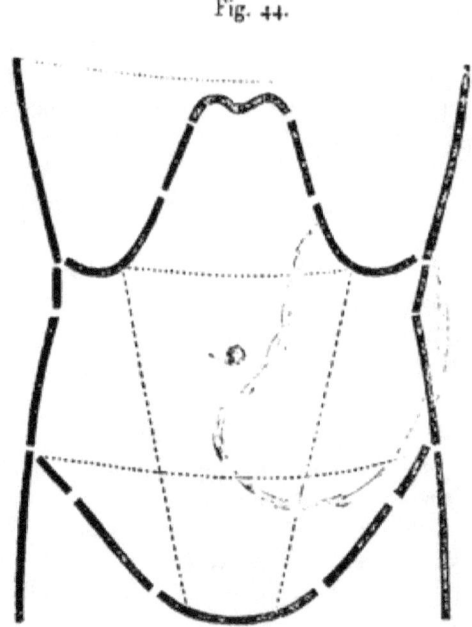

Fig. 44.

Figs. 44 and 45 represent two successive stages of the abdominal tumour in a patient labouring under congestion of the spleen. (Cases 2 and 3.)

Fig. 45.

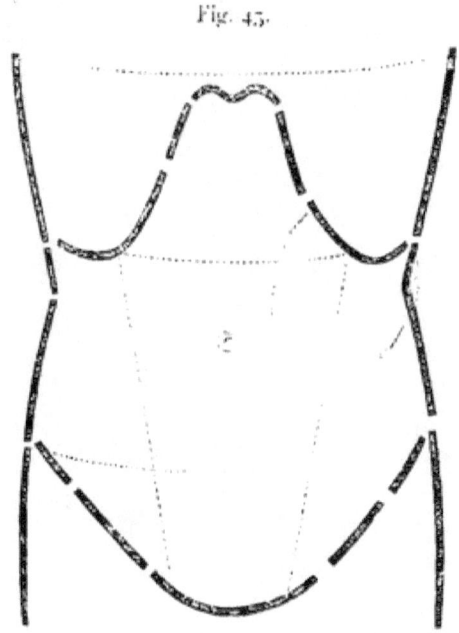

CASE 5.—*Enlarged spleen, occurring in a case of fatal diarrhœa.*—Mary S——, æt. 42, was admitted into Guy's Hospital, under my care, November 24th, 1830, affected with a severe dysenteric diarrhœa, of several weeks' standing. Her complexion was remarkably sallow, her lips pallid, and her eyes glassy, but there was not the slightest tendency to jaundice. The abdomen, as she stood, appeared greatly enlarged; and when in a recumbent posture, there was no difficulty in ascertaining immediately the source of the enlargement, which was evidently the spleen, enormously increased in bulk; it occupied the whole of the left side of the abdomen, and its margin was distinctly to be traced, lobulated in two or three parts, and extending from under the margin of the ribs, inclining rather forwards, so as to advance to the umbilicus, and descend quite into the pelvis. (Fig. 46.) She informed us that she had been subject to a weak state of health for several years, her complexion frequently becoming sallow. She had borne five children; the last was eighteen months ago, the labour being quite easy and natural. Eight weeks before, she was first sensible of the tumour in the

abdomen, which, however, was at that time so large that she thought it had increased very little since. She complained of some pain in the left side, when she lay on the right, and the tumour was frequently tender in some parts.

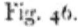

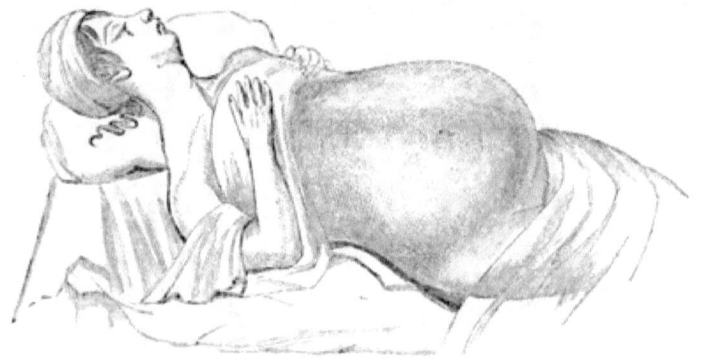

Fig. 46. The abdominal tumour produced by an enlarged spleen. (Case 5.)

I applied blisters over the tumour, and afterwards the Emplastrum Ammoniaci c. Hydrargyro; and under these applications the tumour certainly appeared to diminish; but the condition of the bowels was that to which attention was chiefly directed, for she was constantly subject to diarrhœa and dysenteric symptoms; she had likewise pain running down the left leg, from which she often suffered much.

A variety of remedies were administered; but from none did she receive so much decided relief as from the employment of opiate suppositories and injections, with the occasional use of a combination of tincture of opium and linseed-oil; but the relief was only temporary, and she constantly lost ground.

In the month of March, I began to perceive that effusion was taking place into the abdomen; the fluid was evidently perceptible between the integuments and the surface of the spleen, and in the beginning of May she died.

I greatly regret that I have lost the notes of the dissection in this case; but the enormous size of the spleen, which had acquired a fleshy consistence, was the most remarkable circumstance, together with the ulcerated condition of the intestines, which appeared to be the chief, if not the sole cause of death.

There can be no doubt that a tumour of this unusual size in the abdomen must have aggravated greatly the disease of the intestines, and may have been early a cause of that want of repairing power which prevented the healing of the ulcers in the mucous membrane of the bowels; it might likewise, in a great degree, have contributed to that embarrassment in the circulation which induced ascites, as the general powers of life sunk under continued disease. It is remarkable, in this, and in many other cases, that the enlargement of the spleen seems to make a rapid progress at first; and then to become stationary, seldom increasing by a continuous and progressive growth; but I believe the fact to be, that the organ becomes rather suddenly over-distended; and then, being very little sensible of pain under distension, it is not till some casual circumstance leads to the discovery of the tumour that the fact is detected; and then, probably, the distension has already continued so long, that remedies are incapable of acting, in any considerable degree, to expel the blood; and thus the enlargement becomes permanent and stationary, because it is not so much from the result of morbid growth, as from consolidated natural tissue.

CASE 6.—*Enlarged and fleshy spleen, with chronic disease of the liver.*—Richard D—, æt. 39, was admitted into the hospital, May 12th, 1824, affected with an enlargement of the spleen very obvious to the touch, and ascites; and the veins of the abdomen were much enlarged. He had been all his life a sailor, and much exposed in different climates. He was treated by mercurials and squills, with diuretics, and afterwards by tonics.

He gradually improved; and was so well, that he was about to be presented, when, on exposure to cold, he was affected with peritonitis, and died on the 12th of October.

Sectio cadaveris.—The skin was jaundiced. The peritoneal coat of the intestines was inflamed; there were several pints of fluid in the abdomen. The intestines were covered with a coating of recent coagulable lymph, in shreds. The liver deeply lobulated and puckered; and in some parts presenting an appearance of tuberculation, with vessels ramifying upon it.

The spleen was more than six times its natural size, fleshy and firm, with a cartilaginous patch upon one end.

The omentum, the mesentery, and the mesocolon, were loaded with fat; and besides that, there was a mass, apparently of fat, but almost as firm as cartilage, on the vertebræ, near the brim of the pelvis, to the left side; which appeared to account, in some degree, for the swelling which had latterly taken place in the left leg.

CASE 7.—*Enlarged and fleshy spleen, with chronic disease in the abdomen, mottled kidneys, and albuminous urine.*—In July, 1837, I was requested by Mr. Meryon to see with him, in consultation, a gentleman labouring under ascites and general anasarca. His countenance was slightly suffused with bile, his skin dry, and his urine highly albuminous, and considerably loaded with lateritious sediment. There was no difficulty in pronouncing that the kidneys were diseased, and that the abdominal viscera were greatly implicated. The effusion into the abdomen was too great to allow us to feel any particular viscus. The symptoms had now existed for nearly four months without alleviation, so that we had no expectation of prolonging life many weeks. They, however, underwent various changes; the fluid in the extremities, and at one time the ascites, greatly diminishing; and at another time he was so well, as to get out in a carriage for a few days; but eventually, the ascites increased greatly, and was the chief source of our anxiety; plainly showing, although the urine continued coagulable, that we had other mischief than that connected with the kidney to contend with. He survived to the end of December.

Sectio cadaveris.—A considerable quantity of fluid in the abdominal cavity. Old and very strong adhesions of the peritoneum of the liver to the parietes. The substance of the liver was soft and sodden, but not disorganized. The intestines opaque and thickened. The spleen was full eight times its natural size, and nearly as hard as cartilage. On being squeezed, when cut through, scarcely a drop of blood escaped from it. The kidneys were white, where they were not stained by the decomposition of the abdominal fluid. They were mottled, very decidedly, but by no means in an advanced state of that disease. The lungs and the heart were healthy; there was some effusion into the cavities of the chest.

In cases of chronic disease, particularly of the liver, it is much more usual to find the spleen, if enlarged, in the hard, fleshy, and consolidated state which occurred in the last three cases, than in the almost natural condition in which it was found in the preceding one; but the fact, that sometimes the spleen is to all appearance healthy, when the liver is distinctly indurated and altered throughout its substance—and that occasionally, though enlarged, the structure of the spleen seems natural—and that the most hardened spleens, as in the last case, sometimes accompany livers but little disorganized, proves that there is something more required than the deranging of the liver, to produce this change in the spleen. I may mention, that of the enlarged and indurated condition of the spleen co-existing with a hard, contracted and lobulated liver, we have some very marked specimens preserved in our museum; and it is to be presumed that the change in both bespeaks a state of chronic inflammation.

There is another point, connected with the last case, which deserves remark; and that is, the combination of so much abdominal mischief with albuminous urine; and it is right to mention, that I have known a few cases, besides this, in which enlarged spleen has existed in the same combination, in which the kidneys, though decidedly mottled or granulated, have shown less altered structure than the severity and circumstance of the disease had led me to expect. In such cases, it is possible that the derangement of the spleen is sometimes an accidental coincidence; and sometimes one result, in common with many others, which assists in bringing such cases to a fatal issue. In a great number of cases of albuminous urine, the spleen has been observed in a perfectly healthy condition; and of the 100 dissections detailed in one of the volumes of 'Guy's Hospital Reports,' in 64 of which the state of the spleen is noted, 27 are said to be healthy; and the 37 which deviate from perfect health have no uniform defect, 6 being small, 8 soft, 10 large and more or less fleshy and hard, and 2 small and hard; 1 is mentioned as lacerable, 1 granulated, and 1 tuberculated; and the remaining 8 in variable degrees of softness or hardness, sufficient to attract a casual remark. It is probable that the remaining 36 of the 100 cases presented at least no very remarkable disease in the structure of the spleen, or the fact would have been stated.

Case 8.—*Abscess of the spleen opening into the colon.*—Ann C—, æt. 25, was admitted into the Clinical Ward, November 10th, 1825.

She was a young woman, much emaciated, of peculiarly sallow complexion, and anxious countenance. She complained of general uneasiness and pain in the abdomen, more particularly the scrobiculus cordis and right hypochondrium, at which part there was an evident fulness; pressure, and all ingesta, increased the pain and uneasiness of the stomach, which were relieved by vomiting. The food was often vomited immediately after it was taken; at other times it remained some time before it was rejected. There was also, occasional vomiting of a bilious fluid, and a constant loathing of food. Pulse 120, small and weak; tongue glossy and dry; skin hard and dry; thirst, headache, occasional heats and chills; some pain in the loins; and the catamenia had not appeared for seven months. There had sometimes been œdema of the lower extremities, particularly after exercise, but there was none at the time of her admission. Bowels sometimes costive; at other times, relaxed; and, although much stress was laid upon the diarrhœa, yet, shortly after her admission, we saw some dejections which had a very healthy character. It appeared, from her account, that she vomited blood, to the extent of about a pint, on one occasion, three years ago, but had no return of this since; and her present complaint came on with pain at her stomach, and vomiting, which she dated to the time her catamenia disappeared. I ordered egg, wine, and milk and lime-water for drink, in small quantities, frequently.

    Habeat Ext. Gentian., gr. ij;
    Sodæ subcarb., gr. ij;
    Opii, gr. ½; ter die.

The first two nights after her admission she had paroxysms of shivering, followed by perspirations, almost like fits of ague. Her motions were frequently thin, watery, and very offensive; but she was able to retain a little more food; and nothing was more agreeable to her stomach than an egg beat up with wine.

November 17th.—Feels much exhausted, and has had scarcely any sleep. Pulse not perceptible at the left wrist, and scarcely so at the right; great pain in the left hand; it has a bluish appearance, and is not sensible when touched. The warm poultice which has been applied to the abdomen has given her relief. She vomited once in the night, after taking a powder of the Hydrarg. c. Cretâ. Motions relaxed, and green. She has seemed to relish some soda-water with a little brandy. The affection of the left hand increased; it became livid, and extended above the wrist; then the fingers became black and gangrenous; and, gradually sinking, she died on the evening of the 21st.

Sectio cadaveris.—Lungs and heart sound and healthy. The liver was much enlarged, particularly the left lobe; which, with the spleen, formed an arch, which embraced and pressed upon the cardiac extremity of the stomach. The substance of the liver was hard and granulated, and exsanguine. The right lobe had contracted slight adhesions to the diaphragm. The spleen was enlarged, and firmly adherent to the transverse arch of the colon. There was an abscess in the spleen, involving about half of its substance. On the left side of the abscess, adhesive matter had been thrown out, so as to form a complete partition between the healthy and diseased portions. The abscess, from the adhesions of the colon to the spleen, had ulcerated through the coats of that intestine, and formed a communication with its interior. The contents of the abscess had a grumous chocolate appearance; the spleen had formed adhesion to the diaphragm; and at this part the parietes of the abscess were considerably thinner. There was an abscess in the left ovary, and the cavity of the uterus was irregular in its surface.

It is quite obvious, that, in this case, there was nothing to direct us to a certain diagnosis; and the following short extract, from a few clinical observations which I read to the class the day after I admitted this patient, will show what were my views upon that subject, and serve as a pretty just statement of the extent to which we can fairly venture a diagnosis in cases of such unusual and complicated disease:

"This is a case in which the nature of the disease is not altogether obvious to me. That something is producing the greatest irritability of stomach, is quite evident. The constant vomiting, which for several months past has never been absent for above two days at a time, and the uneasiness she experiences after taking food, until it is rejected, lead very strongly to the belief that the stomach is the seat of organic change; on the other hand, her age, which is but twenty-five years, is much below that at which scirrhous disease of the stomach usually comes on. The character of the vomiting, which is frequently decidedly bilious, is not that which generally attends scirrhous pylorus; in which disease, the matters ejected are often colourless in the early stages; and grumous, or coffee-coloured, in the last stages. Then again, the fulness over the region of the stomach and liver is greater, and more extensive, than is usual in scirrhous pylorus, unless the substance of the stomach be itself involved in the disease. At all events, her countenance denotes plainly visceral organic disease; and her emaciated and weakened frame forbid any but the mildest remedies, or the most gentle administration of the more powerful ones. Speaking to you, as I do, in doubt respecting this case, I could wish each of you to weigh the arguments on both sides. The disease may be in the stomach, or it may be external to it. It may be in the liver; or it may be in the omentum, and the peritoneal covering of the stomach and intestines. It is not unlikely that some extensive and complicated disease of these parts will be found after death."

In the following case, the same great difficulty of going beyond a conjectural diagnosis will be recognised; still, the symptoms are such as connect themselves in a most interesting manner with the appearances after death, and seem to offer much encouragement to our researches into the distinctive marks of disease.

CASE 9.—*Sloughing abscess of the spleen.*—Ann H—, æt. 21, was admitted under my care, January 24th, 1829, into Dorcas Ward. She was a housemaid; and was in a most reduced condition, having been ill for some weeks; during which she had been very actively treated by copious and repeated bleedings, for what had been considered an attack of carditis, coming on immediately after having undergone excessive fatigue by walking upwards of twenty miles.

Her chief symptoms after admission were, great depression, a rapid weak pulsation of the heart, and frequent vomiting; under which she sunk in about ten days, her legs having become œdematous.

Sectio cadaveris.—The body not greatly emaciated; the right leg and thigh very œdematous; superficial veins large, and turgid.

Pleuræ and lungs generally healthy, but exsanguine; some slight adhesion, and some more recent, from the diaphragm to the base of the left lung. The pericardium contained some ounces of straw-coloured serum, with tender films. The heart quite healthy; the blood partially coagulated, deficient in red particles.

In the abdomen, there were some cellular adhesions, of long

standing, between the liver and the diaphragm, and between the liver and the stomach; on the left side were more recent adhesions in the neighbourhood of the spleen, circumscribing a cavity bounded above by the under surface of the left lobe of the liver, to the inner side by the stomach, and to the outer side by the spleen. This cavity contained an offensive dark-coloured matter, with a strong gangrenous odour; which was produced by the breaking down of a portion of the spleen, extending to no great depth into the organ, the remainder of which was firmer than natural, and of a red colour. There was a small circular aperture in the cardiac extremity of the stomach; but a portion of lymph prevented the gangrenous matter from entering. The alimentary canal healthy, but much contracted in many parts. Liver very exsanguine; healthy, except where a part assisted to form the parietes of the gangrenous cavity, and here it was covered with a thick, loose, false membrane. Kidneys and uterus healthy.

The common iliac veins, and the femoral, so far as traced, were filled with firm coagula, almost entirely of a yellowish-white colour, with some puriform fluid. Similar coagula, but accompanied by a larger proportion of puriform fluid, filled the inferior cava to within a short distance of that part where it receives the blood from the liver. As it approached this part, the coagula became considerably contracted; and above this part there was no coagulum.

The lumbar absorbent glands were somewhat enlarged, and of a light-red colour.

In these two cases, we perceive a coincidence in the depressing influence exerted on the circulating, and perhaps more particularly the venous system, as shown by the condition of the extremities in both; but as both patients were in a very exhausted state, we are not allowed to lay too much stress upon this fact, though I shall presently have occasion to mention a third corresponding case.

CASE 10.—*Jaundice from general enlargement of the liver.— Spleen greatly enlarged, and studded with small hard opaque bodies. The glandular and absorbent system much diseased.*—Joseph P— was admitted into Guy's Hospital, under my care, December 20th, 1830. His chief complaint was, the enlargement of his abdomen, which was very considerable. A hard tumour occupied all the upper part of the abdomen; and its edge might be traced distinctly almost into the pelvis. His countenance was a little sallow, and his eyes slightly tinged with bile. He had a troublesome cough, particularly at night, which sometimes went on to produce sickness. It appeared, that three years before he had been first attacked with pain about two inches below the false ribs, on the right side; and since that time had never been perfectly well, though able to pursue his occupation as a shoemaker, for some time. About eighteen months afterwards he went into the country; and it was then that he first perceived his abdomen to enlarge. He suffered no pain; but it increased so much, that seven months ago he was obliged to give up his work, and, in September, 1830, he went into the Marylebone Infirmary; where he was under the care of Dr. Hooper for eleven weeks, and left that institution a week only before his admission into Guy's.

The remedies which I prescribed, during the time he was under my care, were light bitters, with taraxacum, and small doses of blue pill from time to time; in addition to which, I applied the Emplastrum Ammoniaci cum Hydrargyro to the tumour, and afterwards rubbed in the liniment of tartar emetic. Many little changes took place; the urine was occasionally more or less tinged with bile; the stools were sometimes of a drab colour; his cough often required palliative remedies; and the middle of February he experienced frequent epistaxis. His jaundice never exceeded the slightest yellow tinge; and he continued to walk about the ward, when, in the end of February, he left the hospital on account of some domestic losses. I saw nothing of him till June, when he was admitted into Guy's, under Dr. Back. He was now most dreadfully emaciated; the jaundice was much increased; and all along under his jaw was a row of enlarged glands of the size of small plums of an oval form, and only of moderately hard consistence. His cough was very frequent, and he was completely confined to his bed. Serous effusion had taken place into the peritoneal cavity; which, while it rendered the abdomen larger, prevented us from feeling the tumour quite so distinctly as before. His cough was very troublesome; his tongue was red and glossy; his appetite bad, and his bowels relaxed. He had frequent vomiting of frothy bilious matter; and on the 21st of July he sank.

Sectio cadaveris.—The body was decidedly jaundiced, of a dingy yellow colour, and greatly emaciated. The right lung was hepatized, partly from old and partly from more recent inflammation. The liver was greatly enlarged, weighing above eleven pounds. It was flat and smooth on its surface, of an olive-brown colour; and, when cut into, showed a general disease of the acini, which had a tendency to form clusters and masses, resembling, when divided, the cut ends of bundles of muscular fibres. The gall-bladder contained about an ounce of watery mucus, slightly tinged with bile. The kidneys were large; the spleen was at least six times the natural size, rather solid, and pretty thickly studded with very small, light bodies, apparently thickened portions of cellular membrane. The whole of the lumbar glands were greatly enlarged, of a fleshy consistence, and homogeneous in their structure; with nothing of the fungoid structure, and nothing of the scrofulous appearance. Some of them were red, with ecchymosis in their structure; but the greater part were of a flesh colour, with a yellow tinge. The thoracic duct was very large; and was filled with blood, forming a dark, soft coagulum.

The consolidated and granular condition of the spleen which occurred in this case, is, I believe, the result of chronic inflammation; but sometimes an appearance not unlike this is produced by the early deposit of miliary tubercles.

CASE II.—*Spleen reduced nearly to a fluid state, connected with extensive disease of the absorbent glands.*—A woman was admitted into Martha's Ward, under the surgeon, May 17th, 1825, having been long subject to glandular swelling of the neck, and a chronic enlargement of the left mamma. She died after being in the house some time, from erysipelas attacking the neck and the neighbouring parts.

Sectio cadaveris.—The glands of the neck and axillæ, and a set of glands occupying the situation of the thymus gland under the sternum were greatly enlarged, as also the glands accompanying the trachea and bronchi, which formed almost a solid mass; the thyroid gland was hard.

The pleura had evidently been subject to recent inflammatory action; much serum had been effused; and the lungs were covered over, and their lobes stuck together by a thin coating of lymph, but there was not the least tubercular tendency in any part of the lungs or pleura. About two ounces and a half of clear but high-coloured serum in the pericardium.

The abdomen presented considerable evidence of recent inflammation. Vascularity, turbid serum, and shreds of lymph adhering to the peritoneum. The kidneys very remarkable for size, quite healthy in structure. Liver very large, and pale-coloured; it descended below the umbilicus; gall-bladder large. The spleen was twice its natural size; the moment its tunic was broken into the light-coloured grumous contents flowed out, almost like a creamy fluid. Pancreas healthy; mesenteric glands, many of them, enlarged, and of dark colour.

The peculiarly soft condition of the spleen, which presented itself in this case, is by no means unfrequent in a less degree, in acute diseases; it has been particularly remarked as occurring in fevers. In the present case, it was probably to be ascribed to some extension of the inflammatory action which had been lighted up so generally in both cavities of the body, and which was more particularly determined to the spleen from the pre-existing condition of the absorbent glands.

CASE 12.—*Tuberculated spleen, in a case where the tubercular diathesis greatly affected the glands.*—John S—, æt. fifteen months, was affected with the cough, dyspnœa, and quick pulse, which usually accompany protracted inflammatory disease of the lungs in children. He was of an unhealthy aspect, with purple suffusion of the countenance, but not greatly emaciated, even shortly before death.

Sectio cadaveris.—The lungs studded with cheesy tubercles. The bronchial glands were very much enlarged; one at the bifurcation of the bronchi was as large as a pigeon's egg, of a cheesy matter throughout; one higher up, of nearly equal size, was converted into yellow cheesy matter throughout half its extent. Tubercles were discovered in the peritoneum of the liver, and on the lower surface of the diaphragm towards the left side. The spleen was closely covered with omentum, which adhered to it. The spleen itself was tuberculated throughout. The mucous membrane of the intestines presented many small ulcers, resulting from tubercular deposits. The mesenteric glands were greatly enlarged.

CASE 13.—*Tubercles in the spleen, in a case of phthisis, where the glands were greatly affected.*—Patrick H—, æt. 30, was admitted into Guy's Hospital, under my care, June 13th, 1827, in a perfectly hopeless state of phthisis. He was pale and greatly emaciated; he had a troublesome cough, with expectoration and diarrhœa; and the absorbent glands of the neck formed soft and large tumours. He died on the 20th of the same month.

Sectio cadaveris.—Much of the structure of both lungs was still crepitant, but thickly sprinkled with miliary tubercles; other portions were more consolidated, and also sprinkled with miliary tubercles. The peritoneum had, in various parts, formed strong and extensive adhesions. The adventitious matter forming the union was thickly sprinkled with collections of yellow scrofulous matter, most numerous where the adhesive matter was the thickest; but small tubercles were scattered on the peritoneal coat of the intestines, where no adhesion existed. There were some ulcerated tubercles on the mucous membrane of the intestines. The mesenteric glands were much enlarged, and going into a state of suppuration in their centres. The thoracic duct healthy, but small; the liver tolerably healthy, and the bile quite so. The spleen was enlarged to four times its natural size, and indurated; there were a few small yellow tubercles in its substance. Kidneys healthy. The glands of the neck in a state of suppuration at their centres.

CASE 14.—*Tubercles in the spleen, in a case of phthisis, where the glands were greatly affected.*—July, 1826.—A native of Owyhee was admitted into Guy's Hospital with a large mass of suppurating glands in the right axilla, and symptoms of phthisis. He survived but a few days, when the absorbent glands of the axilla were found the seat of most extensive suppuration, which passed under the pectoral muscle to the clavicle. The lungs were sprinkled with miliary tubercles, and the upper lobe of the right lung was in a more advanced stage of disease.

The stomach and intestines tolerably healthy; the liver had one small tubercle on its surface; but on the spleen there were many, and several in the substance of that organ.

The mesenteric glands were much enlarged, forming masses the size of large walnuts, which, when cut into, were found to consist chiefly of soft tuberculous matter. The thoracic duct quite healthy.

CASE 15.—*Tubercles in the spleen, lungs, and liver.*—A black man, admitted under the care of Dr. Cholmely, died with all the usual symptoms of phthisis.

Sectio cadaveris.—The lungs were greatly diseased, particularly at their upper parts. Small tubercles were observed on the surface of the liver, as well as diffused throughout its substance.

The spleen was studded with rounded tubercles; most of which were softened in their centres, so as to leave little irregular cavities when a section was made. (See Fig. 47.)

Fig. 47.

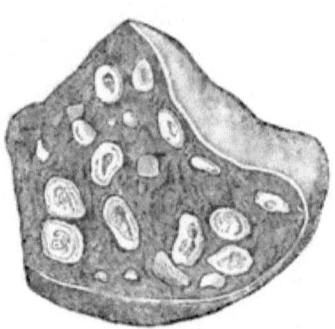

Fig. 47. A portion of the section of a spleen studded with softening tubercles, in a case of general tubercular diathesis. (Case 15.)

It is worthy of remark, that in three out of the only four cases of which I find the notes, where well-marked tubercles have appeared in the spleen of phthisical patients, the glandular system has been more than usually affected, in proportion to the disease of the lungs. In the fourth case the state of the glands is not mentioned.

CASE 16.—*Suppurating tubercles in the spleen, in a case of fever, with ulceration of the mucous membrane of the intestines.*—Jane M——, æt. 18, was admitted into Guy's Hospital, December 3d, 1823, labouring under symptoms of fever, with severe bowel irritation and abdominal tenderness. She lay with her legs drawn up to avoid pain, and was slightly delirious.

It appeared that a fortnight before she had been attacked with cold chills, succeeded by heat, severe headache, pain in the limbs, pain in the right hypochondrium, and sickness. She had been twice bled, and had had a blister applied to her abdomen. The symptoms continued very severe, both as regarded the abdominal tenderness and the tendency to diarrhœa, and as regarded the unsteady and disturbed condition of the sensorium; and although, at one time, there appeared to be, for a short time, a decided amendment, yet erysipelas coming on upon the neck, she sank on the 17th of December.

Sectio cadaveris.—Surface of the dura mater and pia mater very moist, from serous effusion; a small quantity of effused serum in the ventricles; substance of brain, firm; when sliced, exhibiting very florid bloody points. Extensive, but old adhesions of the pleura on the right side, and the same on the left, only to less extent; lungs collapsed, but not disorganized, the blood they contained very florid. The liver pallid, and extremely firm and hard in its texture, containing but little blood, which was florid.

The spleen contained two scrofulous-looking tubercles; one in a state of suppuration, and only prevented from opening into the abdomen by adhesion which it had formed to the omentum; the other was in a state of softening, not having gone to suppuration.

The general surface of the peritoneum and intestines healthy, only here and there exhibiting a florid appearance, and in some parts a green livid hue. The mucous membrane of the lower part of the ileum was in a high state of vascularity, and beset with ulcers of different sizes, which extended to the valve of the colon. Green, feculent matter in different parts of the bowels. The jejunum and upper portion of the ileum perfectly healthy.

CASE 17.—*Tuberculated spleen in a case of fever.*—In the year ——, a young man died in Guy's Hospital with symptoms of fever. He had no appearance of tubercular disease about him; but, on examining his body, the spleen was found much enlarged, and studded with tubercular bodies, each composed of two or three deposits, so as to give the appearance of occupying several cells of the spleen; they were solid, and not undergoing any process of softening. Of this I made a section, and procured a drawing, a part of which is represented in Fig. 48.

It is somewhat remarkable that both these last were cases of fever, and were unaccompanied by symptoms of phthisis.

Fig. 48.

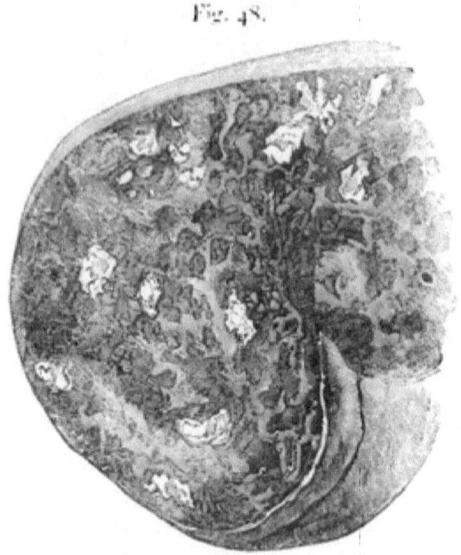

Fig. 48. A portion of the section of an enlarged spleen, studded with tubercles, in a case of fever, without other evidence of the tubercular diathesis. (Case 17.)

The four following cases show the spleen attacked by *malignant disease*. The first two are instances of a somewhat peculiar form of that malady, to which I referred in a former part of this paper, and they are certainly very interesting, as forming a part of the series of splenic diseases. The next is a case of the scirrhous form of malignant disease, developing itself precisely in the same manner in the spleen as it so often does in the liver. The fourth is a case of the cerebriform cancer, showing that the spleen, like the other organs of the body, occasionally becomes the seat of its destructive growth. Of the hæmatoid fungus I do not remember to have met with an instance in the spleen, but I see no reason to doubt its occurrence; and that melanosis pervades this organ occasionally, we have a proof in the very interesting case published, in 1826, by Mr. Fawdington, of Manchester, as likewise in the preparation at Fort Pitt, to which I have already alluded.

CASE 18.—*Spleen pervaded by malignant matter. The absorbent glands very extensively affected.*—Ellenborough K—, æt. 10, was admitted, under my care, into Guy's Hospital, in 1828, the youngest of six children, the rest all reported healthy. He likewise had been considered healthy till thirteen months ago, when his strength, flesh, and healthy appearance began to fail. A tumour was observed in the left hypochondrium, in the situation of the spleen; the glandulæ concatenatæ on the right side were observed to be enlarged; but, by the treatment then employed, the tumours in the neck, and also the spleen, were, at times, considerably reduced. It does not appear that he was ever subject to hæmorrhage; nor, till very lately, to dropsical effusion. His appetite generally good.

After his admission, the tumour on the left side was observed to extend considerably below the left hypochondrium, but was reported to be less than formerly. The glands on the left side of the neck were swollen, as well as those on the right. The abdomen was somewhat distended, and the scrotum œdematous. His complexion was pale and wax-like. He survived several weeks, but no efforts could sustain his powers.

Sectio cadaveris.—The head was not opened. The glands of the neck had assumed the form of smooth ovoid masses, connected together by loose cellular membrane. When cut into, they were formed of almost a cartilaginous consistence, of light colour, slightly vascular, but with no appearance of softening or suppuration. Glands, similarly affected, accompanied the vessels into the chest; where the bronchial and mediastinal glands were in the same state, and greatly enlarged; some old pleuritic adhesions; lungs generally healthy; pericardium and heart healthy, but a slight serous effusion into the pericardium. In the peritoneum, considerable quantity of clear, straw-coloured serum. Mucous membrane of stomach, and intestines healthy. The mesenteric glands slightly enlarged throughout, and but slightly indurated, but those accompanying the splenic artery, the aorta, and the iliacs, were in the same state as the glands of the neck. The liver contained no tubercles, and its structure quite healthy. The pancreas rather firm, and the glands along its upper side enlarged.

The spleen was enlarged to at least four times its natural size; its surface was mammillated, and its structure altered throughout. When a section was made, at least three fourths was seen to consist of white, opaque matter, almost like tallow, pervading every part, and assuming irregular ovoid and spherical masses, very much as if tallow in a melted state had been injected into the cells of the spleen, and then cooled. The glands around the roots of the vessels were all enlarged and hard. (Fig. 49.)

Fig. 49.

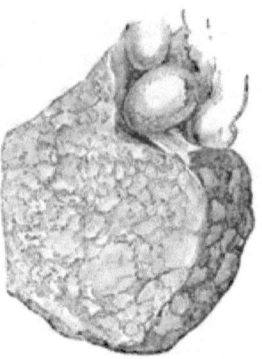

Fig. 49. Section of a small portion of the spleen, much enlarged by malignant growth penetrating its cellular tissue. Some of the diseased absorbent glands are also represented. (Case 18.)

CASE 19.—*Spleen pervaded by malignant matter. The absorbent glands very extensively affected.*—Joseph S—, æt. 9, was admitted into Guy's Hospital, 18th of October, 1826, under the care of Mr. Morgan, on account of a large ulcer on the scrotum, occasioned by a puncture made with a view to evacuate serum from the cellular membrane. It was stated that he had always slept with his brother, who, a few months before, died of phthisis. He was much reduced by an illness of about nine months, during which he had been subject to a pain in the back, extending round to the abdomen. On his admission his belly was much distended with ascites; he had also effusion into the prepuce and scrotum. He died on the 26th of November.

Sectio cadaveris.—There was no remarkable appearance in the head. Slight adhesion, and a little effusion into the cavities of the pleura. Slight trace of tubercular cicatrix at the apex of the right lung, and a very few exceedingly small tubercles scattered through the lungs. Bronchial membrane vascular. Bronchial glands greatly enlarged, and much indurated. Heart healthy.

Extensive recent inflammation of peritoneum, with copious

scrofulous effusion. Intestines tolerably healthy. Mesenteric glands generally enlarged, but one or two equalled the size of a pigeon's egg, of semi-cartilaginous hardness, and streaked with black matter. The substance of the liver generally natural; but a few tubercles somewhat larger than peas, which were semi-cartilaginous, and of uneven surface. The pancreas contained numerous very hard and rounded tubercles, particularly towards its head, which was much enlarged.

The spleen was large; and contained numerous white bodies of irregular ovoid shape, precisely similar to those mentioned in the last case, but not so numerous, the disease not being so far advanced. The absorbent glands about both the two last-mentioned organs were much enlarged.

Both kidneys were mottled, but not indurated. A continuous string of much-enlarged indurated absorbent glands, of a light colour, accompanied the aorta throughout its course, closely adhering to the vertebræ, and extending along the iliac vessels, as far as traced into the pelvis. Thoracic duct healthy.

CASE 20.—*Malignant disease of the scirrhous character affecting the spleen, together with many other organs of the body.*—John F—,

Fig. 30.

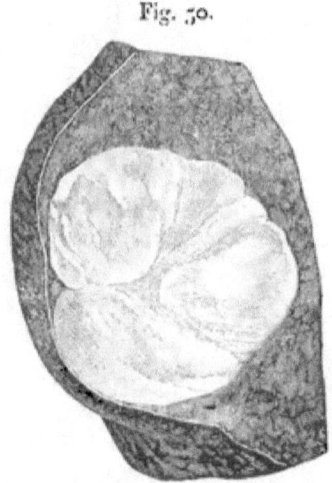

Fig. 30. A portion of the section of a spleen, containing a large scirrhous tubercle, in a case where many of the organs were affected with the same disease. This drawing is reduced to about one third the actual size. (Case 20.)

æt. 30, was admitted into Guy's Hospital, under the care of Dr. Cholmely, with rheumatic pains, quickly followed by paraplegia, under the aggravated circumstances of which he sank in about eight weeks.

Sectio cadaveris.—A malignant tumour was found arising from the ligaments of the spinal canal in its dorsal portion, and pressing on the dura-matral covering of the spinal cord. The substance of the sternum contained a fungoid tumour, and the same disease was found in one of the ribs, the pleura costalis, the lungs, the inner surface of the pericardium, the bronchial glands, and the axillary glands. In the substance of the liver were several whitish-red tubera, one large one in the spleen (Fig. 50), one in the kidney, and one attached to the pelvis. Several small tubera under the pericranium, and one between the bone and the dura mater.

CASE 21.—*Malignant disease of the cerebriform character, affecting the spleen in common with other organs.*—Anne B—, æt. about 35, was admitted, under Dr. Back, on the 10th of June, 1829. She had for some time laboured under an affection of the abdomen, and a hard tumour was felt, attributed to fungoid growth of the omentum. During her illness she appeared repeatedly to suffer from attacks of subacute peritonitis. She became greatly emaciated, and occasionally troubled with diarrhœa, and latterly with vomiting. The case was evidently hopeless, and she sank on the 13th of the following month.

Sectio cadaveris.—The chest healthy. The viscera of the abdomen were matted together by thick peritoneal adhesions, intermixed with tubera of various sizes, composed of cerebriform matter. The omentum was converted into a thick mass of fungoid tumours. There were similar growths in various parts, and, amongst the rest, some which had made their way towards the intestines, on the mucous membrane of which they had ulcerated. One, of the size of an egg, was situated in the small omentum. There were two pretty large and soft tubera, of the same description, imbedded in the under surface of the liver, and a few small tubera, of a similar kind, on the convex surface of the liver. The structure of the organ was pretty healthy, but pale. One, of the size of a pigeon's egg, was imbedded in the spleen, on its convex side. There were one or two small ones on the pancreas, which was in other respects healthy. Similar tubera existed in the mesenteric and lumbar glands. The kidneys were healthy. The whole of the true pelvis was filled, and the viscera matted together, by similar cerebriform tubera.

How far we are authorised in considering the two following cases in any other light than as affording accidental deviations from the healthy state of the spleen, is doubtful; but though this may be assumed with respect to the cellular cysts, yet, in the case where bony deposit had taken place, there was evidence of a peculiar action being set up in the vessels; and it is singular, in connexion with observations which I have frequently had occasion to make, that the same morbid action existed also in the vessels of the mesenteric gland, some of which were likewise ossified, thus supplying us with the third coincidence of this kind—for already we have seen the tubercular action occurring at the same time in the spleen and the absorbent glands, and, also, the malignant action developed together in these two situations.

Case 22.—*Bony deposit in the spleen and mesenteric glands.*—Maria C—, æt. 45, was admitted December 22d, 1825, labouring under anasarca, with feeble and obstructed circulation, great difficulty of breathing, frequent cough, and muco-purulent expectoration tinged with blood. She died on the 23d of January.

Sectio cadaveris.—The form of the chest greatly contracted. Lungs universally adhering to the pleura, and gorged with blood; no tubercles. Heart natural; the pericardium contained four ounces and a half of straw-coloured serum. Kidneys healthy; liver pale-coloured; spleen very small, with two small pieces of bony matter imbedded in its substance (see Fig. 39). Mesenteric glands rather large; one or two ossified.

Case 23.—*Cysts in the cellular membrane of the spleen.*—Charles B—, æt. 45, was admitted into Job's Ward, 23d of June, 1830, affected with general dropsy, ascites, anasarca, and effusion into the chest. He sank about three weeks after his admission, with symptoms resembling apoplexy.

Sectio cadaveris.—Considerable serous effusion was found beneath the arachnoid; the right pleura contained above three pints of clear serum, intermixed with tender flakes; the left pleura adhered very generally; the lungs were sprinkled with tubercles; the pericardium adhered universally by a perfectly formed cellular membrane; slight disease in the aortic valves, and the aorta; peritoneum universally covered with a thin false membrane; the cavity of the abdomen contained a considerable quantity of serum; the liver tolerably healthy.

The spleen was swollen and tuberose at the upper extremity, and evidently contained a fluid; this was found to be in cysts, some of which did, and some did not, communicate (see Fig. 40); they were smooth internally, but yet presented a reticulated appearance; they were quite distinct from the peritoneum, but lay just beneath it. Kidneys slightly mottled. Urine in the bladder albuminous.

The following cases will illustrate some of the changes which take place in connexion with the *peritoneum* of the spleen. It is true that these changes are, in general, such as befal the peritoneum generally; but they must have considerable influence in embarrassing the functions of the spleen, and, according to circumstances, may well be expected, either to prevent the ingress of blood when required, or, by opposing the contractile force of the elastic tumour, to prevent the organ from unloading itself, and thus favour its disorganization.

I do not think it necessary to give cases to show the existence of cartilaginous deposits on the spleen; the instances are very numerous, and I shall satisfy myself with transcribing a few of the statements I have made in various dissections:

"The spleen small, and its external surface rough, with slight cartilaginous deposits."

"The spleen with many small cartilaginous deposits, in spots, upon its surface."

"The spleen, which was very soft and small, had, besides the adhesion before mentioned, numerous small cartilaginous bodies on its surface."

"The spleen afforded a marked illustration of the mode in which the cartilage is often distributed in little lumps or granules on its surface."

"The spleen was soft and light-coloured; a large patch of cartilage was deposited on its surface."

"The spleen healthy, but surrounded by fat, and a patch of cartilaginous substance occupied a part of its surface."

"The spleen four times its natural size; its peritoneum coated with a thin pellicle of recent coagulum, and under that, about half its convex surface covered with a semi-cartilaginous substance."

"The spleen rather soft, with semi-cartilaginous patches."

In other cases the whole spleen is covered in this way with a cartilaginous coating. A fine specimen of this kind is preserved in our museum, having a worm-eaten appearance on its surface, from the irregular deposit, but deficient in no part of the spleen; and two portions of spleens, similarly invested, are preserved in the interesting collection of Dr. Baillie, in the Museum of the Royal College of Physicians.

The cases from which these were taken, varied much; they were cases of epilepsy, apoplexy, dropsy, &c. I may mention, however, that in a considerable majority, though not in all, the large arteries of the body were stated to have been diseased, having atheromatous deposits in their tunics.

I have said that, occasionally, plates of bone are formed in the cartilaginous deposits on the surface of the spleen. To a small extent, this is not unfrequent; but sometimes the whole spleen is found invested with bone; of this I have seen a very fine specimen in the magnificent collection of the Royal College of Surgeons. A spleen of about twice the natural size is covered completely by a thick scabrous coat of bony hardness, presenting small rounded projections of nearly a quarter of an inch in height, over its whole surface.

CASE 24.—*Peculiar appearance of the peritoneal coat of the spleen.* —John B——, æt. 32, a sailor, was brought to Guy's Hospital, November 24th, labouring under most excessive hæmatemesis, which occurred again, with great severity, on the 26th and 27th. He experienced convulsive fits, and fell into a lethargic state, in which he died.

Sectio cadaveris.—Heart and lungs healthy; liver and mucous membrane of stomach and intestines very exsanguine.

The spleen presented a very peculiar appearance; it was covered with a thick, tough, almost cartilaginous membrane, which lay upon it in deep irregular folds. It was evident that the spleen had been greatly distended, and at that time the false membrane had covered it, and doubtless embraced it firmly; but now, by the excessive loss of blood, the spleen had contracted. The covering had not sufficient elasticity to contract with it, and lay folded up upon its surface. The colour of the spleen, internally, was very pale. The splenic vein very large.

The brain was remarkably exsanguine. There was a mass of the size of a large pea, like the pineal gland, attached to the plexus, in the posterior cornu of one ventricle.

In this case, as far as we could discover, the hæmatemesis depended on the spleen, and, in all probability, was owing rather to the state of the peritoneal covering, than to that of the organ itself.

CASE 25.—*Tubercular deposit on the peritoneum of the spleen.*—Mary P——, æt. 14, who was admitted, under my care, with general peritoneal inflammation of a chronic character, died after lingering about two months.

The most extensive adhesions were found, with large quantities of tuberculous matter, in various parts. Those, upon the surface of the spleen, formed a mass of nearly a quarter of an inch thick over the whole convex surface. The lungs were but partially sprinkled with tubercles in this case; but the bronchial and other glands were much enlarged, and in a state of scrofulous disease.

CASE 26.—*Spleen, with the peritoneal covering studded with flat scirrhous growths.*—John W——, æt. 62, was admitted into Guy's Hospital, February 2d, 1833.

In this case, the true scirrhous tubera had developed themselves extensively in the liver and over the whole peritoneum; and the peritoneum covering the spleen was also involved in the disease. Throughout the whole of this membrane, the tubera presented somewhat the same aspect. They were scarcely raised above the surface, and assumed a somewhat circular form, with broken edges, looking by no means unlike drops of tallow let fall into water; some were very superficial, others were of the thickness of a shilling.

As the symptoms and progress of this case presented nothing peculiar, in connexion with the affection of the spleen, it will be unnecessary to go further into its details.

LACERATION OF THE SPLEEN.

The spleen, although protected more than almost any viscus of the abdomen, is liable to be injured from external violence, and not unfrequently death is the result; for though it has been proved that various animals, and even man, can exist, and apparently do well, when the spleen has been partially cut away or has been entirely removed, yet the irritation and inflammation produced by lacerating its substance will, of course, give rise to effects which may destroy life. But the most common way in which this accident proves fatal is in consequence of the hæmorrhage which takes place into the abdominal cavity. When this is very extensive, death is produced by the mere loss of blood; when less extensive, the peritoneal inflammation consequent upon the injury of the organ and the effused blood destroys life in a very limited time; and when the quantity of blood which escapes into the cavity is small, there is every reason to believe, that, by the united efforts of organization and absorption, the extravasated blood may be so disposed of, as to become comparatively inoxious. But there is a still less extent of injury to which the spleen is frequently subjected. In this case, the substance of the spleen only is ruptured, and the blood is retained by the tunic and the peritoneum; by which means a clot is formed, filling up the internal fissure; and from this the red particles gradually disappear, as from an apoplectic clot in the brain, leaving, at last, a yellow mass, which interferes very little, if at all, with the functions of the organ, and is only detected by the peculiar appearance it presents when death takes place from some other cause. (Figs. 49, 51, and 52.)

In the first volume of my 'Medical Reports,' I mentioned two cases of persons who had died of other diseases, but in whom this appearance was casually found; and it is from the drawings made from them that Figs. 51 and 52 are taken. In one of these cases I have stated, that "the spleen, in general pretty natural, had a peculiar appearance in one part, as if, blood having been effused, the red particles had been absorbed, and the coagulum had afterwards become imperfectly organized." But I perceive that Dr. Hodgkin, in his valuable notes to the 'Catalogue of Guy's Museum,' speaks of this appearance as being "a circumscribed degeneration of the

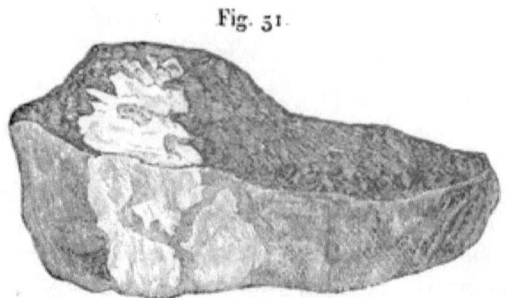

Fig. 51. Section of a spleen which had probably been lacerated; and the blood, having been retained by the tunic and peritoneum, had become partially organized.

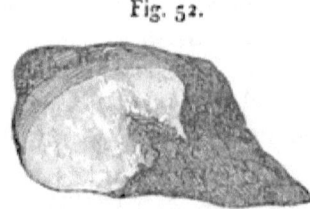

Fig. 52. A similar section from another case.

structure of the spleen, which becomes preternaturally firm and dense, and of a light colour;" which, he afterwards says, he is inclined to think the effect of external injury. I think, however, that the view I had taken of these peculiar hard, yellow-white masses, as being truly altered clots of blood, is probably the more correct; and a preparation in Guy's Museum, where a partial rupture of the kind, to which I have referred, had taken place in the spleen of a child over whom a cart had passed, and who sunk from the complicated and severe injury she sustained, after surviving nearly three days, seems so much in point, that I will give the case from which it was taken.

CASE 27.—*Laceration of the Spleen.*—Ann F—, æt. 9, was admitted into Guy's Hospital, under Mr. Morgan, on the 8th of November, 1826, in consequence of having been run over the day before, a cart-wheel passing over her body so as to produce fracture of the bones of the pelvis, with great general mischief and contusion.

She survived till the following day, having lived nearly three days after the accident.

In addition to all the other mischief, it was found that the spleen had been lacerated, and enough blood had escaped into the cavity of the abdomen to colour the intestines: but there had been no overwhelming hæmorrhage; for it appeared that, though the substance of the spleen had been almost divided through its centre, the peritoneum had retained the blood, so as to form a clot nearly an inch thick across the centre of the spleen, resembling, very exactly, the clot represented in Fig. 51; only that, in this case, the clot, instead of being a yellow substance, was the recent coagulum of blood.

This case, then, seems to present the first stage of that yellow mass which is often found in the spleen; and, under certain circumstances, it is probable that the semi-organized coagulum becomes the seat of abscess, at least such appeared to be the fact in the following case, for further particulars of which I must refer to the second volume of 'Medical Reports,' p. 168.

CASE 28.—*Abscess in the Fibrin left after the Extravasation of Blood in the Spleen.*—Maria L—, æt. 17, was admitted into Guy's Hospital, October 22d, 1829, in an exhausted state; countenance pale and anxious; her eyes sunk; exquisite tenderness to the touch generally; feet and legs slightly œdematous; ecchymosed spots upon the hands and feet; a large abscess in the axilla, and another on the forearm; abdomen tumid, as well as tender; pulse 152; respiration 44, short, difficult, and painful; tongue dry, with a broken fur; much sordes about the mouth and teeth; during last week, some epistaxis and blood in the motions. It appeared that she had been for some time in a declining state of health; but the immediate cause of the external symptoms was supposed to be a prick with a needle on the forefinger, five weeks previously. She died on the following day, under symptoms of great cerebral disturbance, vesication having taken place upon the toes and upon the forearm and hand, containing a bloody serous fluid.

Sectio cadaveris.—There were most unequivocal proofs of very severe recent inflammation of the peritoneum and of the pleura, particularly on the left side, and softening of the brain. But that part of the examination which is more particularly interesting at present is, that the spleen was the seat of extensive disease, appearing to have suffered first by some fibrinous deposit, which was so extensive as to occupy nearly one third of the whole spleen, the greater part deposited about the centre of the organ, nearly crossing its short diameter; and this deposit had lately run into a state of unhealthy suppuration, so that it formed an imperfect abscess; and another smaller deposit of the same kind had undergone a similar change. The arteries and the veins of the whole body were perfectly healthy.

Independently of this case serving to show another step in the progress of this affection, it is interesting, in connection with two other cases of abscess of the spleen already related, in both of which the powers of the circulation had been greatly reduced, leading in one case to gangrene of one of the extremities, as had been distinctly threatened in this.

When we review the cases, which I have selected as forming a fair example of those which occur in practice where the spleen is implicated, we perceive that in the great majority that organ merely partakes with others in some general state of derangement, and does not itself become a separate object of treatment. In other cases the changes in structure are so apparently casual, as neither to be capable of detection, nor, if detected, to admit of any remedial measures. Of the few which remain, the principal diseased conditions are, the congested state of the organ, its consolidation, its inflammation, and its laceration from external violence.

On the treatment of each of these conditions I would now make a few remarks, did I not feel that this communication had already reached to such a length, that it would be right to draw it to a conclusion; but I may observe generally, in reference to splenic disease, that it is probable that the spleen is greatly influenced by the derangement of many of the other organs of the body, and therefore its treatment will often depend on the regulation of their functions; for we cannot doubt, that whatever acts decidedly on the circulating system must in some degree influence the spleen, which obviously, from its structure and appearance, receives large quantities of blood, as subsidiary to the processes of sanguification or circulation. Still, however, it is by no means an organ easily susceptible of diseased action, and withstands the effects of injurious agencies to a very considerable extent. Probably the spleen sympathises in a particular manner with the skin, suffering from suppressed perspiration and cold and damp applied to the surface. It also appears to be affected by certain states of atmosphere, which act as a poison upon the system, evinced particularly in countries subject to marshy exhalations. It also probably suffers from interruption in the functions of the hepatic, the renal, and the absorbent systems, as seen in the organic evidence of their diseases, and partakes of the irregular distribution of blood, caused by the diseases of the heart and arteries.

From reflecting on the frequent combinations of these and other morbid states with splenic disease, we perceive more exactly the mutual relations and unions existing between them, and this is always an interesting light in which to view disease. The chief points of approach or contact to which our attention is directed, are the occasional intermixture of splenic disease with disease more or less extensive and confirmed of the absorbent system; the depressed state of circulation occurring in severe affections of the spleen; the coincidence of splenic with hepatic disease; its connection with derangements of the peritoneum; and some relation, though probably only collateral, between that state of the kidneys which produces albuminous urine and derangement of the spleen. By holding these and such like points in our minds, we shall comprehend more fully the possible value of the knowledge to be derived from following out the history of the derangements of the spleen, than we should by simply considering the morbid states of an organ of which so little is known with certainty; for the enumeration of morbid conditions can at best only be viewed as forming an alphabet for the construction of a language into which we may hereafter translate the complicated and obscure legends of disease.

CHAPTER IV.

RENAL DISEASE.

Amongst the various forms of abdominal tumour, few are so difficult of detection as those which depend upon certain diseases of the kidney. There are many diseases of the kidney which are accompanied by no enlargement, and in some, again, the size of the organ is decidedly diminished. Such forms of disease, which cannot be detected by any tumour of the part, do not, of course, come within the scope of the present investigation; but, on the other hand, the kidney is often enormously enlarged, forming a distinct abdominal tumour. The chief diseases under which I have known this condition to exist are, when numerous cysts have been developed in the substance of the kidney; when puriform matter has collected in the pelvis, and converted the distended kidney into a bag of pus; when fungoid or malignant changes have taken place in the kidney; when fungoid matter or blood has been accumulated in the pelvis.

I have known the enlarged kidney to be mistaken for disease of the spleen—of the ovary—of the uterus—and for a tumour developed in the concave part of the liver; nor is it perhaps possible, by the greatest care and the most precise knowledge, altogether to avoid such errors; and therefore the more necessary it is to prosecute the investigation.

It need scarcely be stated, that the kidneys are placed in hollows on each side of the spine, extending from the eleventh rib to the os ilium, that is, through a space corresponding to the two last dorsal and the two upper lumbar vertebræ; the right being a little lower than the left; they lie behind the peritoneum, from which they are separated by a layer of cellular membrane, which usually contains in its meshes a quantity of fat. They have behind them the diaphragm, the quadrati lumborum, and the transverse muscles of the abdomen; and, to the inner side, the psoas muscles. The right kidney lies under the posterior portion of the right lobe of the liver, and has the renal capsule resting on its upper extremity: while the colon covers it anteriorly, the cæcum lying below it, and the duodenum, with the head of the pancreas, before it, at its superior part. The left kidney has the renal capsule and the spleen at its upper part; and it lies behind the left extremity of the pancreas, which separates it from the stomach, while the descending colon covers it anteriorly.

Although closely attached to the muscles of the loins in its natural condition, yet in those diseases in which it most rapidly increases, the enlargement shows itself much more towards the anterior part of the abdomen than towards the loins; not only because the firm structure of this part is more calculated to conceal a tumour, but also because in the other direction it meets with less immediate resistance; so that it often happens, while we are examining the lumbar region with the greatest care, and obtaining but a doubtful evidence of fulness and hardness by the eye and by the touch, and by careful comparison of the two sides, we can scarcely place the hand upon the anterior or even the lateral part without becoming at once sensible of the existence of a distinct tumour; and then, probably, by pressing that tumour backward, the other hand clearly informs us of its connection with the loins. The part in which the tumour is felt will, of course, vary according to the nature of the disease and to the portion of the kidney which it occupies; and in some cases, where the whole substance of the organ is so diseased as to contribute pretty equally to the enlargement from the beginning, the hardness or tumour will be early detected in the loins. Thus we find, that a rapidly-increasing fungoid disease in the right kidney may be chiefly perceived pushing its way beneath the liver; a large collection of pus, or other accumulation, enlarging the natural cavity of the kidney, will probably be felt most distinctly towards the anterior part, and, from the assistance of gravitation, will occupy a place between the umbilicus and the crista ilii; while on the contrary, a kidney enlarged by numerous cysts, affording a comparatively solid and uniform increase to the whole organ, will be most distinctly felt occupying the lumbar space, and giving solidity and firmness to that part. It will likewise be found, that when inflammation has pervaded the kidney, or attacked the external part, it will be bound down to its natural situation, and completely fixed in the loins, not advancing, as the fungoid kidney often does, towards the anterior part of the abdomen.

The errors of diagnosis into which we may be led are of course different, according as the right or the left kidney is the seat of disease. If the right kidney be so diseased as to make its way forwards, it may be mistaken for an enlargement of the liver, for pyloric disease, for a glandular disease about Glisson's capsule, for disease of the colon or cæcum, or for enlargement of the ovary or uterus.

We may often distinguish it from the liver, by carefully examining its relation to the ribs; when, if the liver be healthy, we shall probably find that the tumour, as the patient lies on his back, instead of passing fairly under the ribs, dips downwards, so as to allow the finger to lie between them and the upper part of the tumour. Again, we seldom have disease of the liver to the extent which is here supposed, without producing some pretty decided symptoms, either in the colour of the eye, or the tinge of the skin, or in the deep colour of the urine, or the diseased secretions evinced by the stools.

When disease of the liver is complicated with that of the kidney —as is sometimes the case, particularly in malignant disease—it may be quite impossible to do more than form an unsatisfactory conjecture; but even here it is possible, that should the urine be altered in its character, more particularly if it contain pus, and, in addition to other symptoms of hepatic affection, should the peculiar hard tubera, which, under such circumstances, often form in the liver, be perceptible under the ribs, we might come to a correct diagnosis as to both the diseases. We may, moreover, in this case, derive much assistance from ascertaining, by the feel and by percussion, the exact situation of the hollow intestines; for although it is true that they suffer great displacement, yet, if we find any of them anterior to the tumour, and lying over it, we may generally infer that the tumour does not form a part of the liver; as it is very improbable that such a growth should arise from the concave surface of the liver, as to have any portion of the intestine in that situation. I have, indeed, once seen the liver, in its normal state, lying posteriorly to many coils of intestine, but this accidental malposition can never enter into our calculation, being of extreme rarity.

The cæcum and ascending colon are liable to disease, and to enlargement both from the presence of flatus and from accumulation of fæces, and occasionally from other accumulations; and as the tumour in such cases corresponds in situation very exactly with the tumour sometimes caused by the kidneys, it will be very likely to lead us into error. In all these instances, although a little time may be necessary before we can convince ourselves of the real nature of the tumour, yet the collateral indications will afford us great assistance, as there will seldom fail to be some very obvious derangement in the functions of the large intestines. We shall, in cases of flatulent distension, ascertain the fact by percussion, and by the rapid alterations which the tumour undergoes. In cases of fæcal abscess, a disease very common from lodgments taking place in the vermiform process, the febrile symptoms generally run much higher than in renal tumours. There is often external inflammation, and much tenderness; and, above all, the tumour is often found too low in the iliac region to be probably produced by the kidney, though I have known such abscesses to discharge their contents almost in the lumbar region. In cases where concretions have formed, occupying a large portion of the cæcum, considerable difficulty may arise in the diagnosis, if we simply look to the tumour; but the disturbance of the bowels, the intense abdominal pains, and tormenting collection of flatus, will be our guide. Perhaps, of all the errors made in the diagnosis of kidney disease, the most frequent has been, to consider the enlarged kidney as an ovarian or uterine tumour. I do not, however, remember to have met with any case in which the converse error has been made; in general, the history of the disease, and the part in which the early growth has been observed, would be sufficient assistants, if we could trust to the observations of our patients; but this is seldom the case, and sometimes, so far from being able to tell us where the swelling began, we shall be the first to announce to the patient the existence of a tumour; then, however, the present situation of the tumour will enable us to discover that it is not connected with the pelvic viscera; and usually there is a distinct sulcus, into which the hand may be placed, between the tumour and the pelvis. Another point to be attended to, is the situation of the hollow viscera; which, by careful examination, will be found to overlap, or to pass over, the surface of the tumour; and this, together with the history of its growth, ought sufficiently to direct our judgment. Occasionally, the ovarian tumour assumes such varieties of form as to deceive the most experienced; and an instance very lately came to my knowledge, when several, who were consulted, altogether denied the ovarian origin of a tumour, and ascribed it to the liver; though, after death, it turned out to be ovarian. In this instance, the absence of any hollow viscera anterior to the tumour would have prevented the supposition of its being kidney at least, though the same might not hold good as to the liver. When the kidney has descended almost to the pelvis, and approached the middle line of the abdomen, it has been mistaken for uterine tumour; but an examination of the neck of the uterus, and of the uterus itself, in the usual way, will come in aid of the indications of which I have been speaking, as applicable to the ovary.

If the left kidney be diseased, the tumour may be mistaken for the spleen, for the descending colon, for the ovary, and for the uterus.

The enlarged spleen is situated more anteriorly, and, in its descent, though occasionally much rounded, generally presents a more defined edge than the kidney, often suffering the fingers to be introduced beneath it; and it is sometimes notched at the edge; it has none of the hollow bowels to interrupt the uniform surface of the tumour. The spleen is sometimes inseparably attached to the tumour of the kidney, of which we have a specimen in Guy's Museum: but when this is the case, the spleen generally occupies the posterior part of the left hypochondrium, and therefore adds little either to the facility or the difficulty of diagnosis. Nearly the same remarks are applicable as regards the descending colon and its accumulations, and also the left ovary and the uterus, as have already been made when speaking of the right.

There are, besides, three forms of tumour connected with the kidney, the possibility of the existence of which must be borne in mind, when attempting to fix the seat of the disease. The one is the real acephalocyst hydatid, which may develop itself in the kidney, or be attached to it, though I do not remember to have met with it in this organ. The next is tumour from disease of the renal capsule. This organ is liable to both scrofulous enlargement, of which I saw an instance in a post-mortem examination very lately, though not of sufficient size to have been detected during life, and it is also frequently the seat of malignant tubera, of which I have seen several cases, and some preparations are preserved in the Museum at Guy's. The third form of tumour arising in connection with the kidney, is the simple distension of the pelvis and ureter with the natural secretion, owing to obstruction in the ureter or bladder, of which illustrations may be found in Guy's Museum. But one of the most striking cases I can at present recall has been published by my friend, Mr.

Estlin, of Bristol. In this instance, the distended ureter produced a large tumour, which for some time excited much anxiety and great doubt as to its nature, till it was found that by a little pressure it was made to discharge its contents into the bladder, under which treatment it gradually contracted; but the ureter was found greatly enlarged and thickened after death, though it had not then been distended for a considerable time.

When hydatids are developed in the kidney, they can only be ascertained by their situation, and by the means applicable to the detection of hydatids generally. The tumour of the renal capsule must at present, from its situation as a portion of the kidney itself, and from our great ignorance of the function it performs in health, be almost beyond the scope of decided diagnosis, but may be suspected from the situation of the tumour in the upper part of the kidney; but the liver lying before it, and the muscles of the back and ribs behind it, it is very improbable that it would be detected. In the scrofulous disease I witnessed lately, the tumour, of the size of a small egg, was fixed to the upper and posterior part of the liver, in which it was almost imbedded. The dilated ureter may be detected by its situation, which may, if not close to the kidney, be sufficiently characteristic, and by its elastic feel, and it will be certainly detected if its contents can be evacuated into the bladder.

Supposing that our diagnosis has been satisfactorily formed, and that a tumour of the kidney has been discovered, it still becomes desirable, if it be possible, to establish the exact nature of the disease to which the increased bulk of the organ is to be ascribed—a problem which is even more difficult to solve than the former. We have often to look back into a long history; and there is every reason to believe that, in many cases, there is a successive or simultaneous development of different diseases, so that it is possible to come to a right conclusion as to part of the disease, and yet not discover the whole. Thus we shall find, by comparing histories with post-mortem appearances, that in one case almost undoubtedly a calculus has been deposited in the pelvis of the kidney, has excited suppuration, and a tumour has been formed, but that after it has existed some time malignant action has been set up. In other cases, we shall find that an injury to the loins has been followed by hæmaturia, and that after a time a malignant disease has established itself. Again, we shall find a calculus to begin, and this followed by a collection of pus in the pelvis, and this succeeded by a granular change in that portion of the renal substance which has not undergone absorption; or we shall have reason to believe that the granulation of the kidney has taken place; and that afterwards, or at the same time, cysts have been formed in the cortical substance, and a tumour of the kidney has been the consequence; and as the post-mortem appearance, in conjunction with the history, is capable of bringing us to such conclusions, so the history by itself, in conjunction with the physical or local and general symptoms, may bring us nearly to the same point. And I will now proceed to refer to some of the data which may serve to guide us in the inquiry.

The two symptoms upon which we can generally look back as most remotely connected with the disease of the kidney are hæmaturia and the passing of small calculi by the urethra. Neither of these symptoms necessarily either indicates or leads to organic change in the structure of the kidney; but both of these, when the change is discovered, throw some light upon particular cases.

It is certain that hæmaturia takes place under a variety of circumstances. Some states of congestion and inflammation, such as often occur in consequence of intemperance, or after exposure to cold, or subsequent to scarlatina, will produce hæmaturia, and this will probably never be followed by enlargement of the kidney, or at all events never to the extent of producing sensible tumour; and of this we may have almost hourly experience. A general hæmorrhagic tendency of the system will often show itself by hæmaturia, in which case, under particular circumstances, extensive ecchymosis will be produced in the pelvis of the kidney, but may subside without causing any tumour of that organ. The more local causes of hæmorrhage, as obstruction to the circulation through the heart or even the large viscera of the abdomen, may produce slight hæmaturia, without any enlargement of the kidney following; but where a profuse hæmorrhage takes place, or a tendency to it shows itself, such mischief frequently follows as leads to tumour of the organ. This hæmorrhage is probably not to be considered so much the result of any one form of disease tending to enlargement, as the source from which irritation is set up. The coagulum forming, and not capable of immediate expulsion, produces irritation, and assists the deposit or the accumulation of calculus; or, by retaining the urine in the pelvis, produces inflammation and suppuration there. Every instance of hæmorrhage which can be fairly traced to the kidney, and in which the entire blood comes away in a form capable of coagulation, must be looked upon with fear, as likely to lay the foundation for some of those organic changes which we are now considering. I am not, however, sure that such an hæmorrhage can be considered as fairly indicating any particular form of disease as likely to follow. I consider it generally, as either the effect of injury or of peculiar weakness of the vessels having no specific character; and whether it is afterwards to lead to the deposit of a calculus, and of what kind that calculus is to be—or whether it is to lead to simple or scrofulous suppuration, or to lay the groundwork for malignant disease—I imagine to depend upon other circumstances existing in the general state of the constitution.

When hæmorrhage occurs in the more advanced state of the disease, I should look to the circumstance of its being pure, or mingled with pus, as important in a diagnostic point of view; when it is pure, forming clots which are perhaps moulded to the shape of the passages—if I found a tumour, I should consider it probable that the kidney was pervaded by cysts, or that in some way great obstruction was experienced to the passage of the blood through the remaining substance of the kidney; still the diagnosis would be modified by the character of the tumour. If it were hard, resisting, and chiefly lumbar, I should be more confirmed in this belief; and if, in addition to this, I found that the urine, when perfectly clear of blood, after the hæmorrhage had for some days completely subsided, was still albuminous, I should very confidently expect some such degeneration in the substance of the kidney as I have described, intermixed possibly with granular deposit.

When hæmorrhage occurs in smaller quantity, but mingled with pus, and generally subsiding rather more slowly than the pus, so as to form a fringe-like deposit on its surface, it probably bespeaks some local bleeding from the pelvis, either depending on the presence of a rough calculus, to a small extent lacerating or rubbing the membrane, or more commonly depending on a tendency to fungoid growths beginning to arise from it.

If small calculi have been passed in the early part of the history of a renal tumour, the natural conclusion to which we come is, that some similar formation having taken place within the pelvis of the kidney, and having been unable to find its way down the ureter, the pelvis has been irritated either by the calculus, or much more likely by the retained urine, and pus has accumulated in the cavity and distended it; but this seldom happens, without pus being actually passed.

When a large tumour is formed by the kidney, and neither calculus nor blood nor pus has marked the progress of the disease, we should be inclined to consider this a fungoid or malignant disease.

There are circumstances connected with the character of the tumour and its growth, which, without any consideration of the discharge, lead us to infer its nature; as, for instance, if the tumour be hard and insensible, and lodged in the lumbar region, we should incline to the supposition that it was neither enlarged from pus nor from fungoid growth, and may probably be changed in structure throughout, or pervaded with cysts.

If the tumour appear to have increased very quickly, and especially to have grown irregularly, projecting in particular parts, advancing upon its upper part towards the scrobiculus cordis, rather than descending towards the pelvis, or increasing regularly towards the mesial line, we conclude that the disease is rather a fungoid or malignant growth, than the product of simple inflammation.

If the tumour have enlarged regularly, or with only certain moderate elevations, forming a somewhat ovoid body, or have become soft or fluctuating in parts, then, even if pus had not been ascertained in the urine, we should be inclined to ascribe the tumour to a collection of pus.

When speaking of the diagnosis of these tumours, it is impossible to pass over in silence the importance of the very valuable test of pus which was first pointed out by Dr. Babington. It occasionally happens, that very large deposits, both of the lithates and of the phosphates, are thrown down from the urine, which on first being seen as they have formed or subsided in the vessel, bear so much the appearance of pus, that not only the patient but the practitioner who has not paid a good deal of attention to the subject has been deceived. The lithates are at once detected by their entire disappearance, if heat be gently applied, or a few ounces of warm water be added to the urine; and indeed we may generally learn, by inquiry from the patient, that the urine was perfectly clear when first passed, becoming turbid only as it cooled. The phosphates, however, are of less easy detection; but if there be any suspicion that the deposit is purulent, by pouring off the clear fluid, and adding to the deposit a few drops of the liquor potassæ or the liquor ammoniæ, and agitating them together, we find that if it be pus it is converted, in the space of a few seconds, into a substance resembling the most tenacious mucus, and this process is often carried on previously to the discharge of the urine; for if the urine become alkaline in the bladder, as it often does in paralysis and in some other cases, this conversion of pus into mucus takes place in the bladder itself; and this has probably often misled the practitioner, who has been in the habit of regarding the large quantity of ropy mucus, which is sometimes found at the bottom of the vessel, as a secretion of the mucous membrane of the bladder, whereas it is in reality very often only a puriform secretion of the kidney which has undergone conversion in the bladder. I have at this time under my care a lady labouring under copious purulent discharge from the kidney, which on one or two occasions has been passed in the form of mucus, owing to the administration of alkaline remedies.

The history of those diseases which induce tumours of the kidney will of course vary greatly, according as they depend on simple inflammation, on a scrofulous constitution, or as they are more or less malignant in their character. The approach is often slow and insidious; and when the tumour has shown itself, or by other indications the established disease is discovered, the patient is often able to refer back to some period when unusual exposure to cold, or some sudden jerk, or some accident to the loins, may here be the presumed exciting cause. Very frequently we find in females, that although some other cause may be discovered, and perhaps some symptoms may have previously occurred, yet the malady had never shown itself decidedly till after pregnancy, and the tumour has first been discovered as the patient recovered from her confinement; and where this is the case, it is reasonable to suppose that the pressure of the uterus having obstructed the passage of urine along the ureters, may have acted as an aggravating, or perhaps as an exciting, cause of suppuration or of malignant disease. There are, however, some other circumstances connected with pregnancy which act, in the first place, as throwing a difficulty for several months over the detection of a tumour in the abdomen, and then calling the attention more directly to its existence. In some cases, we can distinctly trace that the obstruction and irritation resulting from stricture, from disease of the bladder, or from stone in the bladder or kidney, have been the exciting causes of the disease. Diseases of the kidney, tending to the formation of tumour, are confined to neither age nor sex. Scrofulous disease with enlargement, and fungoid diseases of the most remarkable and rapid growth, occur in children of the most tender age; indeed, the kidneys of children are very susceptible of disease, both functional and organic. In more advanced age, the obstructions in the urinary passages increase, and formidable calculous diseases multiply. The further history, however, of these tumours will perhaps be best illustrated by the following cases, selected for the purpose:

CASE I.—*Tumour of the kidney, from numerous cysts formed in its substance.*—In November, 1835, I was consulted by Mr. Iliff on the case of Mr. —, about 30 years of age. His aspect bespoke a man labouring under some formidable chronic disease. He was evidently much emaciated, the muscles of his legs and his arms were shrunk, and the glutei muscles remarkably reduced. He was so feeble, as not to walk a mile and a half without great fatigue. He passed a moderate quantity of urine, which was of a light colour, acid, and albuminous. I learned that his present illness was dated from about two years back, at which period he had decided hæmaturia, which continued at intervals for some time. Since that, he had never considered himself in health; he had, however, pursued his usual occupation till lately, but for the last four months had been more decidedly an invalid. His state of emaciation allowed of a full examination of the abdomen, and a tumour was distinctly to be ascertained in the left lumbar space, where it appeared pretty firmly fixed. (See Fig. 53.) It might be fairly grasped by the hand, so placed that the thumb was near the spine and the finger advanced into the hypochondriac region. The history of the case, the state of the urine, and the situation of the tumour, all led to the easy decision that the tumour depended on enlarged kidney. When felt in front, the spleen, or the descending colon loaded with fæces, suggested themselves; but the fact that it seemed to belong to the posterior rather than the anterior part of the abdomen, and its fixed feel, would have removed these doubts, had not the history of the case pointed so distinctly to the kidney. The exact nature of the renal disease was less obvious. The very considerable enlargement of the organ did not belong to the usual history of albuminous urine, and the general loss of power bespoke some formidable organic disease. He was ordered a well-regulated, nourishing diet. The Emplastrum Ammoniaci c. Hydrargyro was applied to the seat of the tumour; and the uva ursi in infusion, and slight alkaline preparations, were directed to be taken. Under this treatment we at first received flattering reports; but the disease advanced, all the symp-

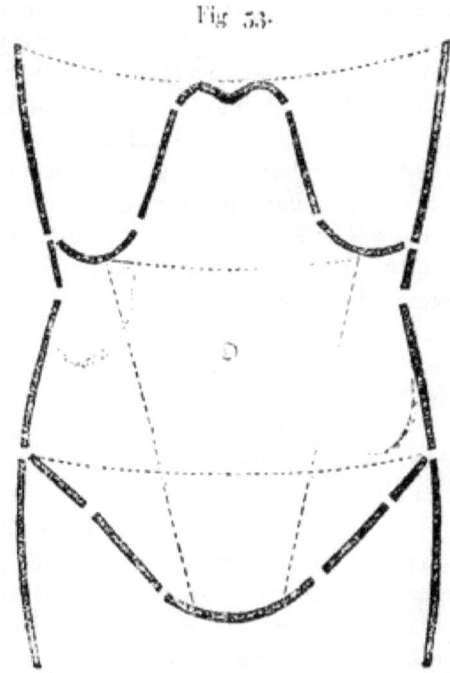

Fig. 53. Diagram showing the situation of the tumours in the case of a patient both of whose kidneys were enlarged by very numerous cysts, distended with fluid.

toms became worse, enlargement of the right kidney also became perceptible, the urine remained moderately coagulable (about a pint and a half in twenty-four hours), and he suffered a great deal of pain at the neck of the bladder, from the frequent passing of fibrinous coagula, of a slight, pinkish-yellow colour, about an inch long, and apparently moulded by the urethra. His emaciation became extreme, and he had frequent returns of hæmaturia. From the middle of February he was completely confined to his bed, expecting death daily. In the first week of April he experienced some slight convulsive seizures, and fell into a state of coma for a few hours before his death, which occurred about the 10th of April.

I was not present at the post-mortem examination, but I had an opportunity of examining the kidneys. They both presented most extreme specimens of the vesiculated kidney; the left was the largest, and was probably eight or ten times the natural size, while the right was at least six times the size of the healthy kidney. The whole appeared made up of a congeries of vesicles, from the size of a pigeon's egg to a pea; and the substance of the kidney was almost obliterated, nothing but a thin layer of secreting structure remaining, and that greatly altered from the natural texture. The pelvis of the kidney and the mammillary processes alone retained a tolerably healthy appearance; the lining membrane of the pelvis had no undue vascularity, and was perfectly smooth; the mammillary processes, though somewhat flattened, showed, when divided, the healthy organization; the ureters were healthy; but the renal vessels, particularly the veins, were large. The other viscera were healthy, and the bladder contained half a pint of urine.

In this case, I believe, we have an instance of the combination of the granulated kidney with the vesicular degeneration. The combination is not at all uncommon; indeed, in the hard, granulated kidney these vesicles occur, to a certain limited extent, more frequently than otherwise. In the present instance, the portion of the kidney which remained was compressed to such a degree, that its texture could scarcely be appreciated, but I considered it granulated. The vesicular degeneration, however, gave the peculiar character of increased size to the organ.

CASE 2.—*Suppuration of the kidney from stricture of the urethra, attended with perceptible tumour.*—I was requested to see, with Mr. Edinburgh, a gentleman who had for many years been subject to urinary difficulties, arising from stricture. During this time he had often retained his urine for many hours, even after he had felt the desire to pass it, and the urine had often been turbid, but for the last four months he had been most decidedly worse; the urine thick, and at times very fetid; he had lost flesh greatly, had suffered from night perspirations, had weakness in the loins, was looking exceedingly sallow, and was quite unable to pursue his occupations in the city. The urine very acid, and of a uniform, opaque-yellow colour when first passed, but on standing, a considerable quantity of greenish-yellow, creamy pus subsided; when rendered nearly clear by filtering, it was still coagulable by heat. He experienced several rigors about six weeks before, after which the urine became particularly thick and offensive. In this case there was a small tumour to be felt, by deep pressure, in the right hypochondrium, corresponding with the situation of the upper part of the kidney (Fig. 54); and we concluded that, as the suppuration of the kidney had made such inroads upon the constitution, the great indication was to support the system, and for this purpose we gave combinations of bitter infusion with muriatic acid and mild sedatives. He was also put upon a more generous, though mild diet; he was even allowed some porter; and under this treatment he gradually but greatly improved, and was able to return to a considerable part of his ordinary occupation. An external irritation was kept up near to the affected kidney for a considerable length of time, by means of the Linimentum Antimonii Tartarizati. After a few months, I heard that relapse had taken place and terminated fatally, but no examination could be obtained.

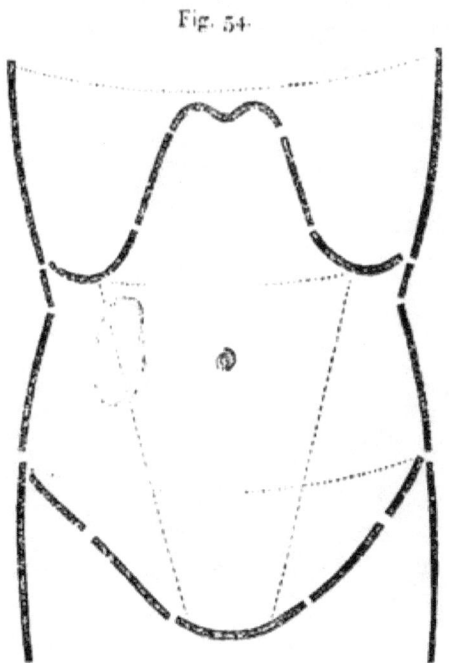

Fig. 54. Diagram of the situation of the tumour in a case of suppurating kidney.

212 ON ABDOMINAL TUMOURS.

This case affords a fair example of a very numerous class of diseases, where fatal injury occurs to the kidney, from the neglected effects of stricture or from other causes, leading to the undue retention of urine in the bladder, and consequently in the ureter and kidney. We had in this case an assistance, in our diagnosis, from perceptible tumour, which is very often not to be obtained, but this was facilitated by the state of emaciation. It is probable that the remaining structure of the kidney was granulated.

CASE 3.—*Tumour formed by the kidney, the pelvis being distended with pus.*—Charlotte P—, a slight, delicate woman, æt. 30, was admitted, under my care, into Guy's Hospital, June 13th, 1832, the subject of a large abdominal tumour, which I very carefully examined as she lay in bed upon her back. It occupied a situation which extended over nearly half the abdomen, not very different from that of a greatly enlarged spleen (Fig. 55), but running back more completely into the lumbar region, and there affording a tense, somewhat elastic feel. It appeared to be perfectly *fixed*, so that it did not admit of any motion; and even when the patient was turned completely on the right side, it did not shift its place. It felt as if

Fig. 55.

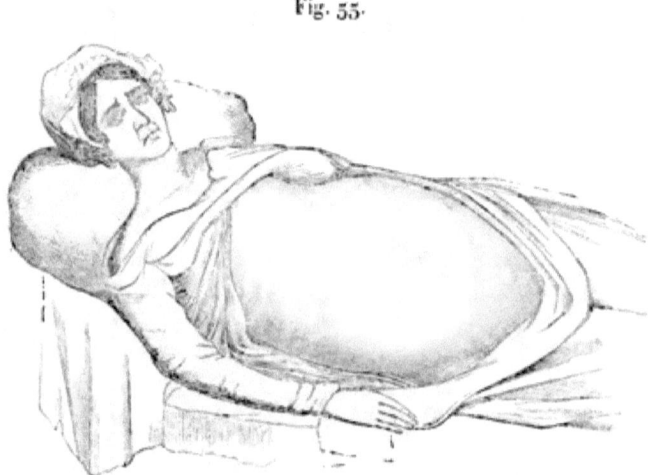

Fig. 55. The external appearance of the abdomen in a case where enlargement had existed in the left kidney, owing to a collection of puriform matter.

fixed to the ribs themselves, under their margins, which were obviously protruded a little by its bulk. Towards the lower part, and particularly below the crest of the ilium, and descending towards the pelvis, the enlargement felt much softer and less tense. I was at once convinced that this tumour depended on a diseased kidney, and I thought that the softness of the lower part might arise from a portion of the intestine, which probably was the colon passing over the kidney.

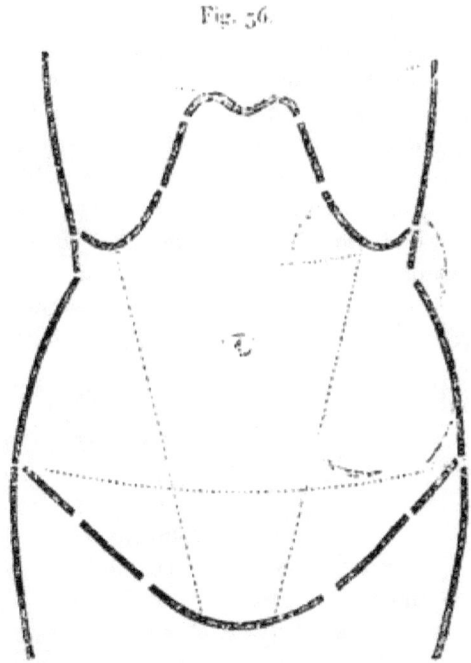

Fig. 56. Diagram showing the situation of the tumour, as felt in the case of Charlotte P—. See also Figs. 55, 57, and 58.

On inquiring into the particulars of her history, we found that about three years before she had frequent calls to pass urine, accompanied with pain and forcing, and that occasionally the urine was slightly tinged with blood; which state of things continued for many months. Eighteen months after, she was put to bed with a living child, and about six weeks subsequently she first discovered the tumour. Since that, however, nine months before her admission, she had borne another living child, and about Christmas she began to pass considerable quantities of what she considered "matter" with the urine. She experienced very little pain, except in the neck of the bladder, till about three months before entering the hospital, when she began to feel pain in the left iliac and lumbar region, and to observe the tumour much more than she had done previously.

At the time of her admission, all her ailments were plainly referable to the state of the kidney, and to her debility, induced by its long continuance; the pulse was 120, and she was thin, looking hectic. She had very frequent calls to pass urine, and complained of considerable pain at the time; seldom more than an hour elapsed without the necessity of passing it. The urine was of a tolerably natural colour, but was often loaded with pus, which subsided to the bottom, and was sometimes like the pure contents of an abscess, at other times was mingled with mucus. The urine was not the least alkaline, but, on the contrary, both it and the pus, when separated, reddened litmus-paper. Some days the quantity of pus was very small, but on other days as much as six or eight ounces, of almost pure pus, were collected from the vessels; and after a large discharge, the tumour was often decidedly reduced for a day or two. The bowels were costive, so that she was obliged to strain very much, but the appearance of the motions was tolerably natural. She was always relieved by having the bowels open, and the irritability of the bladder was rather diminished by the decoction of the Pareira brava with soda and conium, under the use of which the mucus disappeared from the urinary discharge and the apparent bulk of the tumour diminished; but this evidently depended a good deal on the casual increase of purulent discharge. About the 13th of July, her lungs began to suffer; she was harassed by cough; her breathing became shorter, and by degrees a large quantity of puriform expectoration took place, and she sunk under the symptoms of chronic pneumonia, with considerable diarrhœa.

Sectio cadaveris, August 9th, 1832.—On opening the cavity of the thorax the lungs were seen pale-coloured, and rather emphysematous on the anterior part, but on raising them it was found that the posterior parts were much hepatized by recent inflammation, and that about the edges more particularly a hard, puriform, curd-like deposit, not strictly tubercular, had taken place. The pleura was also somewhat inflamed, and a small quantity of puriform lymph thrown out, which lay in flakes, attached to the lower margin of the lungs. The upper lobes had a few puriform and hard deposits, and the whole lung, except the front part, cut firm, and was distended, but was pervious to air through the greater part of its extent.

The heart was natural, but there was rather more straw-coloured effusion than natural in the pericardium.

The parietes of the abdomen were greatly attenuated, and as the body lay there was little appearance of tumour; it was, however, to be felt. When the abdomen was first opened, there was no appearance of disease, the omentum being spread out over the whole abdominal contents; but when this was raised and drawn back (see Fig. 57), the tumour came in sight, occupying the left iliac and lumbar regions, and passing under the large end of the stomach towards the diaphragm. The spleen was seen just showing itself from beneath the ribs; and the descending colon, contracted like a thick cord, ran longitudinally on the surface of the tumour. The colon throughout was much contracted, and the greater part of the small intestines occupied the pelvis. The duodenum and the jejunum were remarkably vascular, but there was no sign of inflammation. The liver was large, soft, and of a pale-drab colour; the gall-bladder thick.

Fig. 57.

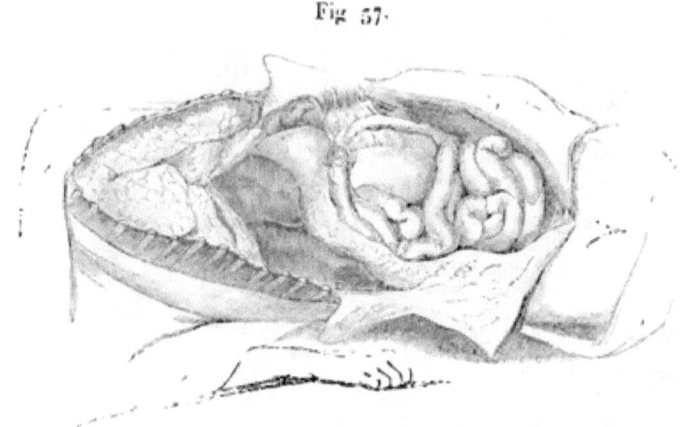

Fig. 57. The appearance of the viscera when the abdomen, represented in Fig. 55, was first laid open, and the omentum turned back. The contracted colon is seen passing over the tumour, to which it is adherent.

When the liver and stomach had been removed—and the arch of the colon divided where it became attached to the tumour, and, with the omentum, had been taken away—the whole extent of the tumour became evident. (See Fig. 58.) It was of an ovoid form, and of a yellow colour, with some few vessels passing over it. It extended from near the brim of the pelvis to the diaphragm, passing under the pancreas, which was seen lying flattened upon its surface; while the superior portion of the tumour passed upwards to the diaphragm, whose crurae were rather pushed to the right by it. The tumour had contracted adhesion to the lumbar parietes and to the colon; and on attempting to remove the mass which was formed by the suppurating kidney, the walls of the abscess were so thin at the back part that they were torn just below the angle formed by the ribs and the spine. The ureter was with difficulty discovered, for it was thickened, and resembled an artery, and its canal was by no means proportionably large. It was traced to the bladder, where its orifice formed a permanent opening, into which a goose-quill could easily have been inserted, and the membrane around was tuberculated. The bladder was exceedingly small and vascular; the uterus natural.

Fig. 58.

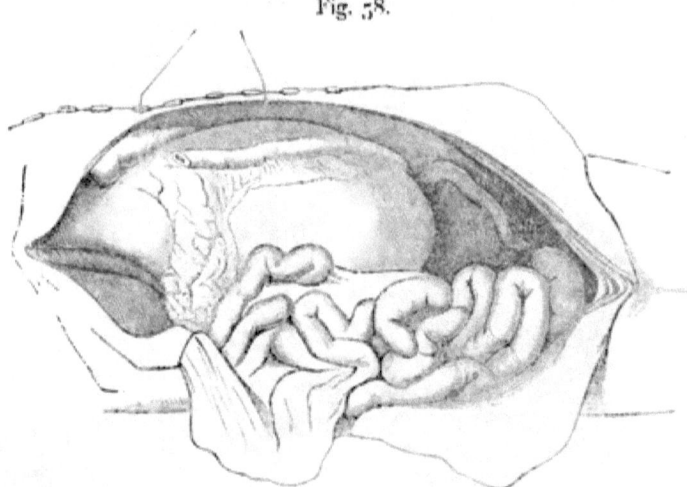

Fig. 58. The tumour formed by the left kidney more fully exposed, by the removal of many of the viscera. The enlarged kidney is seen extending from the diaphragm almost to the pelvis. The pancreas, and the descending colon, and the spleen, are seen attached to the tumour. This figure is on a somewhat larger scale than Fig. 57.

The tumour itself felt tense, but evidently contained fluid, and when opened, first by being torn at the back and then by following up the ureter, proved to contain about a pint and a half of the most perfect, well-formed pus, lodged in cells communicating with the pelvis of the kidney, and apparently formed from the distended infundibula; while a small portion only of what appeared the kidney itself formed thin parietes and septa to these cells. Externally, the whole was covered by a dense tunic. The right kidney was perfectly healthy.

In this case, the situation of the tumour was sufficient to leave scarcely a doubt of its nature; but had any further proof been wanting, it was abundantly furnished by the decidedly puriform character of the matter which passed with the urine, and the circumstance of its being so firmly fixed in its position favoured the supposition that it was the result of simple inflammation.

This tumour was, however, just before the patient came to the hospital, supposed to be connected with the uterus, a mistake to which, most probably, the history of the disease had led, for this was one of those cases where pregnancy first apparently developed the tumour.

It is observable, that in this case, as well as the last, the urine was always acid, and in connection with that was the perfectly puriform character of the discharge, very different from the ropy mucus which frequently occurs when the urine is alkaline. Although this patient was much emaciated when she came to the hospital, and was already confined to bed with symptoms of hectic from the profuse purulent secretion, yet there is no doubt that the suppuration of the kidney was not the immediate cause of death, but that her dissolution was owing to pneumonia and the accompanying diarrhœa.

The following case affords another example of the supposed connection between parturition and disease of the kidney; and there is no doubt, from various cases which I have seen, and one or two which I shall immediately relate, that it is often very difficult to decide between renal and uterine or ovarian tumours.

CASE 4. *Tumour from puriform collection in the kidney, first perceived after parturition, but apparently depending on the presence of a calculus.*—Ann L—, æt. 29, was admitted, August 26th, 1829, into Martha's Ward, with a tumour in the right iliac region, easily felt, and apparently about the size of a fist,[1] attended with pain in the part and in the situation of the right kidney. Her health had become much impaired, and she had suffered from the date of her last confinement, which happened about sixteen months ago, when a suspicion was entertained by her friends that some injury had been sustained. Her urine was thick, and coagulated on the application of heat. Astringents and tonics were prescribed; she was directed to keep her bed, and to observe the recumbent posture. Her appetite was remarkably good. She is reported to have had occasionally a discharge from the bowels, of puriform matter, in considerable quantity, at which times the tumour suffered some diminution. Her health continued pretty firm till the night of the 23d of September, when she was attacked with symptoms of cynanche tonsillaris, which became very urgent by the morning, apparently from involving the glottis, and she died on the 24th, almost suddenly.

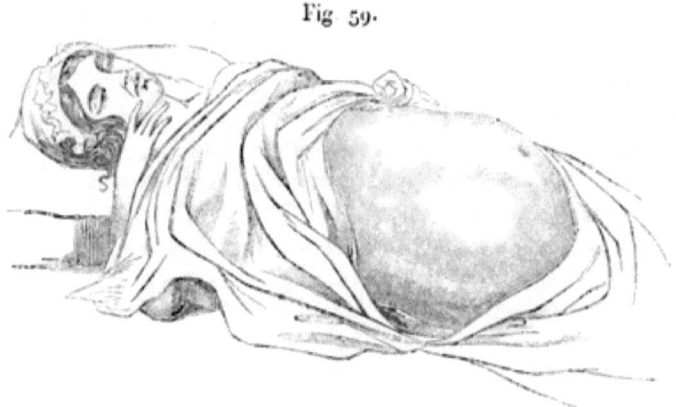

Fig. 59.

Fig. 59. The external appearance of the abdomen, in a case where enlargement had existed in the right kidney, pus being discharged with the urine. This figure is intended to illustrate a very frequent situation of the renal tumour. (See also Fig. 60.)

Sectio cadaveris.—The head was not examined. The contents of the chest were quite healthy. The right kidney was found very

[1] See Figs. 59 and 60, which represent very nearly the situation of the iliac tumour, though taken from another patient.

much enlarged, and on cutting into it, about half a pint of pus escaped. The abscess was in free communication with the pelvis of the kidney, and appeared to have originated there. A small calculus, seemingly composed of the earthy phosphates, was found in the cavity. The walls of this abscess were lined by a thick coating of lymph. The ureter had become firmly adherent to the parts beneath its course, but its canal was still pervious, though contracted. The left kidney was perfectly healthy, as were all the other viscera. The spermatic veins, from their origin to their termination, were considerably enlarged and varicose; this was particularly remarkable on the right side. They seemed in a state perfectly analogous to varicocele in the male. The transverse arch of the colon was passing over the tumour formed by the right kidney, and appeared to have been compressed between that and the parietes of the abdomen.

Fig. 60.

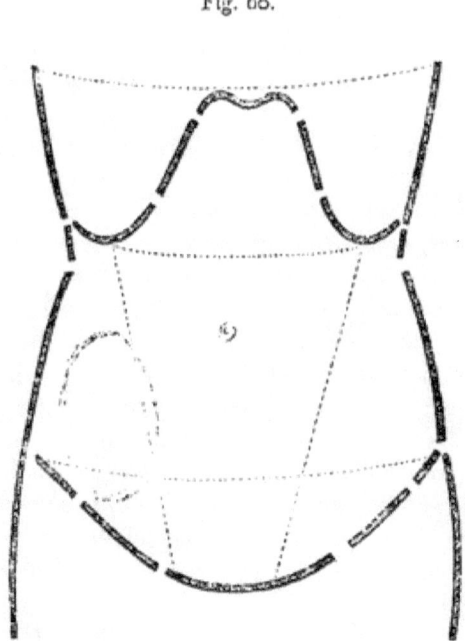

Fig. 60. Diagram representing the situation of the more prominent part of the tumour, in a case where the right kidney was diseased. (See also Fig. 59.)

In this case, as in the preceding, a disordered condition of the bowels had taken place, probably in consequence of the adhesion between the tumour and the descending colon, although it is not stated that any communication was found between the abscess and the intestine; which, however, is by no means an uncommon occurrence.

I was requested to visit the subject of the following case a few days before her death; but having been prevented, I trust to the minute description written by an intelligent student. The morbid appearances I had an opportunity of seeing.

CASE 5. *Large tumour formed by the left kidney, supposed to be uterine, the pelvis being distended with grumous matter, and the substance of the organ suffering, together with the liver, from malignant disease.*—M. A. F—, æt. 42, a tall and muscular woman, whose general health seems to have been good, and in whom the catamenia appeared at the age of fifteen. When about two years of age, she received some injury from a fall, which was followed by occasional paralysis of the bladder and hæmaturia, the latter symptom being present until the age of puberty. Menstruation does not appear to have been regularly performed; the periods of its occurrence frequently being distant, and the intervals marked by a leucorrhœal discharge. Nineteen months ago the tumour was first observed, occupying a portion of the left iliac region, and producing occasional difficulty in micturition and defecation, but no local pain. The tumour continued to increase in size, and, after a lapse of ten months, was found to occupy the whole of the left iliac region, extending as high as the umbilicus, and partly into the left lumbar region. It appeared as if two tumours were present; the one large and in the umbilical, the second small and in the lumbar region; the latter was moveable, and appeared to contain fluid, as it seemed to empty itself partially on pressure. On examination per vaginam the os uteri was found drawn upwards, and on its left edge there was a small induration. The tumour was considered to arise from the uterus.

January 18th, 1839.—Since the time above referred to, the tumour has slowly increased in size, and she has begun to suffer from abdominal pain, and occasional difficulty in passing her urine. Menstruation has not now been performed for the last six months.

The tumour presents a somewhat pyriform outline, the apex of which is towards the pelvis; and although occupying the umbilical region, yet it inclines considerably to the left of the median line, and partly fills the left lumbar and iliac divisions; its greatest diameter is probably about eight inches; it appears to possess a generally even surface, and its structure is yielding and elastic, at one portion affording imperfect fluctuation; the intestines are displaced, being lodged in either hypochondriac region, whilst the ensiform cartilage appears somewhat everted, from upward pressure. Passing across the superior part of the tumour is a band of intestine, apparently held down by adhesions, and which, in some parts of its course, is remarkably distinct.

With the exception of occasional pain in the seat of the tumour, and of difficult micturition, she does not suffer from any immediate effects of her disease; and the most active symptoms are those dependent upon hysteria, a disease from which she suffers considerably. There is some tympanitic distension of the abdomen, and occasional neuralgic pain. There is no derangement of the thoracic viscera.

February 12th.—Is now suffering from considerable constitutional irritation, the pulse being accelerated, and tongue furred; she is complaining of sickness, with thoracic oppression, and some dyspnœa; the abdomen is considerably distended, from the accumulation of flatus; the tumour is evidently enlarged, and appears to be softening, particularly towards the inferior portion, which now occupies the left iliac region, and conveys an indistinct idea of fluctuation (see Fig. 61); the urine is scanty, and upon cooling, deposits a large quantity of the lithates, and if allowed to remain, a portion of purpuric acid is left at the bottom of the vessel.

These symptoms increasing, in spite of the very attentive administration of remedies, she died on the 19th of February.

Sectio cadaveris.—The head was not opened.

On opening the chest, the diaphragm was noticed pushed up on the right side by the liver, as high as the sixth rib.

There were a few adhesions of old formation within both pleural cavities. The lungs were crepitant throughout, though much congested; towards the edges they were emphysematous. The secretion contained within the bronchial tubes of both lungs was rather more viscid than natural; the mucous membrane was also more vascular than in its healthy state. The pericardium was healthy, as was the heart. The abdomen was considerably distended, on account of the left kidney being very much enlarged. The liver was nearly double its usual size, and had encroached very much on the left side of the abdomen. It was extensively affected with malignant disease, forming tubera, from the size of a pea to that of an orange, of a whitish colour, and remarkably hard. The spleen was of its natural size; it was somewhat harder, and its colour darker than natural. The mucous membrane of the stomach, small and large intestines, was congested, otherwise healthy.

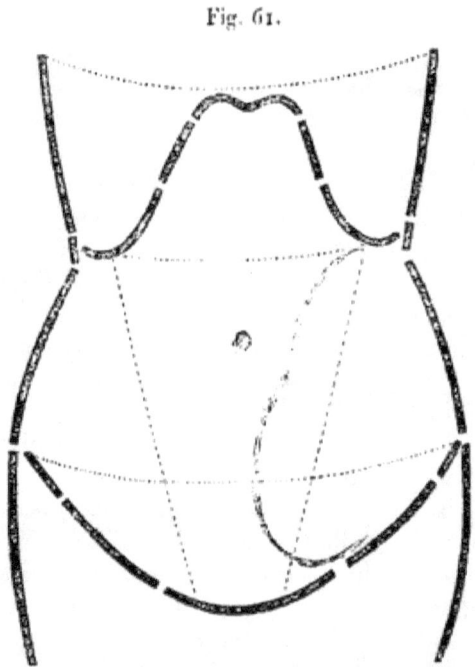

Fig. 61.

Fig. 61. Diagram of the position occupied by the enlarged kidney, where it descends towards the pelvis, and has been supposed to be connected with the uterus or ovary.

The left kidney was much enlarged; it was full ten times the natural size; the upper end of it was adherent to the diaphragm. The pelvis was much dilated, so that it presented the appearance of a large cyst, containing about two pints of fluid, of a brownish colour, resembling coagulated blood of long standing. The infundibula were enlarged, and appeared like several cysts impacted together, communicating with the pelvis of the kidney; each cyst was equal in size to a small pear. Within the pelvis of the kidney there was a mulberry calculus, of the size of a walnut. The left ureter was slightly enlarged. The tunic of the right kidney was easily separable; its structure was slightly congested.

The mesenteric glands were much enlarged, and on cutting into them they appeared affected with the same kind of malignant disease as that noticed in the liver. There was likewise a malignant mass apparently lodged in the substance of the kidney itself, at the upper part.

The following case further illustrates the difficulty which has occasionally been experienced in forming a diagnosis between renal tumour and enlarged ovary. The preparation is preserved at Guy's, though the case did not occur there; and I have copied the report from the records of the museum.

Case 6. *Tumour formed by the kidney dilated with puriform fluid.*—September, 22d, 1827.—Mrs. —, æt. about 34. She was a married woman, and the mother of many children. For about three years she had a tumour on the left side of the abdomen; the exact situation of the part at which it commenced is not ascertained, but it appeared to have been sufficiently low down to have excited a suspicion that it depended on the ovary. It continued to increase, but somewhat slowly; it did not appear to have occasioned constant or severe pain, and the lady bore up against the malady. She gave birth to an infant about four months before her death. Her health continued to decline from the time of her accouchement. Her urine had been scanty and puriform, and a few days before her death she was affected with a most reducing diarrhœa; by the use of sedative enemata it was suspended, and she seemed for a short time to rally.

Sectio cadaveris.—The body had a sallow or rather dusky appearance, and was emaciated.

The head was not opened. The lungs and heart were healthy. The pleuræ were remarkably free from adhesions.

On opening the abdomen, a large but soft tumour was seen occupying the greater part of the left lumbar and iliac regions.

In common with the viscera, it had a dark, dusky, appearance; it had contracted few, if any, adhesions, and having a smooth peritoneal coat, it bore considerable resemblance to a distended stomach. The descending portion of the colon, and part of the sigmoid flexure, passed over it. It was evidently an enlargement of the kidney. Its ureter, which was elongated, and but little dilated, made a tortuous course round it. There was no obliteration of its passage, but the pressure of the tumour had probably been the cause which impeded the escape of the fluid with which the kidney was distended. When cut into, it had the appearance of a membranous cyst; the parietes were in some places scarcely one eighth of an inch in thickness. The interior was of a gray and dusky colour, and though generally, was not universally smooth. The fluid had the appearance of dirty, discoloured, watery pus.

The lining membrane of the bladder was of a deep-livid colour and corrugated; in many parts the rugæ were ulcerated with numerous large granulations, which were soft and appeared to be partially in a sloughing state.

The right kidney was larger than usual, but did not seem to be diseased. Its hypertrophy was probably the effect of the suspension of the function of the left.

The mucous membrane of the intestines was in many places deeply injected, but no trace of ulceration could be discovered.

The uterus and ovaries appeared healthy, and the liver and other viscera offered nothing remarkable.

CASE 7. *Tumour of the kidney, with copious puriform discharge through the urethra, and probably through the bowels.*—April 19th, 1838.—I was requested to see Mrs. B—, in consultation with Mr. Toulmin, of Hackney. I found her an elderly lady, of emaciated aspect, and I was informed that the chief symptom under which she laboured was the passing of pus in the urine, presumed to come from the kidney. Her youngest child was sixteen years of age.

Twenty years before, she had had an attack of gravel, and passed three calculi, larger than peas; from that time forward nothing of the kind occurred, but for the last year and a half she had had some pain in the loins and across the abdomen, with rather frequent calls to pass the urine, and for the last four months some deposit had been observed from the urine, such as at my first visit, with now and then a little streak of blood. For the last month the symptoms had been growing worse, and about three weeks ago she first consulted Mr. Toulmin.

I found her exceedingly emaciated, but able to sit in her drawing-room, as if in tolerable health. The tongue, fauces, and gums aphthous; pulse frequent and weak; complexion and conjunctiva sallow. *She positively denied having any tumour or hardness of the abdomen*, and said there was no sense of bearing down in the vagina. She complained of a little sickness and nausea, and an occasional feeling of chilliness in the loins; she was called up about three times in the night to pass her water, and had some pain in voiding it. Not being satisfied with her assertion, I requested her to go to bed, to afford us an opportunity of examining her abdomen; and I immediately put my hand upon a very large tumour, not less than three large fists, arising probably from the right loin, but *not presenting any great resistance in that part*, advancing forward beyond the umbilicus, and passing down almost to the pelvis of that side. This tumour was hard to the feel, and not the least tender, so that our examination gave no pain. The urine was acid and turbid when passed, depositing copiously a puriform sediment, which, on the application of an alkali, became a thick, tenacious mucus. The remedies we employed were chiefly of a palliative kind, gently to sustain the strength and allay irritation, while a moderately generous diet was adopted. I saw nothing more of her at that time, but occasionally heard very excellent accounts; and these continued, and she gained in flesh and in appearance, never, however, losing the puriform discharge from the urine.

March 16th, 1839.—I again saw Mrs. B——, when I learnt that she continued to do well till near Christmas, when she thought she had strained herself in the loins, since which she had never been well, and for the last fortnight or three weeks had suffered from diarrhœa, and her mouth had again become aphthous; she had lost flesh, but the tumour had not enlarged.

I carefully examined the abdomen; its appearance, at first view, was curious, for the tumour, which was decidedly less than when I saw it before, formed the least projecting part of the abdomen, its inner margin being surmounted by several small coils of intestine, which ran into an irregular knot, and a portion of intestine passed over the part which lay more in the ileo-lumbar region. On applying the hand, it was still more evident that the tumour had rather diminished than increased since I last examined it. The intestines, which could be to a certain degree seen, were more distinctly recognised by the touch; and those which lay on the tumour towards the umbilicus gave a gurgling sensation, and appeared as if fixed to the tumour, and at one point considerable tenderness was experienced; this led me to think it probable that a connexion might be formed in this case between the intestine and the tumour, and in answer to direct questions, we were told that the same kind of matter which used to pass abundantly by the urethra now passed with the stools; a fact, however, which has not been fully ascertained. The tumour, as I have said, was decidedly less than formerly, and evidently lay behind some portions of intestine; it was not very evident in the lumbar space, but still, on pushing the anterior part of the tumour backwards, the motion of the tumour was felt by the hand placed at the loin. The urine was turbid and acid, and on standing, a deposit took place, which, though much less than formerly, was of the same character.

In this case we see some interesting circumstances. In the first place, it presents a very striking illustration of the little dependence we can place upon the observation of our patients, as to facts towards which their minds had not been particularly directed at the time. We should hardly have thought it credible, that a well-informed woman, whose thoughts had necessarily been turned to the state of her health for the last year or eighteen months, and had suffered pain in her abdomen more particularly, should have been ignorant of a tumour as large as the head of a child in that very part; yet, doubtless, this had existed for some considerable time, perhaps almost from the period when her health had first manifestly failed.

A second circumstance worthy of notice was the absence of any great fulness in the posterior part of the lumbar region, leading to the belief that the substance of the kidney had not been so inflamed as to produce adhesion to the lumbar muscles.

In a diagnostic point of view, the manner in which the tumour was traced, situated behind the intestines, is very important, and the probable evacuation of the tumour, by adhesion and ulceration, into the intestines, is an illustration of a not unfrequent portion of the history of such cases.

CASE 8. *Tumour formed by the left kidney, discharging pus copiously both by the urethra and the rectum, depending on a large renal calculus.*—April 30th, 1836.—I was requested to see Mr. A——, æt. about 40, in consultation.

For the last twenty years he had experienced occasional pain in the left side, which he ascribed to a blow; he had likewise, at times, felt pain in passing urine, which was then turbid with deposit; but about three months only before my visit had a tumour been detected or suspected in the left lumbar and iliac regions.

I found him with all the appearances of considerable emaciation. His urine neither acid nor alkaline, with a very disagreeable smell, turbid when discharged, and depositing a thick, heavy pus, on the top of which a little blood was obvious, and sometimes besides this a little clot was passed. The whole quantity of pus passed daily was from four to six ounces.

I had not been informed of any tumour existing, but I immediately detected one, descending far below the umbilicus, hard to the touch, and fixed in the left lumbar and iliac regions. It felt smooth and even, and was rather tender at one point.

June 1st.—The tumour appeared to occupy nearly the situation of an enlarged spleen, but I thought I felt the colon passing over it. (Fig. 62.) The urine passed in twenty-four hours contained only three ounces of pus. The perspirations were profuse.

July 6th.—He had lately suffered a good deal from pain in the left side, and was evidently feverish; he was accordingly directed to leave off the tonic and nourishing medicines and food he had been taking.

15th.—Two days after my last visit diarrhœa came on, accompanied with tenesmus. I now found the tumour greatly diminished, which induced me to ask whether pus had been passed by stool, and though I was answered in the negative, on examining the stools it was quite evident that a considerable quantity was passing. The discharge of pus with urine was undiminished, but there could be no doubt that the abscess in the kidney had ulcerated into the descending colon. For the last two days he had been distressed by a considerable hiccough.

17th.—Hiccough much less during the last two days, but not entirely subsided. The puriform discharge continued, both from the urethra and the rectum.

228   ON ABDOMINAL TUMOURS.

These symptoms were subject to further slight variations; he gradually sunk, and on the 17th of October died, but I had not seen him for six weeks previous to his death.

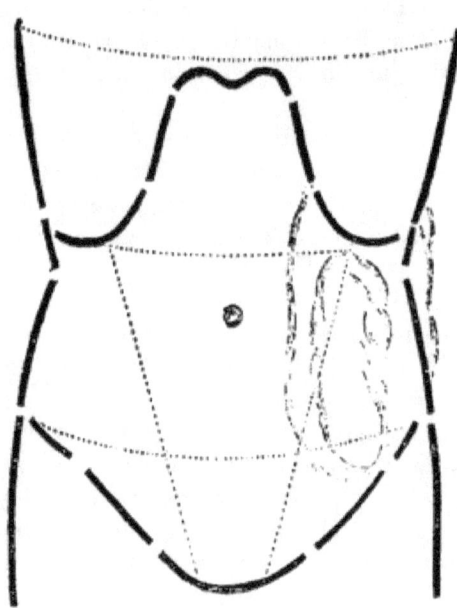

Fig. 62. Diagram of a large suppurating kidney on the left side, showing the relative position of the descending colon.

Sectio cadaveris.—The body was much emaciated, the abdomen sunk in, but the projection of the tumour quite obvious; and fluctuation was so plainly felt in the posterior or lumbar region, that a trocar was introduced, and at least a pint of green pus was drawn off. When the abdomen was opened, the left kidney was seen occupying the space from the diaphragm to the brim of the pelvis, and along its whole length passed the ascending colon, much contracted. The liver very healthy, but the gall-bladder contained very little bile. The small and large intestines were all contracted. The bladder not much distended, and rather thin than in any way thickened, but it was a little vascular. There was a small fistulous opening, not larger than sufficient to admit a goose-quill, from the abscess to the sigmoid flexure of the colon, as it passed over the lower part of the kidney, just at the point where peculiar tenderness had been early observed, and here the intestine looked a little drawn in. The pus was found to have escaped by ulceration into the psoas and lumbar muscles very extensively.

The pelvis of the right kidney was remarkably small, giving the idea that it had never been distended of late, but that, owing to the frequent calls to pass urine, it had been constantly nearly empty. On removing the left kidney, and examining it more accurately, it was found to contain a large, coral-formed, lithic-acid calculus, extending its branches into all the cavities of a sacculated pelvis. The kidney was full of pus, and in several parts cerebriform matter was sprouting into the cavities with most luxuriant growth, into which tufts of vessels were seen entering.

This case affords a very fine example of the ravages inflicted on the kidney, when a calculus of large size is deposited in its pelvis; there is reason to believe that this had been gradually augmenting for nearly twenty years. Here the character of the urine had undergone some change, and it had lost its decidedly acid quality, probably from the constant irritation to which the kidney was exposed, an irritation which led likewise to the development of truly malignant disease in some parts of the pelvis. Here likewise we had a decided communication between the abscess and the descending colon, of which we have one or two specimens preserved in the museum at Guy's. From the mode in which the kidney had enlarged and approached the surface, there would have been no danger in drawing off the pus by means of a trocar, but in all probability it would have been an operation of no permanent utility. I once saw the kidney tapped by Mr. Morgan in a case of this kind, which occurred to him in the hospital, and I lately heard a very interesting case of the same kind related by Mr. Croft, who operated twice or three times, drawing off large quantities of pus, but in neither of these instances was the ultimate result favorable.

CASE 9.—*Cerebriform tumour of the right kidney, supposed to be a tumour arising from the concave surface of the liver.*—October 30th, 1836.—I was requested to see a young woman in the Borough, who had lain-in with a healthy child five months before. The labour had been severe, and protracted through nearly two days and nights. For some weeks she had suckled her child, but had lately been too weak and ill to persist. She was a woman of very delicate appearance, with dark eyebrows and long eyelashes, and was now nearly confined to her bed.

It appeared that, three months before her confinement, she had fallen down stairs and struck her side, and from that time she dated her illness, which, however, was so complicated with the inconvenience of pregnancy that no particular account was taken of her ailments. Soon after her confinement she discovered a small tumour, which she described as having been in the right hypochondriac region, pointing out its situation as nearly on the edge of the liver; but she neglected it altogether till six weeks before I saw her, when she applied to the Surrey Dispensary, and used to be able to walk backwards and forwards to get medicine and advice till within a few days, when her illness increased very much, and new symptoms of an inflammatory character took place, with great pain in the right iliac region and much irritation of stomach, with vomiting; leeches and other remedies were employed, with the effect of reducing the urgent symptoms, but now the tumour excited still greater attention, and soon after this I saw her. It was the only opportunity I had of visiting the patient and I will give the notes I took on leaving the house, in the words I hastily wrote them:

"To the sight, the whole abdomen is large, but the right side projects most; the skin is not in the least distended, but two large superficial veins are seen rising from the right inguinal region, and passing upwards; one lost when it approaches the axilla behind the right mamma, the other disappearing to the right of the sternum. Passing the hand gently over the abdomen, the increased resistance of the right side is evident, and on further examination, it appears that a tumour occupies the lumbar region of the same side and and extends forward nearly to the umbilicus, which seems to be situated lower down than usual, on account of the tumour, which descends almost to the crest of the ilium, where the hand easily grasps it, showing that it has no connexion at all with the pelvis. The tumour forms two large, nearly spherical masses, elastic to the touch. It is not obviously traced under the ribs, because there is a margin of a softer substance which seems there to overlap it. It does not fill that part of the lumbar space precisely which is occupied by the kidney. (See Fig. 63.) It feels to me, all things considered, like a tumour growing chiefly from the under surface of the liver. This, I think, is either hydatid or fungoid, springing from or attached to the concave surface of the liver, but probably not at present disturbing greatly the structure of that organ. Its comparatively rapid growth, and the evident illness of the patient, rather favour the supposition that it is fungoid, and that it is an encephaloid malignant disease of an important organ, probably the liver, though there is no jaundice."

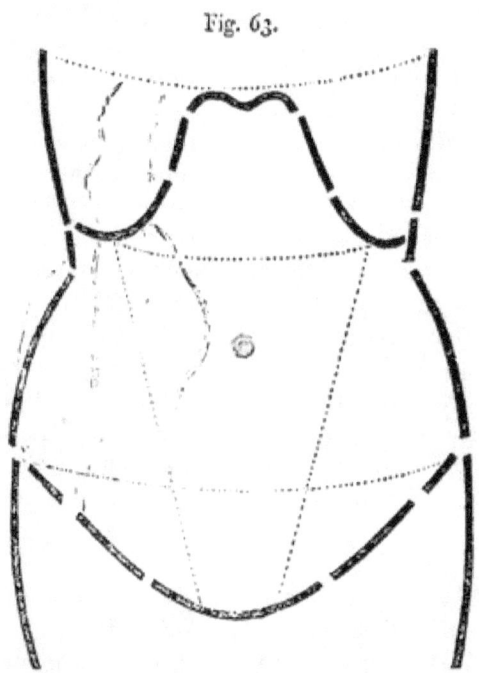

Fig. 63. Diagram of a case where a fungoid tumour of the right kidney was supposed to be connected with the concave surface of the liver. The situation of some large subcutaneous veins is marked.

The only remedies I had to propose were gentle, unirritating laxatives and a supporting diet, which would not increase or re-excite the inflammatory action lately present.

I never saw this patient again, but I learnt that she died exactly a month after my visit, and Dr. Hughes examined the body on the 30th of November. He informed me that, on opening the abdomen, a large encephaloid tumour was found united to the colon and to the duodenum, and on further examination this proved to be entirely the right kidney.[1]

I consider this case as highly important and instructive, showing at once the extreme difficulty of the diagnosis in such cases, and still proving how much may be done, and holding out the hope of more. Here were many facts capable of guiding us as to the nature of the tumour, and had indeed almost led to an exact knowledge of its situation, but that which probably most completely misled us was expecting to find a greater fulness in the lumbar region posteriorly—an indication which I now know to be not always present; on the contrary, the growth of the kidney seems often to take place so much more towards the anterior part, where the soft or yielding viscera afford so much less resistance than the lumbar muscles, that it sometimes happens that very little fulness is perceived in that part. There was another very important indication which was wanting in this case, and that was any unnatural appearance of the urine. Frequently as this symptom is wanting, it is always the most satisfactory when present, and this case is one amongst many which warn us not to infer too hastily, that because there is neither pus nor blood in the urine, the tumour cannot arise from the kidney; indeed, I have learnt, since writing the above, that my friend Dr. Barlow, who saw this case two or three times after I did, actually pronounced it as his opinion that it would prove a tumour of the kidney.

CASE 10.—*Tumour of the kidney from fungoid disease mistaken for the spleen. Death by rupture into the peritoneal cavity.*—Mr. H——, in December, 1828, sent to the museum of Guy's a very large fungoid kidney. It had formed a tumour in the left side of the abdomen of an insane patient. The urine had been

---

[1] In the museum of Guy's Hospital we have a preparation described as follows in Dr. Hodgkin's 'Catalogue': "Section of kidney greatly enlarged by fungoid disease. It contained numerous large, broken-down tumours, of some of which the cysts are ossified. It was taken from a lady between twenty and thirty years of age. The tumour which it occasioned commenced when the patient was a girl, and was at one time thought to be ovarian, at another time it was supposed to be in the liver. A portion of the colon, preserved with the kidney, has tubercles in or immediately under its mucous coat. There are fungoid tubercles in a preserved portion of the liver."

perfectly clear, and the tumour had been supposed to be the spleen. The immediate cause of death had been the effusion of blood from one part of the kidney into the cavity of the abdomen. The pelvis of the kidney was in part distended by fungous matter, and in part by a coagulum, laminated like the coagulum of an aneurism. The ureter and the pelvis were filled with the same grumous matter.

Case 11.—*Fungoid tumour of the kidney, affording the appearance of two tumours.*—In the year 1830, a man was admitted into Guy's, with a tumour which was said to have been first perceived in the left iliac region, and he had latterly been wasting rapidly. He was obviously sinking from visceral disease; his countenance was shrunk, and his whole frame emaciated. It appeared that he had been in the London Hospital about five months before, labouring under fever, and it was on recovering from this that he first perceived the enlargement. On careful examination, the tumour, which lay in the left iliac region, gave to the touch a sensation as if a second, rather smaller, tumour were connected with it, lying a little to the inside. There was a sense of hardness communicated to the touch in tracing the disease upwards, which went almost to the angle of the ribs, but the tumour itself did not seem to go directly to that part. (See fig. 64.) The tumour had been pronounced to be spleen, but from the following considerations I thought it likely that it might be diseased kidney. The patient was positive that he first perceived the tumour in the iliac region, and not under the ribs. The hardness did not run up under the ribs in the manner that the spleen usually does. I felt a division in the tumour, which was marked by softness; and I thought this might be the descending colon passing over the kidney. At the same time the urine afforded no satisfactory indication; for though a little turbid, and even ropy, yet the pressure of any such body upon the kidney might produce irritation in that organ.

He gradually sunk, and in a few weeks he died.

Sectio cadaveris, September 23d, 1830.—Body greatly emaciated; abdomen swollen, and tympanitic.

A small quantity of turbid, brown serum in the abdomen; the intestines protruded forward. The omentum came into view,—a mass of fungoid tubercles, of the size of peas, lying partly above the arch of the colon, and a good deal to the left side over the spleen. The sigmoid flexure of the colon was seen passing into the pelvis, over a large tumour, to which it was firmly glued. The whole peritoneum was studded with small fungoid tubercles, more particularly

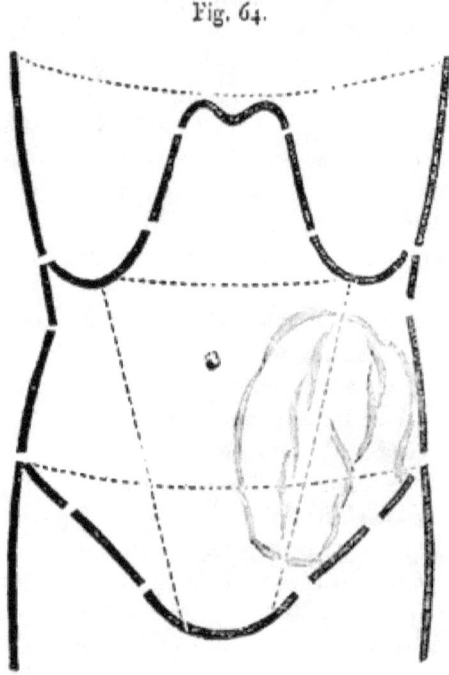

Fig. 64. Diagram of the tumour formed by the left kidney, over which the distended colon was felt to pass. (See Fig. 65.)

the part lining the parietes; the same tumours covered the lower surface of the diaphragm in the same way, and they formed a thick mass along the lumbar vessels. (Fig. 65.) The thoracic side of the diaphragm was affected in the same way. But the most singular appearance was on the surface of the lungs: not only were some hard tubercles seen, of the size of small seeds, but there was a network of the same hard substance beneath the pleura, formed apparently between the small lobules of the lung, consisting of a deposit of the same morbid matter. Spleen small and healthy.

On cutting into the large abdominal tumour it was found to consist of a yellow, fungous mass, into which a few vessels might be traced; but altogether it broke down, like curd which had scarcely been pressed together, or like the fatty matter often found in the ovaries with hair and teeth, but it had no smell. The exact connexion of the mass with the kidney was a matter of great doubt. Part of the kidney was sound, but firmly compressed, and this mass appeared to be at least within the capsule of the kidney, if not in its substance.

Fig. 65.

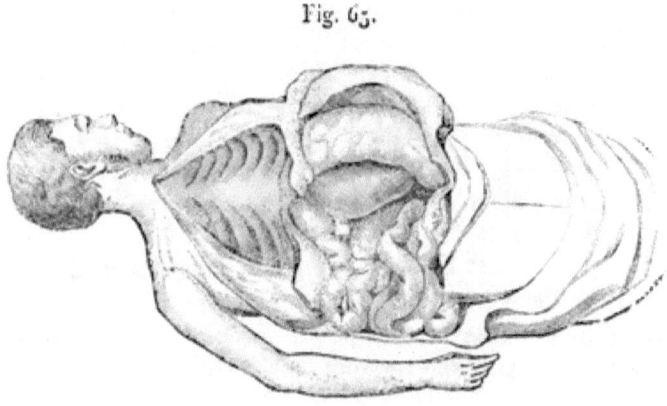

Fig. 65. The appearance presented on opening the abdomen, in a case where the left kidney was greatly enlarged. The descending colon, much distended, is seen passing over the tumour, and dividing it in such a manner as to give to the touch, before death, the impression of a double tumour.

By this inspection, it became evident that the hardness which appeared to go towards the left hypochondrium was occasioned by the diseased omentum lying over the colon and over the tumour, and the second body which was felt was a portion of the kidney separated by the colon.

CASE 12.—*Fungous disease of the glands of the mesentery, resembling enlarged kidney.*—Mr. Hardy brought to Guy's a curious specimen of tumour, from a woman æt. 50, supposed, during life, to be ovarian tumour, and ascribing its origin to a fall from a carriage, on the abdomen, about three years previously.

This tumour had been largest on the right side, and on opening the abdomen the muscles were found glued to a part of it. Dividing these, a little below the umbilicus and near to the pubes, a collection of fetid pus was displayed, extending deeply into the mass; about this part several of the mesenteric glands were white and fungous, and a number of the lumbar glands were involved in the same disease.

On cutting into the principal tumour, at first it appeared that it was an enormously distended kidney, in the pelvis of which, apparently, a large quantity of yellow, cheesy substance, not unlike scrofulous matter, had been deposited, distending it so greatly as to compress the substance of the kidney, giving it the aspect of a cyst, in the sides of which the bundles of the tubular portions could just be discovered. This mass of disorganized matter was going into suppuration; about one fourth was reduced to a greenish pus. On further more minute inspection, it was discovered that this was really a large glandular mass, which had compressed the kidney on the outside into a flattened substance, and was, in fact, quite external to the kidney.

The substance of the uterus was thick, and contained three or four small tubercles. The neck was thickened and diseased, enlarged into a tumour about the size of the natural uterus, projecting into the vagina and pressing on the rectum.

The cases which I have thus brought together will, I trust, be found to contain a pretty faithful record of facts applicable to the greater number of cases of renal tumour which may occur in practice, and will, perhaps, serve both as a guide and as affording lessons of caution. The great difficulty of diagnosis will, I think, be readily acknowledged, and several of the sources of that difficulty have been illustrated by striking examples. And what adds greatly to the perplexity of these cases is the frequent immunity of the patient from many of the constitutional symptoms by which we are apt to expect that renal disease will be accompanied. All those symptoms connected with the stomach—all those symptoms depending on the deranged absorbent system—all those symptoms connected with the brain and nervous system—and even those indications which the urine itself affords, are often entirely wanting during the whole period that the disease is submitted to our care; for the fact is that, in most of these cases, one only of the kidneys is materially affected, while the other carries on all the functions usually performed by both, to a sufficient extent to ward off the mischief which a highly diseased, a greatly diminished, or an inordinately increased secretion of urine never fails to produce. And it is not unusual to find that the healthy kidney has been considerably enlarged, from the fact of its having been called upon for more than its accustomed labour, affording a beautiful illustration of the importance of a double organ, and the compensating power which nature, within certain limits, occasionally exerts.

In the foregoing cases we have instances of suppuration of the kidney of two kinds—where the disease seems to have begun in the substance of the organ itself, and where it has been, apparently, almost entirely a purulent secretion from the pelvis, and this latter is by far the most common in cases which afford any enlargement of the organ capable of being discovered before death. In these cases, the whole kidney becomes reduced almost to the state of a thick, sacculated membranous, bag, the lining of the pelvis being brought so nearly in contact with the external tunic that nothing but a thin and condensed layer of the substance of the kidney separates them; but there is still no apparent breach of continuity or suppuration in the substance of the organ, nor does it appear to have commenced in that way. Frequently, however, after some time, fungoid growths spring from the lining membrane, and frequently the tendency to extend and to suppurate is not bounded by the organ itself; and the most common result is, that an opening is formed into that portion of the colon which passes over it. This process, even before the communication is fully formed, is often attended with diarrhœa, which, in the already weakened condition of the patient, adds greatly to the urgency of the disease; and when the ulceration has extended into the intestines, much puriform matter is evacuated. At other times, the tendency seems to be rather to the formation of an external opening. I do not remember to have met with a case in which it has opened of its own accord in that way; but where the fluid has approached so near the surface as to lead to the evacuation by the lancet or the trocar, it has again and again accumulated. There is at least a third way in which the pus may escape, and that is, by ulceration or rupture into the cavity of the abdomen. It is not very probable that this effusion of pus should take place by ulceration, because it very generally happens that the adhesive process prevents such a result, but it is more probable by accidental rupture, and then would most likely prove fatal. The kidney, it will be seen in the foregoing cases, is very subject to malignant disease; and we have in Guy's Museum specimens of all the various kinds, from the hard, white tuber to the softest form of cerebriform cancer or the genuine hæmatoid fungus, and these intermixed with the true melanotic deposit which occasionally occupies this organ most extensively in its simple form; and it is remarkable that in all these forms of disease, as likewise in the scrofulous affection of the kidney, a large part of the bulk of the tumour is formed by some kind of morbid deposit within the pelvis of the kidney itself. Amongst the cases I have related one will be found, where the fungoid disease had led to a large effusion of blood into the cavity of the abdomen, and in this way had proved fatal. The more common mode, however, in which this form of disease terminates, is by wearing out the powers of the patient, frequently inducing diarrhœa, and favouring the destructive progress of some apparently accidental attack of inflammation.

CHAPTER V.

DISEASED LIVER.

It is proposed, in the present chapter, to follow out the subject of abdominal tumours, drawing the illustrations from the LIVER, as has already been done in previous memoirs from the ovary, the kidney, and the spleen, and from the development of hydatids.

The great and important organ to which I shall now refer has justly claimed the constant attention of the physician; but it is certain that, even in this case, prejudice has occasionally outrun the dictates of sound judgment, and symptoms depending upon the heart, the lungs, the spleen, the stomach, the colon, or the kidneys, have been hastily and pertinaciously ascribed to the derangements of the liver, and hence the value of every diagnostic aid which experience can afford.

In seeking to render our diagnosis as correct as possible in any case of hepatic disease, we are necessarily led to attempt to discover the size and form of the affected organ—a task in many cases difficult, if not impossible; and sometimes, when performed, liable to lead us astray, unless we carefully take many other circumstances into consideration, but at other times affording us the most important information towards the discovery of disease.

One of the chief sources of difficulty in ascertaining the size and form of the liver, depends upon the situation of the organ, for it is so placed, with regard to the ribs and the diaphragm that, in its most perfect state of health it is almost as much concealed from the sight and removed from the touch as the contents of the cranium. Another difficulty arises from the liver being liable to displacement, from causes independent of disease within itself as, from occasional, though not very frequent, deviations from its natural position, and from pressure exerted upon it by effusions within the right cavity of the chest, or from tumours between the liver and the diaphragm.

And a third source of difficulty is found in the induration and enlargement of neighbouring organs, as of the right kidney, the stomach, the omentum, and the colon. But in spite of all these embarrassing circumstances, we are able, in most cases, by the aid of careful examination, by the external appearance, by the feel, and by percussion, to arrive at a very satisfactory knowledge of the size and form of the liver, when it deviates in these respects materially from its normal state; and our diagnosis is greatly assisted by the attendant symptoms and the general condition of the patient.

The large right lobe of the liver, in its healthy state, lies completely in the hollow formed by the diaphragm, not descending below the margin of the ribs, and extending upwards to between the sixth and seventh ribs on the right side. The left lobe usually extends to the soft space below the ensiform cartilage, a short way into the left hypochondriac region, and a portion of its lower margin is thus seen lying across the scrobiculus cordis when the body is opened, and is frequently the only part of the organ which is visible.

As a necessary consequence of this situation, the healthy liver influences very little the sound produced by percussion on the soft part of the abdomen, which, if all the organs are free, healthy, and empty, is usually clear and sonorous, from immediately below the margin of the ribs to the very lowest part of the pubic region. If, then, the sound in any part be dull, it is our business to ascertain the extent and connection of such unnatural sound; and in this way, if we can trace an uninterrupted dulness to the margin of the ribs on the right side, our suspicions may fairly be excited that the liver is the origin of the disease. The more perfect and the more practised the ear, the more likelihood there is of tracing the deviations of sound from their natural clearness; but in some cases of very extensive disease, where the liver or other organs are irregularly enlarged or tuberculated, the investigation is most difficult; and yet, according to my experience, the touch, however tutored, is still more fallible than the ear, in cases of extensive tubercular or fungoid deposit in the abdomen. We must never suffer ourselves to be led into the error of denying the existence of hepatic tumour because the dulness or the hardness are so extensive that they appear to reach beyond the probable bounds of the liver, for, in fact, there is no tumour of which the abdomen will admit so large that it may not be an enlarged liver, and if we can satisfactorily trace the continuity of the dull sound, or the hardness under the ribs of the right side, while no other obvious indication leads us to ascribe it to another organ, we may legitimately consider the liver as the seat of the disease. Still, I confess that we shall not be always right; for such are the difficulties, that infallibility is not to be obtained.

There is another error to be avoided, which is, considering the rapidity with which the tumour has appeared to be inconsistent with the idea that it can have originated from the liver; for we find tumours of the most extraordinary extent generated in the liver in a few weeks; nor are these always attended with such remarkable pain as might be expected under such rapid distension of structure. When the local symptoms or physical signs leave us at fault, we turn to those which belong to the general condition of the body. Thus, for instance, disease of the liver seldom exists long without producing a peculiar appearance in the countenance of the patient. In some cases, as we shall see, actual jaundice, and that of the most decided character, accompanies hepatic tumours; but many of the more formidable conditions of the liver are indeed but slightly marked by this symptom. Still, the approach to the jaundiced state, the sallow cheek and temples, and the lightly-tinged conjunctiva, are most often present when disease has greatly altered the structure of the liver, or gone on to the formation of tumour. To this, however, there are remarkable exceptions, so that the absence of the symptoms should never lead us to repudiate the idea of hepatic disease. Fungoid growths to a very considerable extent may occupy the liver, and yet no jaundice, and no approach to it, may be present; and one very remarkable change of the whole substance of the liver may proceed to the great and obvious intumescence of the organ, without producing a shade of yellow in any part of the body;—I refer to the fatty intumescence of the liver, which, however, has been often traced by its own peculiar effects upon the skin, as pointed out by Dr. Addison.[1]

Gradual or rapid emaciation, with a peculiar cachectic aspect, frequently accompanies disease of the liver, though even this is far from constant; for there are certain forms of disease in which the liver is enlarged, and which are marked rather by an increased deposit of fat in the cellular membrane of the body, and in the omentum and mesentery, than by emaciation. The state of the

[1] 'Guy's Reports,' vol. i, p. 479.

bowels and the stomach greatly assists our diagnosis. Hæmorrhages taking place from the stomach and intestinal canal, and effusion of serum into the cavity of the abdomen, are amongst the symptoms which call our attention to the condition of the liver, and often strengthen our diagnosis.

The tumours depending upon the liver vary greatly in the extent they occupy, as also in their characters; sometimes descending scarcely below the margin of the ribs, and sometimes encroaching upon the pelvis. They are sometimes smooth and even, sometimes lobulated, with greater or smaller inequalities on the surface; sometimes soft and yielding, sometimes hard.

In attempting to describe hepatic tumours, I shall adopt an artificial twofold division, into *smooth* and *irregular*, depending on their obvious forms, as ascertained externally; which will nearly, though not altogether, coincide with the arrangements which might arise from the nature of the several diseases on which they depend. But before entering upon the consideration of these tumours themselves, it will be well to clear away, or at least to point out, some of the more prominent sources of error, with regard to hepatic enlargement.

Amongst the many sources of such mistakes, by which physicians may be misled, and induced to conclude that the liver is the seat of disease when in fact it is not, feculent accumulations in the colon are perhaps the most frequent, and they lead to a deception the more complete, because they occasionally imitate, in the most striking manner, enlargements of this and other organs, and appear to afford a decided and tangible evidence of disease such as few can withstand, even to afford time for making trial of remedies, which, by acting freely on the bowels, might at once show the cause, and remove the tumour. Cases bearing upon this point are of very frequent occurrence; and I have before me the short notes of four, which have taken place in my own practice—three of them within a few months of the time at which I am writing; and although I intend to avail myself of another opportunity of speaking more particularly respecting the tumours which depend upon diseases of the colon, I shall not scruple to introduce these cases now, because intimately connected with a most important consideration with regard to the diagnosis of hepatic enlargement.

CASE 1.—*Accumulation of fæces in the sigmoid flexure of the colon, imitating organic tumour.*—August 1st, 1840.—I was requested to see a young gentleman who had been brought to town a few days before, convalescent from a severe attack of purpura, followed by extensive pleuro-pneumonia. He had been seized in the night with bilious vomiting, great prostration, with writhing pain in the abdomen. The pulse was frequent and small, the countenance sunk and pallid, and I found considerable tenderness on pressure; there had been one small motion the day before, and another that morning, but I could see neither. The first idea which suggested itself was of some serious obstruction of the bowels or hernia, amongst other causes. I inquired for any pain towards the groin, and on placing my hand low down in the left iliac region, not far from the internal ring, I felt a distinct tumour (Fig. 66, *d*). The part of the abdomen between that and the margin of the ribs on the same side was more tender than any other, and somewhat tense. I naturally felt uneasy, lest some mechanical or organic cause should exist. The tumour was more diffused than any ordinary hernial protrusion, and yet its more prominent part felt circumscribed; it did not dilate on coughing.

A poultice was applied over the left side of the abdomen, and two grains of calomel with half a grain of opium were ordered; effervescing draughts, with excess of alkali, were given to allay the sickness; and a large injection of soap dissolved in water, was thrown up. These remedies having been repeated two or three times, we procured before night a large feculent evacuation of solid lumps, and the tumour in the iliac region was quite removed, and all the symptoms subsided.

In this case, the situation of the tumour did not lead to the supposition of hepatic tumour; but had the fæces been delayed in the transverse instead of the descending colon, they would have presented the physical signs of loaded liver, as the following case, which occurred a few weeks before, had done.

Case 2.—*Fæcal accumulation in the colon, imitating hepatic enlargement.*—I was requested by Mr. Baldwin to see an old gentleman in the city, confined for several days to bed, gradually becoming jaundiced; the tongue furred; appetite gone; pulse excited; no sleep; considerable general enlargement of the abdomen, with some tenderness; frequent hiccough, and some retching; the bowels were reported to be by no means constipated; and some of the motions which I saw were well supplied with bile, and not scanty. On examining the abdomen more carefully, there was a distinct hardness discovered, which I concluded to be the liver, extending from the margin of the ribs on the right side to below the umbilicus. (Fig. 66, c.) For some days we continued to treat him on the supposition that some organic change had taken place; and were of course very apprehensive of the result. We gradually, however, began to suspect that the bowels were scarcely enough acted upon, and we increased our purgatives; the compound decoction of aloes with senna and alkali, and the compound galbanum pill with blue pill and extract of colocynth, were largely administered; and the quantity of feculent matter which we daily had the opportunity of seeing was almost beyond belief. All the swelling gradually subsided; the dulness on percussion gave way to the clear sounds of the hollow viscera; the jaundice disappeared; the appetite returned; and in a few weeks the patient was completely restored, and is now in perfect health, without the vestige of hepatic lesion. In this case I have not the slightest doubt, that however much the liver was gorged, as in all probability it was, the greater part of the enlargement and dulness felt in the hepatic region was from feculent matter confined in the colon. In cases such as this, there can be little doubt that a combination of circumstances conspires to the fulness of the hypochondrium; and that the liver becomes congested as a consequence of the loaded bowels; for where the colon is not distended, we sometimes find the hepatic fulness; and we likewise find it yielding to the action of remedies chiefly of a purgative quality, in a most remarkable manner.

CASE 3.—*Fæcal accumulation in the colon, imitating fungoid tumour.*—On October 1st, 1839, I was requested by Mr. Newton to see a patient affected with a tumour on the right side of the abdomen, respecting which there had been much diversity of opinion. The patient was about thirty years of age, of a peculiarly exsanguine aspect, more nearly approaching to the appearance of the most marked case of chlorosis. I learned that, three years ago, he had suffered from an inflammatory attack of the bowels, which had been followed by other attacks; and that his bowels had always continued irritable, yet requiring occasional assistance from purgatives; that about a year ago he had first perceived a tumour in the right iliac region, which had gone on constantly increasing to the present time. I found it now occupying pretty nearly the situation where a tumour at the curve of the duodenum might be supposed to appear; it was of the size of an orange, and was somewhat moveable. (Fig. 66, *b*.) I learned that some months before it had been much more moveable, and had changed its place, as if by gravitation, according to the movements of the body. I felt myself quite unable to give a decided opinion as to its nature and situation, but was inclined to consider it an independent tumour, unconnected either with kidney, liver, or any other organ; perhaps attached to some fold of the peritoneum. As the bowels were very irritable, and generally purged, I ordered fifteen minims of the liquor potassæ to be given in the infus. cuspariæ, three times a day, and the emplastrum ammoniaci c. hydrarg. to be applied locally.

October 18th.—I saw him a second time. The medicine had been taken regularly, and the tumour was rather softer; but though still moveable, found that the space between it and the margin of the ribs was dull to the sound, as if an elongation of the liver were extending to it, or as if a body forming in the omentum had become attached to the liver, for it was evidently close under the parietes. Then I likewise entered in my note-book, as a question, whether it might possibly be a collection of fæces in the colon.

November 22d.—I again saw him. He had suffered from a severe attack of diarrhœa and sickness for the last ten days; he looked pale and thin, and had relinquished the liquor potassæ on account of the diarrhœa. The tumour was certainly much diminished, and was but indistinctly to be discovered; which of course excited our strong suspicion that it was a collection of fæces. Still, however, it did not entirely disappear under purgatives; and we supposed that the fæces formed but part of the tumour. Shortly after he was put upon the use of the tinct. ferri muriat.

March 29th, 1840.—I was particularly requested to call, that I might see the great improvement he had undergone. I found that the chalybeate had been persisted in; but about three weeks ago, the bowels becoming constipated, Mr. Newton, who watched the case most carefully, resolved upon trying a large injection of soap and water. This was immediately followed by the passing of some remarkably hard lumps of fæces, and, encouraged by this, he had repeated the injection every day; and now the tumour was not to be felt. I could just perceive a little knot, probably a slight thickening of the ascending colon; but the tumour was gone.

In this case we have the most striking illustration of the way in which feculent accumulations are calculated to mislead; for this tumour had been most confidently pronounced some months before, by a very high authority, to be malignant. And this case further presents a good explanation of some of those reported cures of tumours to which various localities and origins have been ascribed.

CASE 4.—*Fæcal accumulation in the colon, imitating malignant disease of the liver.*—A. B—, a seafaring man, æt. about 55, was admitted into Guy's Hospital, under my care, with a hard lobulated tumour about midway between the point of the ensiform cartilage and the umbilicus, in which he suffered considerable pain, both from pressure and without it. (Fig. 66, *a*.) His complexion was sallow, his bowels stated to be freely opened. After careful examination, I had very little doubt that the tumour was organic, and connected with the left lobe of the liver, nor did the effect of remedies, or the appearance of the patient, at all undeceive me for some weeks; but I presently began to suspect that the pains, of which he made such frequent complaint, were rather of a spasmodic character, and such as indicated some detention of fæces in the intestine. I therefore put him on a more decided plan of purging than at first, though the bowels had never been neglected. He now took repeated doses of compound extract of colocynth, galbanum pill, blue pill, and small quantities of muriate of morphia. The effect was, after a few days, to bring away a quantity of hardened balls of fæces; and, in proportion, to diminish the supposed malignant tumour, till both pain and morbid growth, and every other symptom of disease, had disappeared.

I could multiply such cases considerably; but those which I have stated, showing accumulation in each different portion of the large intestine, will be sufficient for the present object. I should in general be inclined to say, that whenever an abdominal tumour occurs in what may be considered the course of the colon, we

Fig 66.

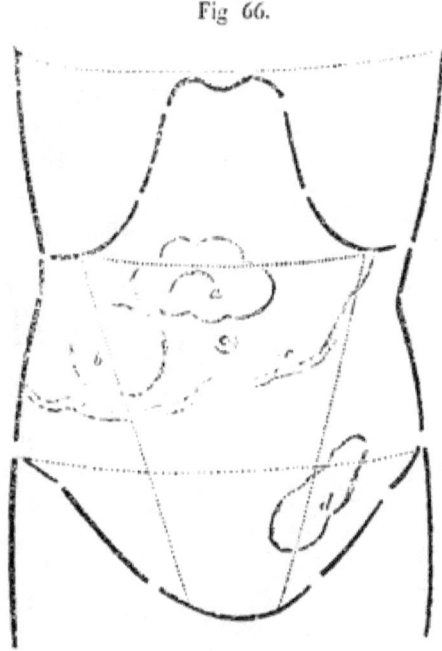

Fig. 66. Diagram representing the situations of tumours in four different cases of feculent accumulation in the large intestines.

    a. A nodulated enlargement, existing for many weeks, from fæces in the arch of the colon. (Case 4, p. 246.)
    b. A round tumour, continuing and slowly increasing for many months, from fæces in the ascending colon. (Case 3, p. 244.)
    c. Extensive hardness occupying the whole space included within the double line, to the scrobiculus cordis: chiefly depending on large acumulation of fæces in the colon. (Case 2, p. 243.
    d. Tumour from recent feculent accumulation in the sigmoid flexure of the colon. (Case 1, p. 242.)

should be very guarded in our diagnosis: and yet this will hardly cover all the possible cases of deception; for the colon is itself, of all the viscera of the abdomen, that which varies most in its course; so that scarcely a month passes in which we have not an opportunity of witnessing some variation; as an illustration of which I may refer to the diagrams (Figs. 67, 68, 69), which represent three sketches, all made by me within ten days of each other. In one, the arch of the colon suddenly descended below the umbilicus; in another, the sigmoid flexure advanced beyond the same point; and in the third the sigmoid flexure performed two complete convolutions, the least of which ascended to the duodenum where it commences in the stomach, and then descended to the pelvis.

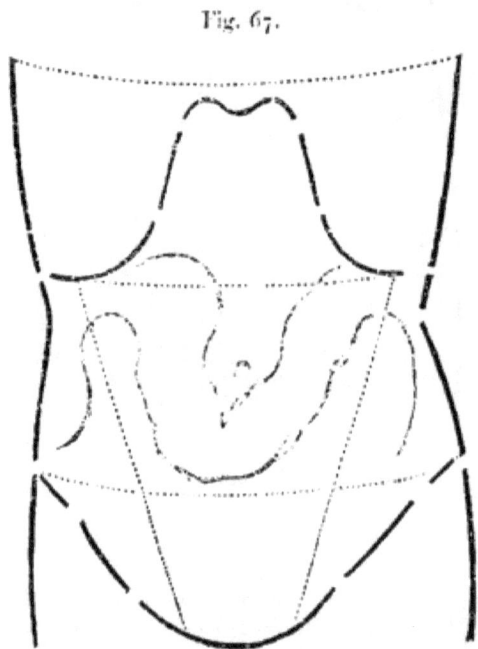

Fig. 67.

Figs. 67, 68, and 69, varieties in the natural position and extent of the colon.

Fig. 67. Diagram, showing the course of the arch of the colon descending considerably below the umbilicus.

I was present at the examination of a child who had died of croup, this week; when we found the sigmoid flexure even more voluminous than in this last case.

Another source of difficulty in diagnosis is to be found in disease of the kidney; and this is a difficulty of frequent occurrence; for though the kidney seldom enlarges in such a way as to push the right lobe of the liver before it, yet it often presents itself as a tumour, proceeding from the under surface of the right lobe; and as it has sometimes attained a considerable size before it has been detected, it has been supposed to be continuous with the liver, and a growth from its substance. There are, however, many circumstances in the situation of renal tumours, as well as of the accompanying symptoms, which afford great assistance in their detection; but I shall content myself with referring to what I have already said pretty fully upon this point of diagnosis, in a chapter especially devoted to the consideration of renal tumours, in a former part of this work;[1] and I would more particularly refer to the observation in p. 210, and the ninth case, p. 237, as affording illustrations of this subject.

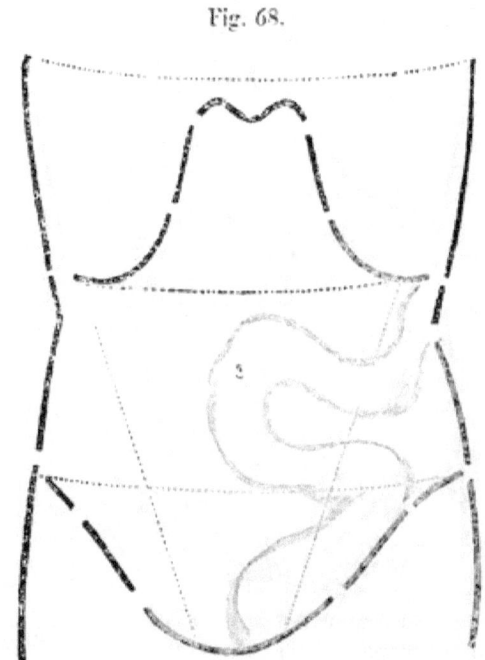

Fig. 68. The descending colon advancing to the umbilicus.

Disease of the stomach might be mistaken for tumour of the liver, particularly of the left lobe; but this will not often occur. The small curvature, when scirrhous, and particularly when fixed by

[1] See previous chapter.

disease to the liver, resembles greatly hepatic tumour. A malignant tuber in the stomach likewise, or a malignant thickening of the whole of that organ, may at first sight deceive; but strict examination, particularly by percussion, will demonstrate the cavity beneath, and show that the disease is situated in a hollow viscus. In general, the pain referred to the stomach, and increased or excited by eating, the frequent nausea or vomiting, the marked emaciation, and the absence of the more remarkable symptoms of hepatic disease, will enable us to determine that the tumour belongs rather to the stomach than the liver.

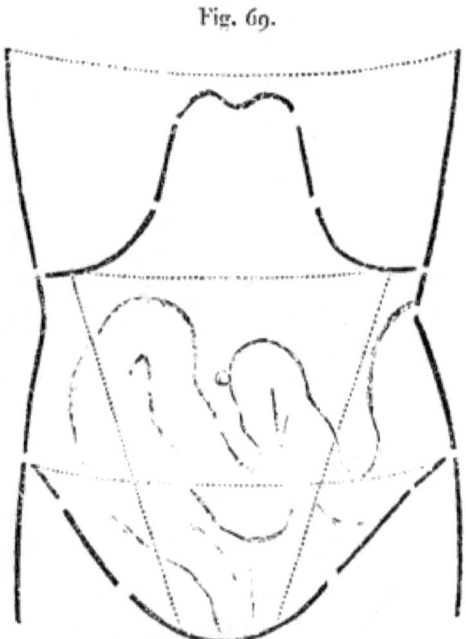

Fig. 69.

Fig. 69. The sigmoid flexure forming two complete convolutions; and extending nearly to the margin of the ribs on the right side, and into the right hypochondriac region.

A much more frequent source of difficulty is to be found in the omentum and peritoneum, which may undergo many changes, and assume a very near resemblance to the liver studded with tubera or enlarged by disease; in most cases there will be found an obvious separation between the tumour and the liver, and a space where the colon or the stomach emits a clear sound on percussion; and the hard portions in the enlarged abdomen will be separated in a manner which will prove that they are not connected with the liver; there will likewise be an absence of many of the symptoms of hepatic disease. I will however detail one case in which the peritoneal change was such as to render it peculiarly difficult to speak positively; and although it might perhaps be better introduced when speaking of the tumours depending on the peritoneum, I have preferred detailing it in this place, as well calculated to illustrate the subject before us.

CASE 5.—*Malignant disease of the peritoneum resembling hepatic tumour.* (Fig. 70.) I was requested on the 22d of November, 1830, by Mr. Fernandez, to see C. R—, æt. 44, a shoemaker by trade. The account we obtained was, that about a year ago he first felt a small lump below the ensiform cartilage; and the hardness seemed to increase across the stomach at the upper part, gradually extending downwards, to the present state; for some months he had occasionally vomited his food, and for the last six weeks this had happened constantly, about half-an-hour after eating,

Fig. 70.

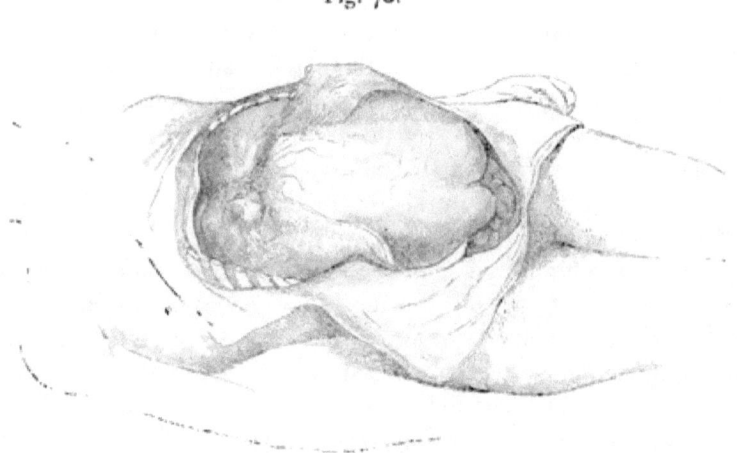

Fig. 70. Appearance of the peritoneal tumour when the integuments were first removed. This mass, closely representing the enlarged liver in its form, was very hard, and of a malignant character.

without pain or difficulty; though the nurse said that what he vomited was of a dark colour, having both the appearance and smell of fæcal matter. The stools were dark. His countenance pallid, but not sallow; and he had never had anything approaching to jaundice. On examining the abdomen, there were two or three projecting lumps, of the size and nearly the shape of half an egg, near to the scrobiculus cordis; and the whole upper part of the abdomen presented one uniform hard substance, almost as firm as cartilage, giving a general and equal fulness to the abdomen; this hardened condition extended almost to the pelvis, where there was a distinct lobulated margin to be traced, in the form of the lower margin of the liver; this descended lowest on the right side, but also was low on the left, where one or two lumps were to be felt, like independent tubers separated from the general mass.

I afterwards saw this man once or twice; but no material change took place, except increasing exhaustion. He died on the 9th of December; and on the 11th, Mr. Fernandez kindly afforded me an opportunity of being present at the examination.

Sectio cadaveris.—Body emaciated and pale, a general hardness over the whole abdomen, almost to the pelvis; and at the pit of the stomach, a distinct rounded projection. On removing the external integuments and muscles, the peritoneum remained thickened to nearly a quarter of an inch in some parts; and when this was thrown back, a large mass, very firm, and nearly the colour of fat, presented itself, descending into the pelvis, and there assuming the form of the liver, with a division between its lobes. This mass extended upwards, so as to push the diaphragm before it, and assume nearly the form of that muscle, in expiration. Raising this mass from below, the intestines came into sight, pushed chiefly to the left side, and covered with rounded masses of a semi-gelatinous form and appearance, assuming quite the disposition of fungoid disease, sprouting up, and growing in botryoidal forms, and giving an indistinct vesicular appearance, when cut through. Many of these fungous masses were arranged near the point where the mesentery joins the intestine, and some were quite pendant by threads not less than half an inch; and some had three or four such threads supporting them, apparently vessels. Many were seated upon the mesentery, or on the intestine. A large mass had formed between the rectum and bladder.

On examining more carefully the large mass which filled the

greater part of the abdomen, it was found to be almost entirely formed of the adventitious structure, and the liver and stomach were both included in its substance; the liver not greatly altered in its colour or texture, but dwindled in size; and the stomach greatly contracted, and rendered quite irregular through its whole internal surface, so that the cavity bore no resemblance to the natural form or appearance. This mass likewise descended to the kidneys, which were partially imbedded in it. It could be raised from its lower margin like an enlarged liver, and then the intestines were displayed; but the fungous granulations from the different parts had produced some adhesion. The texture of this mass was quite vesicular, and though it seemed formed of numerous cysts of almost equal size, not larger than sweet-peas, so that great part of it presented a rather uniform texture, it was evident that it assumed, in some of its loose and less-restrained portions, the structure which Dr. Hodgkin has ascribed to malignant growths, and in many of the cavities a gelatinous matter had collected, as in the ovarian dropsy.

The lungs were remarkably healthy, collapsing most completely when the chest was opened; but on the pleura were several little transparent fungoid bodies, like those in the abdomen, which particularly arranged themselves, in one or two instances, in lines along the inferior margins of the ribs. On the upper surface of the diaphragm also, which, below, adhered to the liver, several fungoid bodies of the same characters were growing.

The peritoneum covering the diaphragm was greatly thickened by the same morbid growth, and adhered to the liver; but this adhesion was rather from close apposition than from a welding together of the substance; for they were easily drawn asunder, and the projecting vesicles from the one seemed then to fit into the depressions of the other.

I procured a portion of the intestine, to be injected; and the size ran into the tumours so as to colour them; the size being very distinct in vessels, particularly near the peduncles and junctions with the intestine. On dissecting the tumours, it seemed that the peritoneum covered the lower parts; but it was so much attenuated on those more distant from the origin, that it was not demonstrable; from the appearance, however, of many parts where the disease looked like a nodulated thickened transparent peritoneum, and did not rise up in highly-projecting tumours, there was reason to think that the disease began beneath the peritoneum; and it was confined to the two great serous membranes of the abdomen and thorax.

I sent a portion of the tumour formed on the peritoneum surrounding the liver to Dr. Babington, requesting his opinion as to its composition, and the following was the answer I received:

"My dear Doctor,—I have examined the substance with which you have furnished me, and find that it consists almost wholly of inspissated mucus. It is, with the exception of the cellular tissue in which the substance is contained, soluble in water at the common temperature, also in alcohol; soluble, however, with difficulty, as mucus usually is. When in solution, it is not precipitated by heat or alcohol, or acids, or tincture of galls, or oxymuriate of mercury, or sulphate of zinc; but subacetate of lead, which is Dr. Bostock's test for mucus, throws it down abundantly. The mineral and vegetable alkalis dissolve it, producing a dark, nearly opaque solution; which, on dilution, has a dirty reddish-brown colour. From this solution a neutralization of the alkali does not again precipitate it. It does not contain a particle of albumen, if we except the cellular tissue; and, in short, comports itself exactly as that tough transparent mucus from the bronchi which is often coughed up in little masses, and is called, I think, by Laennec, 'pearly sputa.'

"The odour of this substance, as it is now beginning to putrefy, is peculiar, resembling stale though not yet putrid fish, much more than putrefying meat.

"Believe me ever yours,
"B. G. Babington."

Previously to death, it had been a question, in this case, as to what organs were the seat of disease; and the general history of the gradual development of the tumour lead to a conclusion that it was either the liver or the omentum, but no decided opinion could be formed.

On reviewing the circumstances, there seem to have been some which might serve as diagnostic in this case.

The two tumours near to the ensiform cartilage were rounded and egg-shaped; not flattened in the centres and circular, as is usually found with large malignant tubera in the substance of the liver. The general surface of the mass was tolerably smooth; certainly presenting no nodular bodies, as in tuberous diseases of the liver. The tumour was unusually hard and unyielding. There were one or two rounded masses to be felt in the left iliac region, which were separated from the original mass. There was at no time jaundice, or even icteric sallowness.

All these circumstances, when compared with the appearance, become at once explicable, and might certainly have assisted in the diagnosis.

Another source of error exists in the displacement of the liver, by disease in the right side of the chest; for it frequently happens that extensive effusion, or consolidation of the lung, either from pneumonia or malignant disease, depresses the liver so much as to render the sound of the right hypochondrium most remarkably dull for several inches below the ribs; and then it is by no means uncommon to find the medical attendant fully convinced that the liver is enlarged; and probably now, if not before, he is induced to doubt whether the previous inflammatory attack did not belong to the liver, rather than to the lung or pleura.

Case 6.—*The liver pushed down by fluid in the right side of the thorax.*—Mr. — came under my care June 14, 1836. He had been affected with pleuritis six months before, and though somewhat relieved, was labouring under all the symptoms of effusion into the right cavity of the chest. There was a hard tumour in the abdomen, occupying the situation of the liver, but descending almost to the umbilicus. There were no hepatic symptoms; and finding the right side of the chest without vesicular respiration, and perfectly dull on percussion, and at the same time hearing the history of the case, I had no hesitation in concluding that the tumour depended upon the liver having been pushed down by the fluid in the chest. And accordingly, in proportion as by diuretics, mercurials, and other means, the fluid was absorbed, the tumour in the abdomen receded.

In October, a severe relapse took place, with a return of the same symptoms, with irregularity of pulse, swelling of the legs, &c. He became again better, but in February had an attack of influenza, with renewed inflammation of the lungs and pleura, and ultimately sunk; the liver being at that time to be felt slightly below the ribs.

Sectio cadaveris.—On opening the abdomen, the liver came into sight, descending an inch or two below the margin of the ribs. Its surface appeared unhealthy, owing to an opalescent thickening of its peritoneum, which was perfectly smooth, but showed lines of greater opacity, as if marking out an incipient stage of the hobnail degeneration. On cutting into its substance, however, no such change was discovered, and the only altered appearance was the coarseness of structure which follows the frequent congestion of the vessels.

The heart was large and dilated, with thin parietes. The two auriculo-ventricular openings were large and dilated, so that the valves must have acted imperfectly. The aortal semilunar valves also slightly deranged, but not decidedly diseased. Half an ounce of dark-coloured fluid in the pericardium.

The whole of the right cavity of the chest filled with a puriform fluid, enough to fill a wash-hand basin. The lung compressed to the size of an orange, of which the upper half only admitted air very imperfectly; the remaining portion was pressed together, so as not to admit any air; and it sunk immediately in water. It felt soft, tough, and yielding; and was surrounded by a thick layer of lymph. The pleura was universally covered with a very thick deposit of successive layers of lymph, which on the outside was flocculent, and imbued with pus. The left lung healthy, but unusually adherent.

In this, as in almost all similar cases, there will be a combination of causes, bringing the liver below the margin of the ribs; for we seldom find extensive effusion into the cavity of the chest without the liver having suffered in its substance from congestion, which produces an actual, and not a mere apparent, enlargement of the liver; and such was, in fact, the case in the present instance.

CASE 7.—*Apparent tumour of the liver, owing to that organ being pushed down by pleuritic effusions.*—George S—, æt. 45, was admitted into Guy's Hospital, under my care, October 17th, 1832. He stated, that he had suffered from cough above a year and a half; and that he had got much worse since January last, now nine months ago. For the last month he had experienced anasarca, both of the legs and face. His extremities were cold; his countenance sallow and bloated; his lips purple; his mind bewildered; right side of the chest quite dull on percussion. There was an obvious tumour occupying the scrobiculus cordis nearly to the umbilicus, and extending to the right side. It was not very hard, giving way, however, bodily, on pressure. It did not yield the slightest tympanitic sound on percussion, while all other parts of the abdomen did. Pulse 112, rather sharp.

  Pil. Scillæ cum Hydrarg., No. i, et Pulv. Digit., gr. j, o. n.
  Mist. Camph., ʒij, et Liq. Ammon. Acetat., ʒss, ter die.

19th.—Has passed a number of loose, green stools during the night.

  Mist. Camph. cum Sp. Æth. Nit., ʒss, et Tinct. Camph. Comp., ♏. xx,
   ter die.
  Rep. Pil. o. n.
  Applicetur Emplast. Lyttæ inter scapulas.

20th.—He had a sudden attack of dyspnœa, which was relieved by powerful doses of æther, squills, and ammonia; but he died the next day.

Sectio cadaveris.—Heart large; aortal valves bony; one valve lacerated and bony; several thin opaque, almost cartilaginous spots on surface of heart; aorta pretty healthy. Left lung—bronchial membrane irritated. Right cavity of chest filled with a large quantity of serum, so that the lung was compressed into a very small space, and a portion was carnified; liver not unhealthy in structure, but rather enlarged from congestion, presenting a good specimen of the nutmeg liver, in which the internal portions of the acini had become comparatively light coloured, while the external portions, or the interstices, were highly congested. All the intestines were of a deep colour, from congestion; the spleen hard, large, and loaded with blood; kidneys hard and fleshy.

In this case, as in the last, but in a still higher degree, the tumour felt in the region of the liver arose from combined causes; partly from the congestion of the organ itself, though chiefly from the large quantity of fluid with which the right cavity of the chest was filled.

The same effect, but almost in a greater degree, may be occasioned by tumours, or unnatural growths, or deposits of any kind, situated between the upper part of the liver and the diaphragm.

CASE 8.—*Abscess situated between the diaphragm and the liver, producing apparent enlargement of the liver.*—August 6th, 1834. —A boy was admitted into Luke's Ward, under the care of Dr.

Back, labouring under bronchitis. He became rather suddenly the subject of a very large swelling in the situation of the right lobe of the liver; but passing over, in a cushion-like tumour, towards the left side. No hepatic symptoms presented themselves. It was leeched and other remedies employed; and at a time when it seemed to threaten great mischief, it rather suddenly diminished to a great extent; and then it very naturally became a question whether this had been a highly congested state of the liver from the bronchitis, or whether it might have been fæces in the colon, or whether some abscess in the liver had found means to discharge itself. The relief obtained was very temporary, and on the 11th of August he died.

Sectio cadaveris.—The lungs bore decided marks of bronchitis and of pneumonia; the right lung was adherent to the diaphragm. A large abscess was situated between the diaphragm and the liver, pressing down the latter. Its parietes completely insulated it from the general peritoneal cavity; but it had so compressed the right lobe of the liver, as to produce the complete appearance of an excavation in that organ, as an empyema seems to scoop out the lung with which it lies in contact. The surface of the liver, however, was not broken; so that there was no trace of bile in the abscess.

In this case, there is no difficulty in understanding the apparent tumour of the liver, which was itself perfectly healthy. It is not quite so easy to say why the tumour became suddenly diminished, as there was no evidence that any quantity of pus had made its escape.

The deviations from the natural position of the liver, with which I have met, have been very few; but where they do occur, they must necessarily present difficulties in diagnosis scarcely to be overcome. I have never been present at the examination of a body in which the organ was transposed, but I have seen the left lobe so much elongated and enlarged, without any disease in the structure, as to vie with the right in size; and in other cases to extend across to the left hypochondrium, reaching quite to the spleen. I have also seen, in one case, the liver placed behind several coils of intestine, so that whatever had been its size or extent, percussion would have yielded a clear sound.

Case 9.—*Small intestines situated anteriorly to the liver.*—Mr. B——, a man of about 50 years of age, with sallow complexion, had consulted me frequently, in the last two years, for a loathing of food, and a sense of sickness of stomach without vomiting. Bowels costive, but he suffered much from the action of purgatives. He spoke of pain at the scrobiculus cordis, running back to the spine, and up the centre of the chest. He obviously became emaciated, and his symptoms were altogether such, that I suspected for some time malignant disease, though I could not specify its situation. In the last year of his life, cough affected him, and symptoms of phthisis pulmonalis were plainly developed.

In March 1835, I was apprised of his death; and an opportunity was afforded of examining the body. On viewing it, there was marked emaciation; but the most careful examination through the integuments afforded not the slightest trace of tumour or glandular enlargement. In the apex of each lung were old phthisical cavities, and some tubercles in other parts. The heart healthy, but small and flaccid. Towards the pyloric extremity of the stomach were two or three small round ulcers. Pylorus healthy; duodenum granulated. There were several ulcers in the ileum, particularly near the valve, and also in the colon. The mesenteric glands, near the ulcers, slightly enlarged; liver healthy; pancreas congested; spleen twice its natural size; kidneys healthy, but discoloured by congestion.

Such was the condition of the several organs; but the most remarkable circumstance was, the relative position of the abdominal viscera, when the abdomen was laid open. Neither the liver nor the colon presented itself to view, but, in their stead, the convolutions of the small intestines, which were found to have come completely in front of the liver, the colon and the omentum doubling over the liver, and pressing it back, so as to have made deep furrows in its anterior surface.

With this curious malposition of the organs, it is quite obvious, that no clue could have been derived from touch or percussion, whatever had been the diseased condition of the liver. And in this case, had a tumour formed in the right lobe, one important aid to diagnosis would have failed; for upon finding, on percussion, that the hollow viscera lay in front of the tumour, the legitimate deduction would have been, that it belonged to the kidney, or, at all events, originated from the lumbar region.

I have seen great difficulty arise when the left lobe of the liver alone has been involved in disease, or where the disease of that lobe has been greatly disproportioned to the disease of the right lobe; of which the following case furnishes a good example.

CASE 10.—*Malignant tumour confined entirely to the left lobe of the liver, and ascending towards the thorax.*—A. C—, æt. 59, was admitted, under my care, into Guy's Hospital, November 6th, 1839. She was a widow, and her health had never been robust, as she had frequently suffered from rheumatic and dyspeptic complaints. She dated, however, her present illness only six weeks back, at which time she had been wet through, and was attacked with rigors, flushes of heat, and great thirst, with pain in the left side, which she says had existed in a less degree for some time before. This pain was aggravated by a cough and deep inspiration.

At the time of her admission, her countenance was expressive of much suffering; and she complained of great pain in the left side, near the angle of the ribs. In the left hypochondriac region, just below the margin of the false ribs, there was a tumour of the size of a large fist; very tender on pressure, and protruding, in a very obvious degree, the lower ribs. Tongue brown and dry; urine passed in moderate quantities, depositing the purpurates, and not coagulable by heat.

The right side of the chest, anteriorly, yielded a clear sound on percussion, and the respiration was natural. On the left side, anteriorly, it was dull on percussion, as high up as between the second and third ribs, and no respiration was heard; posteriorly, it was dull on percussion, the respiration tubular, and there was bronchophony. The sounds of the heart heard more to the right of the sternum. She died in ten days; and the following account of the appearances after death was furnished me by Mr. Noyes:

Sectio cadaveris.—The body was slightly emaciated, and somewhat tinged with a yellow colour. Brain was healthy, as far as regards the structure; but the arteries were thickened.

On opening the chest, the diaphragm was noticed to be pushed up by the liver, as far as the third rib on the left side; but on the right, only as far as the sixth. The left lung was pushed up very high, as far as the seventh rib; but there was a small portion which was situated lower down, posteriorly, and which appeared much compressed; they were otherwise healthy.

The heart was pushed up, and more to the right side than natural.

Abdomen.—On opening this cavity, a large tumour presented itself; this was situated in the left hypochondriac region, and originated within the left lobe of the liver, which pushed the stomach to the right side. The tumour within the liver was of the size of an adult's head, and of a rounded form; its external surface was firmly adherent to portions of the lower surface of the diaphragm, and posteriorly to the spleen and kidney. (Fig. 71.) On cutting into the

Fig. 71.

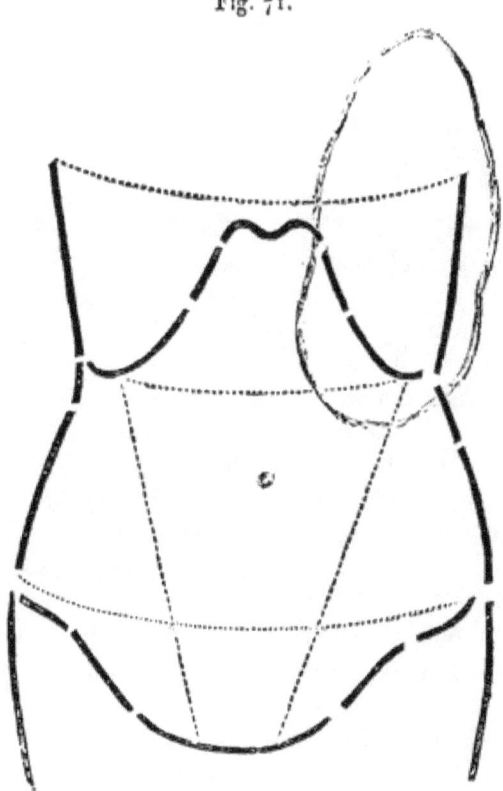

Fig. 71. Diagram, showing the position of a tumour in the left hypochondrium, and encroaching upon the left lung, depending on disease of the left lobe of the liver.

tumour, it was found to be of a fungoid nature (fungus hæmatodes), originating within the structure of the left lobe of the liver, internally; it was in some parts rather soft, of a dark-red colour, resembling a clot of extravasated blood; whilst in others its structure was of a pale colour, resembling cerebriform cancer. In other places, the surface of the liver presented a hob-nailed appearance; it also contained a small portion of fat. The gall-bladder was healthy.

The spleen was firmly adherent to the tumour; much pressed upon so as to be elongated, and its structure fleshy.

The left kidney was much pressed upon by the tumour, so as to be flattened; tunic easily separable, and the structure healthy. The right kidney was of the natural size, but the tunic was quite adherent, and the structure somewhat granular.

The other viscera were healthy.

The difficulties which a case like this presents to accurate and decided diagnosis are but too obvious; for the stethoscopic signs resembled very closely those which consolidation of the lung would have furnished, while the protrusion of the ribs might have originated from effusion within the cavity of the chest; nor did the imperfect history of the painful attack in the left side, by which disease was ushered in, serve much to diminish the difficulty. The continued and increasing pains were not, however, likely to be the accompaniments of the ordinary results of pleuro-pneumonia, although they were not inconsistent with malignant disease in the chest; and the hardness of the tumour to be felt below the ribs was unlike anything which is usually produced by pleuritic effusion, and could scarcely have been referred to disease in any other organ but the left lobe of the liver, the spleen, or the stomach. The complete immunity of the right lobe of the liver tended greatly to obscure the diagnosis.

Besides the difficulties which have already been enumerated, as opposed to unerring diagnosis, we must not omit to mention, that the spleen, when diseased, has occasionally been mistaken for the liver, and the liver for the spleen; errors into which we may easily fall, when the left lobe of the liver is particularly affected, or is supposed to be so: nor is it an unusual thing to find both liver and spleen enlarged at the same time. It must likewise not be forgotten, that ovarian tumours encroaching in their progress upon the right hypochondrium, and on the upper portions of the abdomen, have not only by careless and ignorant men, but by the skilful, been pronounced hepatic. I shall not, however, enlarge upon these topics, but rather refer to what has been said in two former memoirs, in which I have endeavoured to point out the diagnostic symptoms of ovarian and splenic tumours.[1] And I shall now proceed to describe some cases of actual enlargement of the liver, adopting, as I have said, a division into the SMOOTH and the IRREGULAR forms of tumour.

In the first of these diseases may be included enlargement from the passive congestion of blood—from acute or subacute inflammation; from retention of bile; from chronic hypertrophy; from fatty changes with intumescence; and from diffused malignant disease.

In the second division—tumour of irregular form—may be included abscess, both acute and chronic; hydatids; the result of chronic inflammation, producing irregular contractions in the cellular membrane of the liver and permanent roughness of its surface; malignant disease in the several varieties of the scirrhous, cerebriform, and melanotic deposits.

SMOOTH TUMOUR, OR TUMEFACTION OF THE LIVER FROM SANGUINEOUS CONGESTION.

The most simple form of hepatic enlargement is that which results from sanguineous congestion, where the increase in size is entirely owing to the unnaturally distended condition of the blood-vessels. This form of disease is by no means unfrequent in its less aggravated degree, apparently connected with loaded bowels making pressure upon the returning veins; and probably, with the deficiency and sluggishness of the peristaltic action of the intestines, encouraging delay in the circulation of the blood; which again, when once collected in the liver, proves an additional impediment to the onward progress of the stream. When the liver is thus loaded with blood, it gives rise to many of those ailments which are variously denominated dyspeptic or hypochondriacal, interfering with the digestion;

---

[1] See Chapters III and IV.

and oppressing the nervous energies of the whole system, and sometimes mechanically impeding the action both of the heart and lungs. A slight fulness is perceptible on the right side, and the ribs are a little raised. To the hand, the space below the ribs is more resisting, and even hard; and although there is no defined tumour, the edge of which admits of being traced, the dull sound which is elicited by percussion an inch or two below the margin of the ribs contrasts strongly with the clear sound of the hollow viscera which ought to occupy that space.

The enlargement from sanguineous congestion, in the limited degree of which I have spoken, may be difficult to ascertain; but there is a degree of congestion betraying itself most manifestly by the enlargement of the organ, which descends several inches below the ribs, and may be felt as a hard, full cushion, with a defined margin, sometimes on a level with, and sometimes below the umbilicus. In cases of this kind, besides the defined character of the tumour, we have usually a peculiar sallowness of the complexion, which more especially directs our attention to the liver; and that sometimes to such a degree, that experienced physicians have been led away entirely from the primary disease on which the hepatic congestion depended, which is generally some obstruction of the circulation in the heart; and I have known, in this way, a patient supposed to sink under hepatic disease, while ossified valves and enlarged and distended heart have been the true cause of all the symptoms. In such cases, it is true that the liver, from being simply gorged, becomes gradually disorganized, passing from the nutmeg liver of distension, to the permanent yellow and red liver, in which probably some adventitious deposit or some permanent change of character has taken place; but this is most decidedly a consequence of previous appreciable disease in another organ.

The following case affords a very marked example of the secondary affection of the liver, which frequently follows obstruction in the circulation through the chest.

CASE II.—*Liver enlarged, and altered in its structure, from frequent congestion.*—Jane K—, æt. 30, was admitted, under my care, into Guy's Hospital, labouring under anasarca and ascites, with great dyspnœa. The lower extremities were swollen and purple; and both feet and hands were cold. There was a purring sensation communicated to the ear, applied to the heart; but no distinct bruit. The abdomen contained much fluid, and the liver was plainly to be traced nearly as low as the umbilicus; it was tolerably smooth and even to the touch, but unyielding and hard, and decidedly tender, on pressure. The countenance was slightly jaundiced, but the cheeks, nose, and lips, purple. Urine high coloured, in moderate quantity, and not albuminous; dejections bilious. Pulse 104, and irregular.

It appeared that she had borne one child, about twelve years ago, and was in good health till about seventeen months ago, when, in consequence of some quarrel, she ran a distance with violence, under great alarm, and was exceedingly exhausted and out of breath; since which time her chest has never been well, and to that unusual exertion she ascribed all her after-ailments.

I acted freely on her bowels with calomel and colocynth, and applied a poultice to the right side. She passed daily two or three stools, tinged with bile, but irregularly mixed. The urine was generally loaded with lateritious sediment. On one occasion, ten ounces of blood were taken, by cupping, from the right side. The tumour was still very distinct, but not so extensive; the countenance still retained its orange tint, and the tongue was dry; but the rest and quiet of her situation had diminished the anasarca, and removed the severe oppression of the chest; and on the 24th of August she left the hospital at her own request.

October 24th.—She requested me to see her at her own house. She told me, that for a month after leaving the hospital no particular change took place; but she always suffered much pain in the right side, just below the margin of the ribs. She then had a bowel attack; the stools became very frequent, her calls almost constant; the matter passed was of various appearance, sometimes like soap-suds, sometimes red, sometimes brown; never like ordinary feculent matter. During a whole week this discharge continued from the rectum, at the end of which time she had passed at least a pailful, and her abdomen was reduced to its natural size. I could not find out that any tumour was discovered when she was so reduced; except she says it felt hard at that part where she complained of pain. At the end of a week the discharge ceased; and since that time her bowels have been always costive, though daily there is some relief. Her condition, when I visited her, was most distressing; the abdomen very large and shining; the fluctution most distinct throughout, although there was some anasarca in the integuments. The legs swollen, almost to the utmost; the feet and knees purple; the hands a little swollen, also purple; anasarca very great about the loins.

She was quite unable to lie down; she could hardly incline to either side; her countenance greatly distressed; cheeks purple, lips more so; in respiration, all the muscles of the neck were called into action. She said, at times, for half an hour she was obliged to "fight for her breath;" then for an hour or two, was rather better. Four days before, rather suddenly, she had first been troubled with cough, which had since been a most troublesome symptom, with some mucous expectoration; there was considerable mucous rattle in her chest; the action of the heart very irregular, tumultuous in the highest degree; pulse at wrist of same character, but very weak, and often quite lost.

She struggled on but for a few days, and then sunk.

Sectio cadaveris.—General anasarca, more particularly of legs and thighs; some lividity of the hands and depending parts of the body.

The lungs adhered closely in almost every part; they were a good deal gorged with blood, and contained some serum. There was a serous cyst, of the size of a small egg, in the fissure between the lobes on the right side.

The heart presented a most extraordinary appearance, occupying a very large portion of the space opened in the chest, when the sternum was removed; and as it lay undisturbed, the right auricle formed at least half of the whole which was exposed. (See Fig. 72.)

On opening the cavities, the right auricle was found to contain about eight ounces of coagulum, like currant-jelly; and several masses of fibrin, mixed with clot, were fixed between the muscular fibres of the appendix. The whole muscular structure of the auricle was prodigiously enlarged, so much so that it had more the appearance of the columnæ carneæ of the ventricles, forming complete fleshy pillars.

The left auricle was quite small and contracted, the foramen ovale closed, the ventricles both contained some rather loose clot; there was nothing like separation of fibrin. The parietes of these cavities were thin, and rather flabby.

The semilunar valves of the aorta were healthy, except that the corpora Arantii were rather large. The tricuspid valve, and the valves of the pulmonary vessels, were healthy.

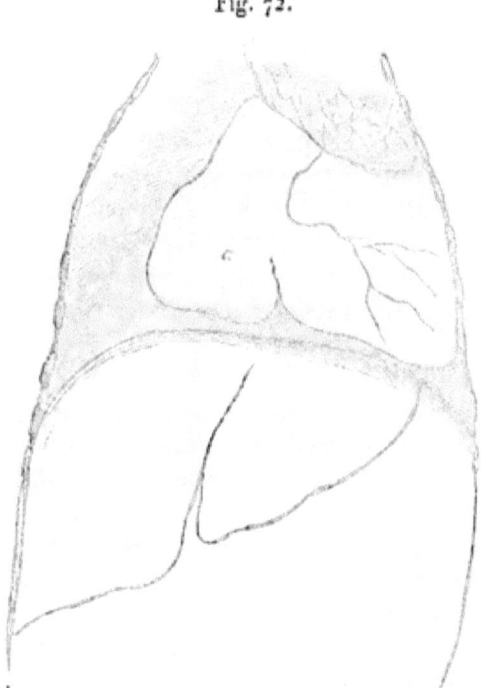

Fig. 72.

Fig. 72. Sketch representing the relative positions of the heart and liver, in the case of Jane K—. The liver gorged with blood, and pushed down by the heart, which occupies an unusual space in the thorax.

a. The situation of the right auricle, greatly distended with blood.

The opening of the mitral valve was contracted to a slit, into which the point of the little finger was with difficulty introduced; and at the corners of the slit, where the two curtains united, was a peculiar appearance, as of some rupture or abrasion of the surface; the whole was thickened, hardened, and congested, but not ossified.

In the abdomen there was nearly a bucketful of pale serum, in which were many shreds of lymph, some of which adhered to various parts, but more particularly the upper part of the intestines, evidently the product of inflammatory action.

The liver was considerably enlarged, and somewhat uneven on its surface; and was throughout mottled, and somewhat granulated. The whitish-yellow specks looked almost like miliary tubercles; but they were only the acini, enlarged and degenerated, set off by the red interstitial parts loaded with blood, owing to the difficult transmission of that fluid through the chest.

The gall-bladder was moderately distended.

The spleen was small, considering the general state of congestion.

The intestines were of a pinkish colour, from inflammation, and the mucous membrane was evidently irritated.

The most careful investigation, carried on with the view of discovering whether there was the least probability of any rupture or false passage having been formed, through which the fluid could have passed from the cavity of the abdomen into the intestines, convinced us that nothing of the kind could have happened; there was no unnatural adhesion, or appearance of ulceration or rupture, throughout the whole alimentary canal. There was a slight adhesion of the gall-bladder, but it was quite superficial.

In the pelvis, the bladder was contracted, the uterus rather round and thick, but healthy; the ovaria congested, almost cartilaginous. The Fallopian tubes appeared pervious, and the fimbriated extremities were red, and I could well have imagined that the fluid had found its way through the uterus; but both the patient and the friends were so positive that it passed by stool, that it was hardly possible to doubt their correctness.

In the spaces between the bladder and uterus, and between the uterus and the rectum, there was a slight ecchymosis under the peritoneum, looking like the effect of bruises, probably from pressure of the fluid.

Kidneys healthy.

This case, while it serves as an example of one of the most frequent causes of great and often-repeated hepatic congestion—disease of the heart—shows the change which is ultimately produced on the liver. That organ had here become permanently altered, so as to present a finely tuberculated appearance throughout, and some roughness on its surface, not perceptible by external examination. The case is very analogous to two which I have just related (Cases 6 and 7), but in which the organic change had made little, if any, progress; and in this, as in other cases, there was a mechanical cause of pressure in the chest, which probably augmented the size of the tumour during life.

INTUMESCENCE OF THE LIVER FROM INFLAMMATION.[1]

It is to be presumed, that in most cases of inflammatory action the bulk of the liver is more or less augmented, in the early stages at least. But it often happens, that the evidence of inflammatory action exists in the pulse, the skin, the tongue, and the altered secretions both from the bowels and the kidneys, and yet no very decided fulness is perceptible in the right hypochondrium; but more frequently we find, on passing the flat hand gently over the part, that it experiences a little more resistance, and a little more sense of fulness, as it arrives at the right side; and, on careful examination with the points of the fingers, we discover the margin of the liver descending from one to two inches below the cartilages of the ribs; and, on applying percussion, the sound is dull over a corresponding space. Sometimes the part is so tender that these investigations can scarcely be borne; while, at other times, the patient complains little at the moment pressure is made, but suffers considerably from aching pain in the part for some time afterwards. The tumour thus produced is somewhat resisting, but not indurated, and it gradually subsides, as the general symptoms of inflammation are subdued. Leeches and the assiduous application of poultices are the local remedies indicated, while bleeding from the arm, mercury with or without opiates, and antimonials, together with free action on the bowels, are the constitutional remedies, which can scarcely be safely dispensed with, where so important an organ, and one so apt to run into suppuration, is inflamed.

I shall not think it necessary to advance cases in reference to this particular form of hepatic enlargement; it forms a single and, as I have said, not a constant symptom in hepatic inflammation; but is, I think, more frequent in those cases which tend to suppuration, and the formation of abscess, than in those on which simple jaundice so often depends.

[1] See 'Guy's Hospital Reports,' vol. i, p. 604.

INTUMESCENCE OF THE LIVER FROM ACCUMULATION OF BILE.[1]

A third form of smooth enlargement of the liver is produced by the bile being retained, so that it accumulates in the biliary ducts. In such cases, the liver gradually enlarges, and may be felt as a tense smooth tumour, descending toward the umbilicus, and proceeding onwards almost to the pelvis, while it nearly fills the right lumbar space. Pressure is productive of some pain, which often lasts for many minutes. In such cases, we are usually directed in our diagnosis by the very decidedly yellow suffusion of the skin; and, in many cases, by a peculiar rounded tumour projecting from the lower margin of the liver. This will, however, depend upon the cause of the detention of bile in the liver. I believe that it very rarely, or perhaps never, happens that the liver is greatly gorged with its own secretion, unless some decided mechanical obstruction exists. When sanguineous distension takes place to a considerable degree, the bile is certainly more or less retained in the small tubes, and produces a jaundiced tinge on the skin; but here the obstruction is only partial, and is not fixed, and the degree of bilious congestion, compared with the sanguineous, is but small.

The circumstances under which I have seen the liver decidedly loaded with bile to distension, so that the bulk of the organ has been enlarged, and manifest swelling produced, have been tumours, or morbid deposits, pressing on the large excretory ducts, or biliary concretions impacted within them. If the obstruction thus produced occur in the hepatic duct, the tumour of the liver takes place, and the organ is distinctly to be traced gradually descending from the margin of the ribs, towards the pubic and the iliac regions, presenting a smooth and even surface. The whole, dull on percussion; and this dulness ascending to the sixth and fifth ribs of the right side. If the obstruction be lower down, occupying the common duct, the same enlargement of the liver takes place; but gradually we perceive the margin of the liver deviating from its even line, and a globular projection protruding itself downwards, of the size of a small egg. This projecting portion of the tumour yields, on pressure, the elastic feel of a deep-seated fluid; it increases, and becomes more tense, and often seems to project above an inch beyond the distended line; in which case it descends almost to the

[1] See 'Guy's Hospital Reports,' vol. i, p. 606.

pelvis, being generally situated somewhat to the right of the mesial line, and on a level with the crest of the ilium. This tumour is the distended gall-bladder. In both these cases, the surface of the body is of a deep yellow colour, but I have suspected that it has not been so deep when the obstruction has been in the hepatic as when in the common duct; of this, however, I am by no means confident; but if it be so, the difference must arise from the change which takes place in the bile after it gets into the gall-bladder, to which, when the obstruction is higher up than the entrance of the cystic duct, it of course never gains access.

In one of the cases I shall now detail, a singular combination of obstructions was discovered after death, and while the enlargement of the liver, and the strongly-marked symptoms of jaundice, depended upon obstruction in the common duct, the distended state of the gall-bladder was immediately owing to a gall-stone in the cystic duct; so that the fluid which the gall-bladder contained was not bile, but the mucous secretion of the gall-bladder itself.

CASE 12.—*Tumefaction of the liver from retention of the bile.* (Fig. 73.)—Jane S—, æt. 56, was admitted into Guy's Hospital,

Fig. 73.

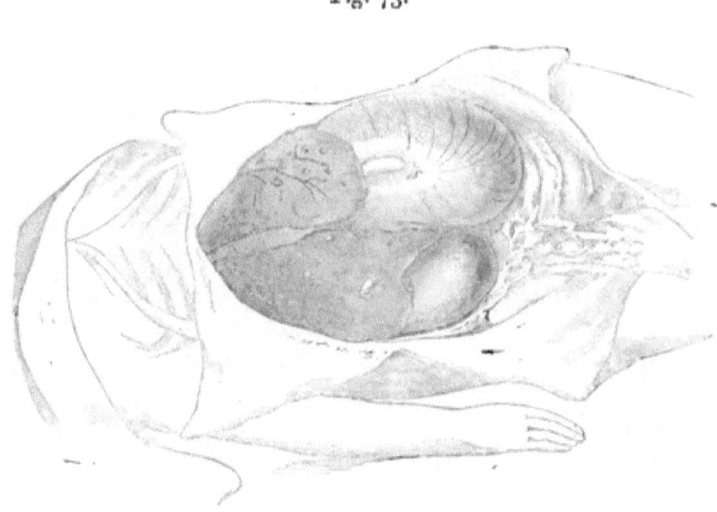

Fig. 73. The liver gorged with bile, descending below the umbilicus; its surface marked by some vesicles from distended biliary ducts. The gall-bladder excessively distended, forming an oval tumour near the crest of the ilium.

November 28th, 1832, afflicted with jaundice, of a dark, rather dingy character, though by no means the olive green of some diseased livers. Her skin flaccid; and it was evident she had lost much flesh. Pulse 84. There was no obvious tumour in the upper part of the abdomen; but as she lay on her back, a pretty distinct tumour, about the size of a walnut, was felt midway between the crest of the ilium and the umbilicus, rather below the direct line passing between the two points, near the outer edge of the rectus muscle. This tumour, though very distinct at times, often seemed to sink in under the pressure of the finger; and I often stated that it seemed like a tumour in the coats of an intestine. She said she had perceived it ever since she had received a severe strain in lifting something. There was some tenderness, though no tumour, in the region of the liver. The urine was most deeply tinged with bile. Stools very small and figured, exceedingly white, and floating in the urine, of very low specific gravity.

It appeared, that about five years ago she was under medical care for spasmodic pains in the stomach and bowels; but that she was never jaundiced till about three months ago, having previously experienced great pain in the lumbar vertebræ, extending on both sides under the ribs; and she still experienced much knawing, stabbing pain on each side of the spine, just at the bottom of the dorsal vertebræ.

Decoct. Aloes comp., ℥j;
Extracti Taraxaci, Ɔj, ter die.
Haustus Sennæ ad sedes.

November 30th.—Copious stools of a very pale drab colour.

December 5th.—Bowels much confined; only one very light stool in three days; and there is a very slight doubtful pellicle of fat on the surface of the urine in which it floats. At the bottom of the urine is some dark gritty matter, which looks much like inspissated bile.

Mr. Rees analysed the fæces, and found the quantity of gritty matter, such as usually exists in fæces, to be about 3 per cent. The black matter was lost.

7th.—Bowels pretty freely opened by castor-oil; the stools, as before, quite untinged with bile.

17th.—Much sickness of stomach; and during the last night, two stools almost white.

Julep: Acidi Nitrici, ter die.

29th.—Has had great sickness, and some purging, and represents the motions to have been of various colours. The tumour in the iliac region has been sometimes more and sometimes less distinct, sometimes quite wanting; but now a tumour is to be felt nearly in the same place, which appears harder, and there is a feeling of solidity the whole way intervening between this and the scrobiculus cordis, as if the liver descended in this direction.

> Opii, gr. i, o. n.;
> Aquæ Mephit. Alkalinæ, oct. j, quotidie.
> Cataplasm. Sinapis scrobic. cordis.

January 1st.—

> Adde Extracti Col. Comp., gr. x, singul. dos. pilulæ.
> Applicetur Empl. Picis Burgund. lumbis.

3d.—

> Aquæ Calcis., oct. ss, quotidie;
> Acet. Morphiæ, gr. ½, quater in die.

4th.—No change has taken place in the jaundice, but she lowers now obviously in her general powers.

> Hydrarg. Submur., gr. i;
> Ext. Hyoscyami, gr. ij, ter die.

8th.—The yellowness of the skin has become evidently more brilliant the last two or three days. She is very drowsy. Pulse 108. Occasional sickness. Specific gravity of urine, 1·014.

> Mist. Mag. cum Mag. Sulph.; et Rep. Hydr. Submur.

9th.—Is very drowsy and helpless; and when she awakes, seems almost lost.

> Pil. Colocynth cum Cal., gr. xv, statim.—Pergat.

11th.—The tumour lately felt in the iliac fossa is now obviously the gall-bladder greatly distended; and the liver can be traced, though obscurely, passing up to the right side.

13th.—Vomiting dark grumous matter. Stools past in bed, with some blood. Some blood in the urine, and from the nose. She emaciates, and the gall-bladder increases rapidly, or becomes much more distinct.

14th.—Omitte Pilul. Hydrarg. Submur.

16th.—She gradually sunk.

Sectio cadaveris.—January 15, 1833.—Considerable emaciation; whole skin of a vivid yellow colour; abdomen flat; the tumour, so plainly perceived before death, was scarcely perceptible. On opening the abdomen, the stomach was seen descending considerably below the umbilicus, on the left side, of a green yellow colour. The liver, looking thin, with no rounding of its acute margin, descended almost to the umbilicus; but this was probably rather lower than in life, owing to the falling in of the parts below. The omentum was doubled back, so that it lay upon the gall-bladder, and being removed the gall-bladder was seen, containing at the least, eight ounces of dark bile, projecting downwards towards the pelvis. This was evidently the tumour which had lately been felt; but, owing to the subsidence of parts, it had fallen a little more over to the left side. The intestines were very irregularly contracted and dilated, and just below the enlarged gall-bladder was seen a small oval distended portion of intestine, which proved to be the caput coli, which had evidently, at some former period, been the seat of peritoneal inflammation, and was thickened and rough; and from the situation it held, I have no doubt it was the tumour occasionally felt during the first part of the time the woman was in the hospital. (Fig. 73.)

Such, then, was the general situation of the viscera which first came into sight; the stomach and liver occupying a very large proportion of the cavity.

There was some undoubted appearance of peritoneal inflammation having preceded death; for the surface of the stomach had a yellow creamy purulent fluid thinly spread upon it, and there were several ounces of turbid green fluid in different parts of the abdominal cavity. The whole peritoneum of both intestines and parietes deeply tinged with bile.

The liver bore a remarkable appearance; it was of a green colour, and had, particularly on its left lobe, many green vesicular projections, from dilated and probably ruptured gall-ducts; these vesicles, which contained bile exactly similar to that in the gall-bladder, varied from the size of a pea to that of a broad bean, and were chiefly seen just above the gall-gladder, on the convex surface of the right lobe; and there were still larger ones on the concave surface of the same, near to the fossa in which the gall-bladder is lodged; and on the edge of the left lobe, both on the convex and the concave side. Cutting into the liver, it was generally quite healthy in its structure, but there were a few very small yellow white masses distributed through its substance, the largest about the size of a pea, much resembling those in Barns. All the substance was pervaded by tenacious bile; and in many parts were small collections of bile, and effusions of it staining the substance around the large ducts.

The pancreas was soft, and pretty natural in texture; but the duct was enlarged into the appearance of pouches, and contained a fluid like thin gruel, of which two or three drachms were collected, and much more made its escape; for the duct being wounded by an accidental cut early in the examination, so much of this white gruel-like fluid escaped that we supposed we had cut into an abscess, which was not the case. No part of the pancreas was scirrhous.

The common, the hepatic, and cystic ducts were so much enlarged, that they were almost the size of the healthy gall-bladder itself. The orifice of the duct in the duodenum was very singular; it projected, in a kind of neck, a full quarter of an inch into the duodenum, and was pervious; for on squeezing the duct, the bile flowed slowly into the duodenum. It was, however, certain that obstruction the most complete had existed during life; for the ducts, the gall-bladder, and the ducts in the substance of the liver, were dilated to the utmost.

There was no hard enlarged glandular substance to make pressure on the ducts; but the parts about the entrance of the common duct into the duodenum were hardened and matted together by what appeared to be a fibrinous deposit from old adhesive inflammation, making a rather hard knot at that part, but simply of hardened cellular membrane.

Towards the fundus of the gall-bladder a hard mass was felt, which, on examination, proved to be an infiltration beneath the mucous membrane of the bladder into the sub-mucous cellular tissue, of a dark fluid, either blood or bile; if the former, certainly much tinged with bile. This mass was not much less than an inch in thickness.

The mucous membrane of the stomach was covered with a thick layer of tenacious mucus, which came off in large flakes; the mucous membrane below presented many little bloody points. The mucous membrane of the whole intestines was carefully laid open and examined—the duodenum, jejunum, ileum, cæcum, colon, rectum, and in no part did organic disease exist; in some parts, a little sanguineous congestion, with redness of the valvulæ conniventes, and the feculent matter slightly tinged with red; even in the lower part of the ileum, the aggregate glands were scarcely perceptible, and throughout there was no trace of bile.

The lymphatic vessels about Glisson's capsule were tinged with pink-coloured transparent fluid, which some thought very slightly tinged with bile; and the thoracic duct seemed divided into several branches in the angle between the aorta and spine, turgid with the same fluid, which had no tinge of bile. The spleen healthy. The kidneys healthy, but throughout their whole structure tinged with bile; the tubular part rather green.

Thorax.—The lungs were much contracted, but quite healthy in structure, except one or two puckerings, from what appeared old healed tubercles. The blood which the lungs contained was thought more florid than usual. The bronchial tubes of a light yellow within, not having the least red or inflammatory appearance. The blood-vessels also tinged with yellow.

Heart.—Its ventricles rather weak; its auricles, particularly the right, distended. The blood in the heart of usual dark colour; and a large jelly-like clot, of a bright yellow, had separated in the cavities of the heart. The pericardium, as well on its adherent as its reflected portions, deeply stained with bile. The internal lining of the heart also of a full yellow tinge.

The aorta rather distended.

The œsophagus very large.

I have detailed this case rather more at length than may be thought necessary; but there appeared some interest connected with the way in which the first small abdominal tumour sometimes appeared, and sometimes could not be felt; as well as the circumstance, that no hardness or tumour was found uniting this tumour with the right hypochondrium. The second tumour which sprung up near the first was connected with the liver, and the post-mortem investigation showed that these two tumours, though occupying so nearly the same situation, were, in fact, of very different origin.

The mode in which the obstruction to the flow of bile was caused from simple cellular thickening is likewise interesting. There is reason to believe that the tumour of the gall-duct made its appearance between the 28th of November and the same day of the following month. The state of the pancreatic duct is also unusual, and it was the suspicion of some pancreatic disease, excited by the slight traces of fatty matter I had observed in the dejections, which led me to request Dr. G. O. Rees to endeavour to ascertain the degree to which it existed. The result, however, was not altogether satisfactory.

CASE 13.—*Tumefaction of the liver from retention of bile.—The gall-bladder distended with its own secretion.*—In the course of the spring of the present year, I was requested by Mr. Holding to see Mrs. T—, the subject of jaundice; but the more immediate object of our consultation was a tumour which had been discovered in the abdomen, and respecting which some diversity of opinion had arisen, though Mr. Holding himself had no doubt as to its nature.

I found an elderly lady, between sixty and seventy years of age, who had been affected with jaundice for several weeks. The colour was a deep yellow, the stools were white, or occasionally of a pinkish-white or drab. The urine very high-coloured yellow, and loaded with lithic deposit. On examining the abdomen by the hand, and, by gentle percussion, the liver was traced of a large volume, going back towards the loins, and descending to the umbilicus. It was smooth and tense, but not hard, and following its margin towards the right side, and between the umbilicus and the crest of the ileum, a large rounded projection was to be plainly traced, which, in connexion with the other symptoms, I had no hesitation in pronouncing to be the fundus of the gall-bladder (Fig. 74); and my opinion was, that there was some mechanical obstruction preventing the escape of the bile down the common duct, and thus producing that gorged condition of the liver and gall-bladder on which the form and situation of the tumour depended. The symptoms by which the disease was chiefly marked, besides those already noticed, were anorexia, flatulency to the utmost degree, occasional vomiting, and considerable depression of spirits. Pressure made upon the liver was not immediately very painful, but left a wearing pain for some time after an examination.

We employed a variety of remedies with no permanent advantage, though we were able to obviate a great many of the most unpleasant symptoms, and render her for some weeks so comparatively comfortable, that she rose, sat on the sofa, and went out airing in the carriage. Still the essential evidence of disease remained; she emaciated and grew weak, and at length, some weeks after my last visit, she sunk.

Mr. Holding obtained permission to examine the body, and found the parts exactly as we had anticipated. On opening the abdomen, the liver was seen descending below the ribs, and the gall-bladder projecting from beneath it. The gall-bladder was not of a dark colour, but was so thin, from long distension, that, while trying to raise it, it burst, and a large quantity of light, dirty yellow, glairy fluid escaped. It was therefore obvious that the distension of the gall-bladder depended on something else besides pressure on the common duct, and it was presently found that a biliary calculus was impacted in the cystic duct, so that nothing could obtain an entry into the bladder, except its own secretion; but this would not account for the jaundice; however, this was also soon accounted for, the entire obstruction of the common duct by induration of the head of the pancreas.

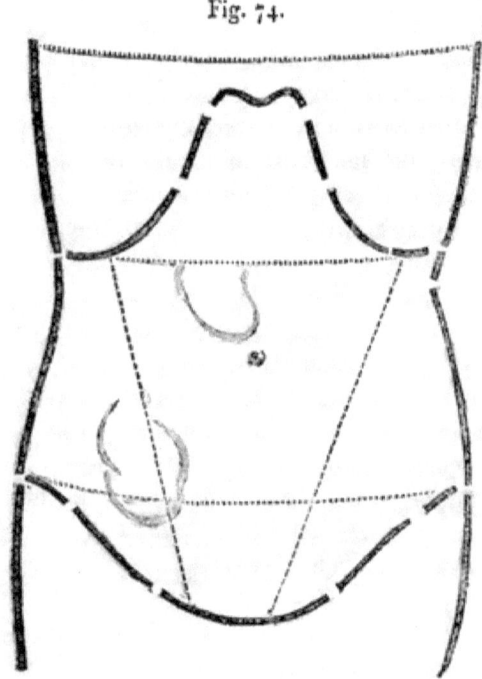

Fig. 74. Diagram, showing the position of rounded tumours depending upon the distended gall-bladder.

This case, then, presents a combination of disease which it was impossible to discover during life; for the liver was itself gorged with bile, and formed a large tumour so that it was most natural to refer both the tumefaction of the liver and the distension of the gall-bladder to a common cause. In the case, however, which I shall next detail, it would have been very possible to predict the obstruction of the cystic duct, separately from any other cause of jaundice.

One practical point is suggested by the examination in this case. I refer to the caution inculcated by the state of attenuation to which the gall-bladder was reduced. It actually gave way under manipulation; and the same might have happened during life, in which case peritoneal inflammation would have been almost infallible. And this struck me the more, because I had several times during my attendance taken the tumour in my hand, and made gentle pressure upon it as upon an elastic bottle; observing, that if I dare to make bold pressure, it felt as if I might possibly overcome the obstruction to the duct.

CASE 14.—*Gall-bladder forming a tumour.—The liver not gorged with bile.*—A woman had been in the hospital for a considerable time, labouring under the most marked jaundice; the dejections white, and urine high-coloured. The usual prostration, both mental and bodily, accompanied the disease, and rapid emaciation took place. The only remarkable circumstance was a tumour, which was felt during the whole time, situated just below the margin of the ribs on the right side. It was quite circumscribed; and changed its place a little, according to the different positions of the body. (Fig. 74.)

Sectio cadaveris.—On the surface of the liver were five or six distinct round indented tubercles of malignant matter, which broke down with ease between the fingers. The tumour which had been so remarkable was the fundus of the gall-bladder, which was greatly thickened, and distended with a mucous matter, and contained eight dark-coloured gall-stones.

In this case, the liver was not remarkably gorged with bile, and had not descended below the ribs; for the tumour of the gall-bladder was found immediately below the margin of the ribs, and resulted from its own secretion retained within it by biliary calculi. It is probable that the jaundice might have arisen in part from the pressure made by the gall-stones on the hepatic duct, and partly by the malignant disease, which could not be discovered during life, because the liver had not descended sufficiently from its natural situation.

CASE 15.—*Liver and gall-bladder distended with bile.*—I have elsewhere referred to a case in which the tumefaction of the liver, and the projection of the gall-bladder, were still more marked than in either of the foregoing. The patient was the subject of diabetes, as well as intense jaundice, the jaundice depending on scirrhous disease of the head of the pancreas. The liver was so gorged with bile, that it was throughout of the darkest olive colour; and the bile poured out from the cut surface, as blood does from a highly congested liver. The gall-bladder contained at least eight ounces of the darkest bile. Here there was, no doubt, cause of obstruction. The impediment was placed at the end of the common duct; and all the three ducts, as well as the gall-bladder, were enormously distended.

While speaking on the subject of tumours caused by the gall-bladder, it is right to observe, that occasionally the gall-badder loaded with calculi is brought into a state of suppuration, and in this way, adhering to the parietes, forms an external abscess, and the calculi are discharged. In this case, a tumour generally presents itself near the margin of the ribs, as in Case 14.

HEPATIC TUMOUR FROM CHRONIC HYPERTROPHY OF THE ORGAN.

There is a state of disease into which the liver is very apt to pass, when it has been long over-stimulated by habits of intemperance. The whole structure becomes uniformly changed, so that the appearance it presents is that of a yellow granular substance, like a coarse-grained sandstone; and at one period of the disease the whole organ is greatly enlarged. Whether it sometimes contracts in a later period I am not quite sure, but if it does, it then passes into a state approaching to the hob-nailed liver; at all events, at the period of which I speak, it forms a large hepatic tumour of a smooth character; for the granules of which it is composed are not perceptible through the parietes, which are usually, in this form of disease, rather loaded with fat, than reduced by emaciation.

The two cases which I shall now detail are examples of this form of disease; as I should be inclined to suppose, in two successive stages of its progress. In one, the enlargement of the liver was very great, and plainly discoverable: in the second, that enlargement was to a much less degree; and the surface was becoming lobulated in a slight degree, as if contraction had taken place.

Case 16.—*Hepatic tumour from chronic hypertrophy of the organ.*—I was requested by Mr. Thurlow to see Mr. T. D—, æt. 34, a man of short stature, indolent and inactive body, mild temper, with great want of energy of mind; rather addicted to study, and of confined sedentary habits from inactivity of constitution; for many years in the habit of indulging freely and even inordinately in the use of wine and spirits; sitting for hours and whole nights with his cigar; and latterly becoming dreadfully inebriated, whenever an opportunity occurred; his appetite for food always small: for a few years past he has been growing stout; though, when young, rather thin.

I was first requested to see him on account of a considerable discharge of blood by the rectum, coming away in clots; his countenance was sallow; his conjunctivæ slightly yellow; his abdomen appeared tumid, as he sat; and, on examination, the liver was found descending quite to the umbilicus, its margin distinctly to be traced round into the left hypochondrium; some tenderness, on pressure in various parts, but not acute; a doubtful sense of fluctuation was perceived, and some tympanitic distension of the intestines; ankles slightly œdematous; pulse rather sharp and frequent.

Leeches were applied two or three times; very gentle aperients were used; and we did our best to limit the quantity of his drink.

In the course of two or three weeks he was so much better, in every respect, that he went into the country. Here, however, he fell into his old habit of drinking to great excess, and he returned in a fortnight, in a state more alarming than when we first saw him; his manner more hurried; his tongue dark, furred, red at the edges; his abdomen more tumid, now evidently containing fluid; and a general light-yellow suffusion over the skin and conjunctiva. The liver was still to be felt, but scarcely so low as before; blood occasionally in stools.

The same remedies, with the addition of the hydrarg. cum cretâ, and afterwards small doses of calomel and squills, were employed. But it was quite impossible to restrain his desire for wine and spirits; he continued, in spite of all the vigilance we could employ, to get more or less intoxicated nearly every second day. His stools varied a good deal in appearance, but contained some bile, and occasionally blood; his urine likewise varied, sometimes quite clear, and partly light-coloured, but more frequently tinged slightly with bile. His countenance became more and more yellow, but never exceeded a moderate light-yellow tinge, more than sallowness, and, for the last day or two of his life, the urine was rather highly tinged with bile. The abdomen swelled by the accumulation of water, but, by accurate measurement, we found this proceeded slowly; his legs swelled more rapidly. He took to his bed about three days before death, and was always able to lie on either side, or flat on his back, though for some time he experienced inconvenience from the pressure of the abdomen upwards, when he first lay down. He was inclined to be drowsy, and refused food.

On the 16th of August, early in the morning, he sent in for Mr. Streeter, to know whether he had not got the rattles. Slight mucous rattle was found, and dyspnœa; pulse rather faltering; he spoke, however, distinctly, and Mr. S. had not left the room half-an-hour, when he died.

Sectio cadaveris.—August 17th, 1828.—Considerable accumulation of fat, half an inch thick, on abdomen, the same observed, in great masses, round the kidneys; the mesentery and omentum rather loaded; the pancreas imbedded in fat, many fatty appendages to the large intestines.

Cavities of chest contained one or two ounces of water. Lungs decidedly œdematous; the serum running out very freely, when cut into, particularly on superior and posterior parts; otherwise quite healthy. Heart fat, and the fat tinged slightly with yellow; otherwise quite natural.

Stomach.—Mucous membrane scabrous, and thickened a little.

Peritoneum, and external appearance of intestines, natural, except one or two patches of vascularity about the meso-rectum; internally in the rectum the mucous membrane thickened, and some patches of vascularity; the same observed in the colon; the cæcum mottled with gray, like lime-seed; one or two parts of the mucous membrane of the small intestine, even in the jejunum, vascular, as if small vessels had given way.

Pancreas and spleen healthy. Kidneys also healthy; a little yellow, from bile.

Liver, a decided specimen of the small granular yellow drab-coloured, rough to feel, and, when cut into, throughout of the same texture, and of the colour of pickled mangoes. In the gall-bladder about two drachms of bile of a dirty appearance, with some pulverulent deposit of bilious matter, yet retaining somewhat of the yellow colour of bile.

CASE 17.—*Hepatic tumour from chronic change in the liver.*—I was requested by Mr. Griffith to see a man æt. 44, an habitual drinker to a very large extent; he had been several times subject to sickness and vomiting, and was attacked very severely in this way three or four days ago. Yesterday morning, Mr. Griffith was suddenly sent for, as he had vomited up blood, filling two chamber-pots with the blood and grumous matter from his stomach. In this state he died.

Sectio cadaveris.—The whole countenance and surface of every part was of a light-yellow colour, between what would be called sallow and jaundice. No apparent emaciation, and, as the body now lies on the table, no tumour is perceptible to the touch. On inspecting further, the fat was found to be very considerable over the whole integuments, and in the anterior mediastinum.

The lungs and heart perfectly healthy; but a slight serous effusion, tinged with red, in the left cavity of the chest.

In cavity of abdomen, about half a pint of serum of brownish tinge. The omentum fatty, drawn up, and forming a mass across the scrobiculus cordis; but not to be felt externally, nor become unnatural, except by fatness. The mesentery very fat, and numerous large fatty appendages hanging from the descending colon and rectum.

The liver, rather thicker than natural, was completely destroyed in its texture; formed of rounded yellow masses, so that it looked throughout of a light, rather bright yellow, and was hard, tough, and on its under surface lobulated; the lobuli quadratus and Spigelii, &c., forming hard lumps. Its general surface nearly smooth, yet feeling uneven to the finger passed over it. The gall-bladder was white, thick, opaque, containing about three or four drachms of a very light glairy fluid, evidently mucus, scarcely tinged with bile. The ducts were quite pervious. When a portion of the liver had been macerated four or five weeks, all the yellow granules became white, like adipocere, and could be shaken out of the substance, leaving a beautiful tissue of vessels, like a puff of threads; and this is preserved.

The pancreas healthy; spleen rather large, but quite healthy; kidneys healthy. In the stomach, about half a pint of clotted blood, slightly grumous. The surface of the stomach was stained throughout with blood; but no vascularity could be traced, and the only mark of disease was here and there a small petechial spot, as from extravasation, under the mucous membrane. The pylorus was quite healthy; and in opening into different portions of the intestines, it appeared that the stain of blood became fainter and fainter as we proceeded down the canal, till it was quite lost in the ileum.

In this case, the cause of the hæmorrhage appears to have been the pressure of the liver, perhaps the smaller lobes, upon the portal vessels. No large ruptured vessels could be seen.

The chief circumstances I would remark are, that this kind of liver appears the legitimate result of dram-drinking; that it was accompanied with the same *slight, imperfect* jaundice which accompanied three or four other cases; that the fat, as in other cases, was abundant; and that, although there is reason to suppose very little bile to have been secreted by the liver, yet it had been remarked in this, as in other cases, that a few weeks before death he passed a large quantity of curdy and flaky matter, which was considered bile.

HEPATIC TUMOUR FROM FATTY DEGENERATION OF THE LIVER.

That very peculiar change to which the liver is subject when its whole substance seems converted into a mass of fat, supported in its form by the usual vessels and cellular membrane, has been known for many years, and has particularly attracted the attention of the French pathologists, who have traced it as connected in many cases with the phthisical diathesis more or less developed. I am not aware, however, that any one had pointed out a diagnostic mark of its existence during life, till Dr. Addison took up the subject, in a communication to 'Guy's Hospital Reports.' And to this I must refer, as I introduce the disease in this place only as affording one instance of hepatic tumour, which, however, is not a constant attendant on the disease in its early stages.

CASE 18.—*Fatty liver descending below the umbilicus.*—Matilda S—, æt. 25, was admitted into Guy's Hospital, under my care, April 11th, 1832, affected with phthisis and diarrhœa. She had experienced cough for a year; but she dated the more decided and severe accession of her illness to a certain time, one month and two days before her admission, when she was obliged to give up her occupation, and confine herself to bed. Since this period the cough had been greatly aggravated, and accompanied with frequent spitting of blood; and the diarrhœa had been severe. When admitted, the diarrhœa was constant, and the evacuations watery. The expectoration was decidedly puriform, and all the physical symptoms led to the belief that cavities existed in the upper lobes of the lungs. She lay with greater ease on the right side. And upon examining the right hypochondrium, it was found that the liver descended below the umbilicus. The whole of that portion of the abdomen was dull on percussion, and presented the resistance of a smooth cushion-like body to the hand; and although no abrupt edge could be plainly traced, the resistance of the liver could be followed far towards the left hypochondrium.

She was ordered to take the chalk mixture, with aromatic confection, after each dejection, and half a grain of the acetate of morphia at bedtime.

April 13th.—The diarrhœa still continued; the dejections, consisting of large quantities of watery feculent matter, decidedly coloured by bile. The expectoration puriform, and part of it rose-coloured. Four drops of the tincture of opium were added to each dose of the mixture, and the acetate of morphia was repeated three times a day.

Under this treatment, the bowels very rapidly recovered a more natural action, the motions becoming consistent; but the cough continued, and on the 30th of the month she died.

Sectio cadaveris.—Both the lungs were attached by old adhesions to the ribs, but were separated without laceration. In the superior lobe of each lung was an old cavity, of the size of a small orange, marked by irregular septa, from vessels not completely eroded. The remaining portions of the upper lobe were interspersed with small cavities, containing fetid pus, which appeared to be the result of a combination of pneumonic inflammation with phthisis; for though there was a good deal of genuine tubercular deposit, the consolidation occupied whole lobules.

The heart was small, flaccid, and most universally adherent by very old close adhesions, like cellular membrane.

The liver was very large, descending two inches below the umbilicus, and reaching quite round into the right lumbar region; while the other lobe extended towards the left, so far as to be firmly attached, by old adhesions, to the spleen.

The liver afforded the most perfect example of the fatty degeneration, with a general hypertrophy of the organ; its colour, of a light pinkish yellow, perfectly smooth, with its lower edge as acute as in the most healthy liver. The acini were exceedingly distinct; and I never saw a liver which, without injection, displayed so much of its structure. On breaking through it, bile, of a light yellow colour, was detected in some of the larger ducts; and the gallbladder contained enough to tinge its internal coat completely yellow.

Spleen healthy, but adherent. Pancreas healthy. The mucous membrane of the stomach soft.

In the lower part of the ileum, and in the cæcum, there were a few spots of ulceration, in which tubercular matter was deposited; and one or two tubercles, not ulcerated, immediately beneath the mucous membrane.

The uterus was healthy; but both the Fallopian tubes and ovaria were attached to the broad ligaments, by unnatural bridles of adhesion.

The remarkable similarity between this case and one which has fallen under my observation since the above was copied out for the press induces me to add it, as a case of tumour from fatty liver; although the urgency of the diarrhœa had drawn the attention so much to the ulceration of the bowels, that the enlargement of the liver, which must have been very perceptible to the touch and to percussion, was not detected during life.

CASE 19.—*Fatty change in the substance of the liver.*—A young lady, æt. 17, was in apparent excellent florid health in November

1839, except as regarded the catamenia, which came at twelve years of age, and were never regular, being frequently absent for six months at a time; but it was observed that she had grown remarkably stout. In November, she first began to feel pain in the bowels, particularly about the right iliac region. In January, she went to Brighton, on account of a disease which had taken place in the first phalanx of the great toe; and while there, diarrhœa came on to such a degree, that for twelve weeks she never had less than six or eight stools in the day; and she generally experienced a little pain in the right iliac region, and some griping over the whole abdomen.

I first saw her on the 17th of July. She was extremely emaciated; and as she lay in bed, my first impression was, that I was called to a case of advanced phthisis. However, I soon found that there was no cough, no perceptible dulness at the apex of either lung, and no other pulmonary symptoms; but that all the disease referred itself to the abdomen; on examining which, I was struck with the circumstance, that though it was generally soft and yielding, yet it did not present the same appearance of emaciation as the other parts of the body; and I could feel what appeared a glandular body, low down in the right iliac region, probably near the head of the colon. Tongue red, with some elongated papillæ; stomach so irritable, that she vomited almost all her food; pulse from 100 to 120. I saw six stools which had been passed that morning; most of them were of a remarkably healthy, brown, feculent appearance, scanty, loose, but not watery, with some small lumps in them; and in one or two I fancied I could perceive the treacle-like tinge which a slight admixture of blood sometimes presents. I considered this a case in which tubercular deposit had taken place in the submucous tissue of the intestines, particularly about the ileo-colic valve, and had probably gone into extensive ulceration; and of course I saw no hope, in that case, of a good result. We made trial, in addition to the many remedies which had been already used without success, of small doses—first, of sulphate of copper, then of chalybeates combined with astringents; but the good effects produced were very temporary; and although at one time, on a diet of mixed food not prescribed by her medical adviser, she appeared to lose in a remarkable degree the irritability both of her bowels and her stomach, so that for two days she had neither vomiting nor diarrhœa, yet this apparent improvement passed off, and the diarrhœa returning with increased violence, she died the last day of August.

Sectio cadaveris.—On laying open the abdomen, the omentum was seen, by no means destitute of fatty matter, spread over the abdomen, and attached at one part in the right iliac region. The liver came at once in view, of a yellow-drab colour, and much enlarged; it descended at least three inches below the cartilages of the ribs, and across the whole scrobiculus cordis, quite to the spleen on the left side; it ascended to the interval between the third and fourth rib on the right side, and occupied a considerable space in the left hypochondrium. It was a perfect specimen, throughout, of the advanced fatty liver. The scalpel was covered with grease, a portion, on applying heat, yielded drops of fat, and made an oily stain on linen; and a piece of the liver, thrown into water, floated readily. A considerable quantity of blood flowed from the incisions of the liver. The gall-bladder contained about two drachms of healthy bile, and a gall-stone, of the size of a small filbert, of crystalline cholesterine.

The Intestines.—The whole peritoneal covering perfectly healthy, smooth, shining, and free from any effusion; but on following out the course of the intestines, we came in the last two or three feet of the ileum, to some dark discoloured spots, where the bowel was contracted, evidently corresponding with internal ulceration; and on arriving at the termination of the ileum in the cæcum, the intestine formed a mass of the size of an egg, in which the vermiform appendage was glued with a portion of the omentum to the cæcum. On laying open the intestines, we found about ten separate ulcers in the lower part of the ileum, some of which embraced the whole calibre of the tube; but the chief ravage was about the ileo-colic valve, which was involved in a mass of ulceration, as was the pouch of the cæcum and the cavity of the vermiform process. The other parts of the mucous membrane were healthy, and the whole lining membrane of the colon was perfect, except one small ulcer about the sigmoid flexure; and in the rectum the membrane was red, but not ulcerated. It was obvious that much tubercular deposit had taken place in the ulcerated patches, previous to their ulceration; for some such deposits lay around them, to which the ulcer had not extended.

The mesentery still contained some fat; and the glands were much enlarged, some of them going into a state of softening and suppuration.

The spleen was healthy, but rather large.

The uterus and ovaria small, and one or two little pendulous cysts hanging from the Fallopian tubes.

The kidneys were healthy in their general appearance, but rather light-coloured, and separated from the tumours so easily that there appeared to be scarcely any union between them. One small tubercle was detected in the substance of the right kidney.

The lungs collapsed quite freely on opening the chest, but the apex on each side was attached, over a small space, by adhesions to the first rib, and in the upper lobe, close to the apex in each, was found the remnant of a former small cavity, now not much larger than a pea, and filled with cheesy matter. A few lobules also were hardened, as if hepatised from inflammation; and in one or two lobules, a scarcely appreciable deposit of tuberculous matter was traced. All other parts of the lungs healthy.

The heart was very small, flaccid, and pale, but without disease.

In this case there can be no doubt that percussion would have yielded a dull sound over an unusual extent of the upper part of the abdomen, as it did in the former case. Indeed, the similarity was so striking, that we ought almost to have inferred the nature of the hepatic enlargement. Such a diagnosis, however, should always be given with caution; although, in a case of decidedly irregular catamenia, with obstinate diarrhœa, and a large smooth tumefaction of the liver, the probability would be greatly in favour of this form of disease; and more particularly before the meridian of life, for I have more than once had reason to believe that the state of amenorrhœa was connected, either as cause or effect, with the existence of fatty liver. It may be a matter of surprise that I did not detect the disease by that state of skin pointed out by Dr. Addison, but in the distressing state in which the patient was, no striking peculiarity in this respect was observed.

CASE 20.—*Liver large, from the fatty change in its substance.*—June 21st, 1828.—A woman, æt. 33, was examined, who had died in consequence of an extensive burn on the upper part of the chest, which she had suffered five months previously. There was a large open wound on each side. The lungs were perfectly healthy, except that the left lung had on its surface, apparently answering to the external burn, a thin, gelatinous, yellow effusion, underneath the pleura. There was no effusion of importance in either cavity; but on the right side a most beautiful display of vascularity on the pleura costalis. There was no material emaciation, and it was observed that small globules of an oily substance floated in a small quantity of serum in the chest.

The liver was large, and the most perfect specimen of the fat liver I have seen; of a light-yellow colour, with a few markings partially on its surface, from which it appeared that the acini were enlarged; but when cut into, no longer could the least mottled appearance be discovered. A few indentations, as if from vessels or spaces between the acini, were to be seen; and from these a complete yellow oil drained, of its own accord. When a portion of this was put by for twenty-four hours, in a bladder, the quantity of oil which drained out was some teaspoonfuls.

A piece, as nearly one square inch as possible, was put into a clear bottle, without any fluid.

A portion was put into New-river water; it floated completely, and globules of oil floated on the surface.

A portion was put into a bottle with rectified spirits of wine; immediately large globules of oil collected at the bottom.

A portion was put into a solution of carbonate of potash; the whole shortly became a saponaceous mass.

A considerable portion was left freely exposed, in an open vessel to the air; by the end of a month, it had become putrid, but had assumed all the character and smell of rancid bacon.

A portion, about a quarter of an inch in thickness, was placed between folds of blotting-paper, and submitted to gentle pressure; the blotting paper was soaked through a great many folds with the fatty stain, and in two or three days the portion of liver formed but a thin film.

The gall-bladder contained a small quantity, perhaps half an ounce, of light-green bile, of a dirty hue, and which, when spread upon a white surface, gave rather an olive colour, than a yellow stain.

The spleen and pancreas were healthy.

The intestines also appeared so, but were not examined internally.

The kidneys were of very pale yellow, but did not contain any white deposit.

Head not opened.

It was remarkable that, with so much hepatic derangement, it was only within the last day or two of her life that the bowels were at all disturbed; diarrhœa then coming on.

It appears that before the accident she was subject to epileptic fits, in one of which she fell into the fire, and thus met with her accident; from that time there was no return of fits.

Mr. Foggarty assures me the alvine evacuations have been very natural.

Although malignant disease for the most part induces tumours of the irregular form, yet it occasionally happens that it is otherwise, more particularly when the disease develops itself very generally through the structure of the organ, forming a great number of small and almost confluent tubera, and thus producing an even surface.

Case 21.—*Malignant disease, producing a regular smooth enlargement of the liver.*—April 13th, 1834.—I was requested to see Mrs. S—, who had been delivered, by Mr. Thorn, of a living and healthy child, two days previously, and had since been seen by Mr. Dunn.

The circumstance to which my attention was chiefly directed was the continued enlargement of the abdomen, which had scarcely diminished since parturition. On examination, a hard smooth tumour could be distinctly traced, occupying all the upper part of the abdomen; rendering the lower half of the right chest dull, and descending some way below the umbilicus. Although the situation of the tumour pretty plainly pointed it out as the liver, yet some who examined it, finding it pass quite over to the left side, had been inclined to think that the spleen was also involved in the disease. The uterus was also distinctly felt in the pelvis. The skin was sallow, there was no peritoneal tenderness.

I learned from her that she was thirty-nine years of age, had been the mother of nine living children, five of whom were still alive; and the last, before the present, about three years old. She had enjoyed excellent health, and her times had been generally very good. During this pregnancy, she had spoken of a peculiar dead weight; and had complained of pain, as she supposed, from flatus; but no idea had been entertained of the existence of a tumour.

I considered this an enlargement, probably fungoid, of the liver; and, of course, nothing but palliative remedies could be proposed. She continued to get lower, her mouth was covered with aphthæ, and the stomach became excessively irritable. She died on the 10th of April.

Sectio cadaveris.—The surface of the body sallow, rather than jaundiced. Adipose matter not wanting on the abdomen. About two quarts of yellow clear serum in the peritoneal cavity. Lungs healthy, except a strong adhesion of the pleura at the upper lobe of the right. Heart healthy, with a few spots of ecchymosis on its surface. The lungs were pressed upward by the liver, which, in the recumbent posture, and with the lungs empty in death, had encroached on the chest, as high as the fourth rib. The liver, when the chest and abdomen were both laid open (Fig. 75), occupied full half of both the cavities; it spread from one side to the other completely, and extended from the fourth rib to considerably below the umbilicus. It was diseased in almost every part; presenting, on its surface, circular white masses, which were not the least elevated, but rendered the whole mottled with white spots, varying from the size of a shilling to a pin's head, irregularly distributed, but occupying by far the larger proportion of the whole. The peritoneum itself was very little influenced. The gall-bladder contained a small quantity of green bile. Pancreas healthy. Spleen healthy, but large. The stomach and intestines, and kidneys, healthy. The omentum loaded with fat. The uterus about the size of the fist.

Fig. 75.

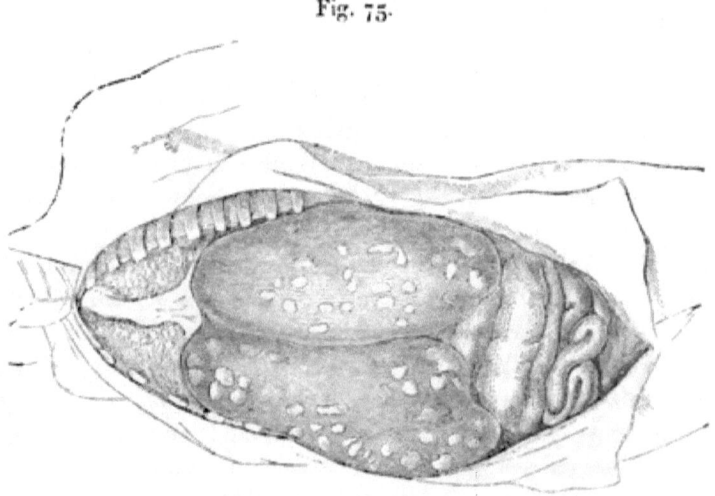

Fig. 75. The liver enormously enlarged by malignant deposit diffused through its substance, encroaching on the chest, and descending below the umbilicus, and forming a large smooth tumour in the abdomen.

HEPATIC TUMOURS OF IRREGULAR FORM.

I regret that the space devoted to the present memoir will not allow me to go so fully, at present, into this department of my subject as I should wish; but I will still attempt to illustrate the irregular tumour by some few cases.

The tumours of this class are, abscesses in the liver, in various conditions, some other results of chronic inflammation, hydatids, and the different forms of malignant disease.

HEPATIC TUMOUR FROM ABSCESS.

When inflammatory affections of the liver have gone on to the formation of abscess, it depends entirely upon the situation in which the suppuration takes place, whether it produces a tumour externally or not. In general, however, some enlargement of the liver follows almost necessarily; and if the abscess does not point sufficiently, or if it be placed completely under the vault of the diaphragm, still it pushes the liver down, so that its margin is perceptible some way below the ribs; this produces an even smooth enlargement, rather than an irregular tumour, and usually the dulness of the right side of the chest extends higher than in health. When the abscess is so situated as to point externally, a distinct tumour is induced; sometimes protruding the ribs, and even pointing between the costal spaces, at other times appearing either immediately below the cartilages, or at some distance from them; the situation, of course, varying according as the right or left lobe is affected. A tumour arising from such a cause is easily to be traced as connected with the liver, of which it obviously forms a part; the dulness, on percussion, being continuous, as well as the resistance on pressure. The resistance, however, is not very great, as the whole organ rather gives way under pressure; and the sensation to the touch is comparatively soft, or it yields an elastic tenseness. More or less pain, and that often acute, is experienced when pressure is made; and generally symptoms of an active, febrile, and inflammatory character have preceded the appearance of such a tumour. It must, however, be borne in mind, that the approach of an abscess in the liver is often so obscure and so insidious, that the inflammatory symptoms have sometimes not been recognised, or have, if not overlooked, frequently been ascribed to other organs; so that the appearance of the tumour has first suggested the mischief which had been going on. Its progress, too, has often been insidious; and an abscess has become chronic, producing an enlargement of a still more striking kind than I have just spoken of, remaining for months as a tangible tumour, almost defying diagnosis; and at length destroying life, by wearing out the constitutional powers, or by some accidental effusion of the pus into the peritoneal cavity (Case 22). Still further than this, however, an abscess of the liver may produce an uneven lobulated condition of the liver, possibly by absorption of the pus; or, more probably, by the escape of the greater part of it through the gall-ducts, and a consolidating change of what remains, which becomes insulated in the thickened cellular membrane. What we then find is a deep cicatrix marked on the surface of the liver; and when we cut through this, a yellow deposit, of a more or less purulent character, or of a chalky consistence, is lodged at the bottom. Such cicatrices are not matter of doubtful existence, but deep and tangible indentations on the surface of the liver; and though generally concealed from the touch by the ribs, yet if the liver were brought down below the ribs by its own enlargement or by external pressure, the nodulated liver would present a very perplexing variety of tumour, which would most likely be mistaken for malignant disease, till sufficient time had elapsed to prove its comparative innoxious nature, and its little disposition to increase.

CASE 22.—*Chronic abscess presenting great difficulties in its detection.* (Fig. 76.)—I was requested, in August, 1839, to give my opinion of a tumour in the abdomen of a lady about sixty years of age. It had existed above two years, during which time she had become emaciated and sallow, had suffered much from dyspeptic symptoms and occasional sickness of the stomach, with a good deal of pain. I was told that several years before she had a most obstinate obstruction in the large intestines, and was under Dr. Carrick, of Clifton, at which time she passed balls, supposed to depend upon the habit of taking magnesia; and also, at another time since, she had obstruction of the colon. The tumour presented some peculiar characters; the most prominent part was just to the left of the umbilicus, where it might be grasped when the abdominal muscles were well relaxed, and followed downwards, and to the right, till it seemed to be lost in the substance from which it arose. There was dulness to be traced by percussion, between it and the margin of the right ribs. It was moveable in a mass, and evidently not adherent to the peritoneum. Its situation was such, that it might have been attached to the liver, the colon, or the omentum; but, considering all its apparent connections, and its peculiar tense elastic feel and its chronic nature, I gave it as my opinion that it was an hydatid cyst in the liver, possibly making pressure on the pylorus and the colon, developed apparently immediately under the edge of the liver. I stated it as probable, that the reason of its not materially increasing was, that the bile had killed the hydatids.

The lady was also seen, separately, by four of the most eminent surgeons and physicians in London; one agreed with me; another declared it to be pyloric; another, that it was a disease of the stomach, but not of the pylorus; and another considered it ovarian.

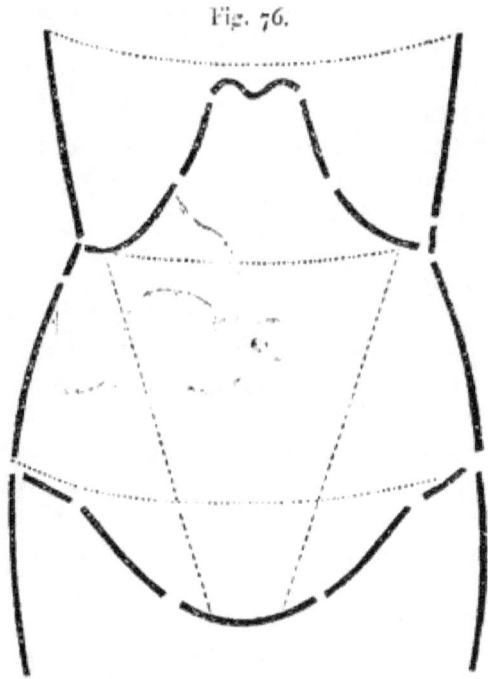

Fig. 76.

Fig. 76. Diagram representing the situation of a tumour depending on chronic abscess of the liver. (Case 22.)

a. The point projecting considerably beyond the substance of the liver.

Of course there was very little to be done, in the way of treatment, beyond such means as would best sustain the powers and give tone to the stomach. She returned into the country, and in about six months afterwards died. I never received a very full account of the post-mortem appearance; but the tumour was considered, by the medical gentlemen who examined it, as a chronic abscess of the liver. There was a cyst arising from the right lobe, of the form of a pear; the base towards the liver, the apex at the umbilicus. This contained one ounce more than a pint of muco-purulent fluid, besides three biliary concretions, one of which weighed two ounces. The whole right lobe was altered in its structure, and become fleshy. The liver, with the cyst and its contents, weighed four pounds. It was supposed that the gall-stones had ulcerated out of the gall-bladder, and excited inflammation, producing chronic abscess in the liver.

The above case is interesting as an instance of very chronic suppuration, in which the difficulty of the diagnosis was sufficiently testified by the diversity of opinions given by the most competent authorities; yet it is equally evident, from the conclusion to which some of us had come, that, by careful examination, it was possible to ascertain the exact situation, which we did; and though we did not detect its precise nature, we made a close approximation to the quality of its fluid contents.

CASE 23.—*Deep cicatrices in the liver from former abscesses.*—I was requested to meet Dr. Budd and Mr. Bell, in the case of a gentleman sinking under the effects of granulated kidneys with albuminous urine. He had made several voyages to India in his youth, but had retired from that service above fourteen years. During his Indian voyages and residence, he was supposed to have suffered from liver disease; and he has always asserted that he was sure his liver was still diseased; one reason for which belief had been, his great tendency to dysenteric diarrhœa and derangement of the bowels.

I was present at the post-mortem examination, and the first thing which drew our attention was the singular appearance of the liver; which was divided by several deep fissures, some of them a full inch in depth, rendering the whole liver irregularly tuberculated. These fissures were the cicatrices of abscesses, and on cutting through them, we found at least twenty small deposits of puriform matter, contained in little cyst-like cavities, formed by the induration of the cellular membrane of the liver; and some of these deposits, though apparently locked up in these cavities for several years—for there was no sign of recent action—still retained the character of most perfect recent pus.

This case may be considered an extreme instance of what often occurs; and had the liver been a little more within reach of manual investigation during life, its broken and irregular surface would have produced the greatest perplexity; but, independently of the object for which it is immediately introduced, it is curious and interesting, as showing the frequent termination of hepatic abscess, and the way in which the remaining portions of pus may become so insulated as to be productive of little or no inconvenience, locally or on the system.

IRREGULAR SURFACE OF THE LIVER INDUCED BY CHRONIC INFLAMMATION.

Under this head I would arrange the numerous cases in which, from contraction of the cellular membrane, the liver becomes deformed and lobulated, either in large proportion, or in that more uniform manner which marks the hobnailed liver. As in this form of disease the liver is generally contracted rather than enlarged, we are frequently deprived of an opportunity of ascertaining its state with certainty, though the general symptoms frequently lead us to correct diagnosis. These conditions of the liver are very apt to be marked by the effusion of blood into the stomach and intestines, leading to most severe and repeated hæmatemesis, as was very well pointed out by Dr. Law, of Dublin, and also to serous effusion into the peritoneum. It is owing to this last circumstance that we are often lead to search for the liver, and to detect it even when its bulk is rather diminished than increased; for as the ascitic patient lies on his back, if the liver be indurated and contracted, it tends to gravitate of its own accord, from its attachments; and thus, falling downwards and forwards, sinks, suspended under a certain quantity of the serum; and thus we find it below the margin of the ribs, so as to be plainly felt. For this purpose the attention of the patient must be drawn away, if possible, to prevent the almost involuntary tension of the muscles; and then, the points of the fingers being placed on the surface, by a quick movement are brought down with the integuments so as to displace the serum and receive the impulse of the liver; and then, taking advantage of a favorable moment, the irregularities of the surface may be felt. Thus I have before me cases where the abdomen is described as loaded with serum, and the liver to be distinctly felt below the ribs; and yet, when the examination was made, after death occurring in a few days, the liver is stated to be rather small, its whole surface granulated, and its texture hard and unyielding.

There are a few other cases of tumours, of a more casual kind, formed on the surface of the liver; as cartilaginous deposits, and even bony tumours, the result of morbid actions, which are generally not progressive. The possible existence of such tumours should be carefully borne in mind, as pointing out the propriety of abstaining from the use of violent remedies for the removal of any internal tumour, whose stationary condition, and the little effect it produces on the constitution, seem to point it out as less likely to prove injurious than our efforts for its removal, which at length will probably be of no avail.

Hydatids afford another source of irregular hepatic tumours; but I have already entered so fully into this subject, that I must content myself by referring to the chapters of this work on hydatid tumours.

IRREGULAR TUMOURS OF THE LIVER FROM MALIGNANT DISEASE.

The different forms of malignant disease must be considered amongst the most common sources of hepatic tumour. We frequently find the liver alone the seat of such disease; but, on the other hand, we still more frequently have instances of the successive or simultaneous attack of several organs. When the disease is confined to the liver, the situation of the tumour is most easily ascertained; for as there is no complexity of diseased organs, we are of course less liable to be led into error; but the nature of the disease is often more easily ascertained when other parts are affected; more particularly such as present facilities for external examination, as the mammæ, the uterus, or the superficial glands; which are all very frequently implicated, and, being far removed from the liver, afford no room for confusion; and the very circumstance of the organ being involved strengthens the probability of the malignant nature of the disease. On the contrary, however, the greatest sources of difficulty, as to the situation of the disease, occur when the right kidney, the ascending colon or its arch, the stomach, the pancreas, or the peritoneum, are involved in the same disease with the liver.

Malignant disease varies considerably in the forms it assumes; but in general, when developed in the liver, shows itself as rounded masses or tubera, approaching more or less to the spherical shape. I shall not enter into the subject of the intimate structure, situation, or mode of development of the malignant growths, but, referring to a memoir in 'Guy's Hospital Reports,'[1] I may say, that I regard them as generally originating in the cellular membrane connecting the essential portions of the organs in which they are found; often, at first, merely displacing the structures which are employed in the proper function of the organ, and interfering, therefore, but little with its duties; but ultimately entering so minutely into these structures, as to effect an apparent conversion, or an obliteration, of the whole. Three very distinct varieties present themselves;—cerebriform disease, and that running into fungus hæmatoides; the hard scirrhus; and the melanosis. Or perhaps the hæmatoid form of the disease might deserve a separate place; making, in that case, four varieties.

Of these, the cerebriform, with or without the hæmatoid, is often the most rapid in its growth, and forms the largest and most distinct tumours in the liver; next to that, the melanosis; and the scirrhus, though apt to attack a great number of organs, and to develop itself in a great many points simultaneously, is the slowest in its progress, and often the least easy to recognise as a distinct irregular tumour.

CASE 24.—*Tumour in the abdomen, from cerebriform tubera in the liver.*—I was called in consultation to see a lady, somewhat advanced in years, who, in consequence of a painful affection resulting from injury, had contracted the habit of eating opium to a large extent.

---

[1] 'Guy's Hospital Reports,' vol. i, p. 638.

Her countenance was sallow and distressed; and she had been long subject to great irregularity of the bowels, and painful affections of the abdomen. Her present illness had existed but for a few days; and consisted in a return of the pain in the abdomen, which seemed very urgent; and she looked greatly reduced by it. On examining the abdomen, I found a tumour, which, as she then lay, occupied about the situation of the cæcum; and I felt a collection of flatus under my hand, with a gurgling, as if air were passing the valve. As she altered her position and lay flat, the tumour seemed to rise to the margin of the ribs; when under the margin of the ribs, it felt more solid, and we thought it arose from the liver; though I had a strong impression that the painful affection, and other knotted parts we felt, depended on a loaded state of the colon; and by colocynth, galbanum, and morphia, we brought away a considerable quantity of fæces; but still the upper tumour remained, and evidently belonged to the liver. The irritability of the stomach was greatly relieved by the cajeput-oil in calcined magnesia and cinnamon-water; but she evidently grew worse; the abdomen became tympanitic, large coils of the small intestines showing themselves; the mind was enfeebled; and she gradually sunk, about a month after the tumour was first discovered.

Sectio cadaveris.—The lungs healthy, but the right was forced up by the liver. Heart rather large.

The liver was full twice its natural size, of a pale-drab colour, and decidedly fatty. Two large massive cerebriform tubera had developed themselves in the right lobe, one under the hollow of the diaphragm, the other near the lower margin, and this had been the source of the hepatic tumour we had felt.

In the abdomen, when first opened, the liver was seen descending some way below the ribs; and the stomach, with several large convolutions of the small intestines, filled almost all the rest of the space exposed, except that occupied by a small part of the colon, and a diseased mass at the cæcum.

The stomach had evidently been distended.

The cæcum was glued closely to the parietes of the abdominal muscles, and formed, with the ascending colon, a deformed and thickened mass. On tracing it further, it was found to be glued down; and it appeared that a mass of glands near the head of the pancreas had become affected with the malignant disease, and had involved in close adhesion both the duodenum and colon, and had ulcerated through the latter. There was imbedded in this mass a gall-stone of the size of a marble.

The only other viscus obviously diseased was the uterus, in the fundus of which a single hard, round cartilaginous body was discovered.

In this case, the examination explained most accurately the cause of the tumours which had been felt; showing, that we should not, in such investigations, reject or neglect those slight variations which the touch is able to detect, and which, as they cannot exist without a sufficient cause, must depend upon real differences in the nature or situation of tumours. It must, however, be confessed, that although we may have approached very near in diagnosis during life, examination seldom fails to bring circumstances to light which we then think ought not to have escaped our research.

This case presented a combination of disease which cannot be very common—the cerebriform tumour with the fatty liver.

CASE 25.—*Tumour in the abdomen, from cerebriform growth in the liver.*—May 17th, 1836.—I was requested by my friend, Dr. Ridge, to give him my opinion of a tumour, under which a connection of his own was labouring. I found a man, of about thirty years of age, now nearly confined to bed. Countenance pale, not jaundiced, nor was the conjunctiva yellow, yet I fancied a slight tinge; he was considerably emaciated; tongue furred; pulse somewhat accelerated. On examining the abdomen, a large rounded tumour presented itself, occupying the whole of the right side from the ribs, under which it passed, nearly to the pelvis, and extending laterally considerably beyond the umbilicus; the intestines were ascertained, by percussion, to be on the left side and at the bottom of the abdomen; and they rose up so as to overlap, in some degree, the rounded tumour. The tumour itself was elastic, almost like a football, without any distinct fluctuation, rapidly increasing, and extending towards the loins. There was no marked irregularity in its form or consistence, but it was most tender towards the lower part. The urine was reported to be in sufficient quantity, and letting fall the lithates on cooling. The stools tolerably healthy, and bilious. I learned, that so long ago as the previous August and September he had complained from time to time of pain in the right side, after writing long; and in October, after a walk of three miles, the pain was so violent as to render necessary full bleeding, followed by leeches; but after three weeks he appeared quite restored. After a short time, he had another still more severe attack, apparently in consequence of a long ride on horseback. This attack was considered decidedly hepatic; and bleeding, leeches, blistering, and mercury, were employed. In three weeks he was able to resume his duties as a clergyman, but he was looking pale and ill; and on the evening of the third Sunday of duty he went to bed, feeling well, but awoke in the morning early in violent pain, and the physician who then saw him detected very considerable enlargement of the liver, under the ribs. Leeches, blister, cupping, and a mercurial course, to salivation, for a fortnight, were employed; after which, all pain was removed, and strength gradually returned. In January last the patient first discovered a swelling in the side, directly below the ribs; it was about the size of a tea-cup, and quite soft and puffy; and from that time had continued to increase, in spite of iodine and other remedies which had been prescribed.

I felt great difficulty, from the examination of the tumour, in coming to any conclusion satisfactory to myself; and I told Dr. Ridge, that it appeared to me to be attached to the liver, and yet might possibly be the right kidney; if the liver, it was either fungoid or hydatid; that there was no evidence of renal obstruction or disease; and, upon the whole, I should lean to the supposition of its being an hydatid cyst attached to the liver, and containing a great many more, so as to account for the elastic feel without fluctuation, for the peculiar globular form, for the absence of jaundice, and for the absence of all ascertainable fungoid tubera in other parts of the liver, or externally. I said, however, that I should like to have another opportunity of examining it, before I formed a decided opinion. I never saw this case a second time; but a month after, I heard that the tumour had greatly increased, and all the symptoms were much worse, and, more particularly, that frequent delirium manifested itself. He lived, however, till September; when, on a post-mortem examination, it was found that the whole substance of the right lobe of the liver was in a most advanced stage of cerebriform disease, the texture was broken down to the consistence of soft brain, and could only be removed by handfuls; no hydatids; a portion of the left lobe retaining the appearance of liver, but with small tubera. The lungs, spleen, heart, and all other viscera, healthy. The left kidney large, but healthy in appearance. The right kidney could not be found, nor any trace of it.

In this case, then, although an error was made in the diagnosis, no real discouragement seems to be thrown upon the correctness of our diagnostic symptoms. I saw this case but once, and was led away by the examination of the tumour, and its obvious appearance, to ascribe to it a wrong cause, though its situation was very accurately pointed out. I believe, however, that the symptoms ought to have led me to conclude that some malignant, and therefore cerebriform, disease existed, rather than hydatids. The extreme pain occasionally suffered, and the obvious constitutional derangement, certainly belonged rather to such a form of disease, than to the hydatid.

CASE 26.—*Tumours in the abdomen from cerebriform growth in the liver.* (Fig. 77.)—The following case has already been given in the 'Guy's Hospital Reports,' vol. i, p. 642, where a full account may be seen of the structure of the fungoid tubera; but the history I have thought it well to repeat here, as an example of very rapid progress in disease, and as being necessary, in order to explain a drawing which I have introduced as an illustration of cerebriform tumours in the liver.

Fig. 77.

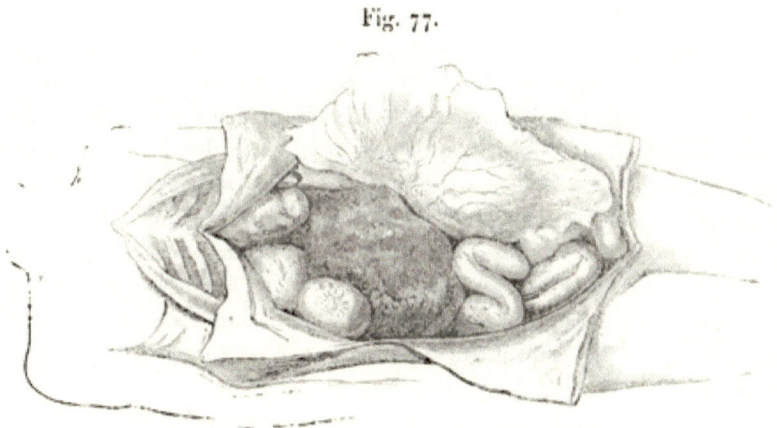

Fig. 77. The liver greatly enlarged from malignant cerebriform disease of very rapid growth. A tumour of similar character, but not connected with the liver, is seen beneath the omentum to the left.

March 28th, 1833, I was taken by my friend Mr. Streeter to see C——, a policeman. His aspect was delicate; his countenance pallid, respiration hurried; pulse 100. Several tumours were easily felt in the abdomen; some apparently in the liver, others below it. They felt rather soft and elastic to the touch, and pressure on them gave no pain. The urine was loaded with a sediment of the colour of rose-pink, which disappeared by heat; it was not tinged with bile, and contained no albumen. He complained of very little pain, but of a most dreadful sensation of sickness. About four years before, he first began to feel out of health; and at that time he used frequently to vomit at night, not apparently in consequence of anything he had eaten. He continued, however, to discharge his duties till nine weeks ago, when he was suddenly seized with a severe pain in the right side, just below the margin of the ribs. It was little more than a week before I saw him, that Mr. Streeter, who was then called in, detected the tumours in the abdomen. I never saw him, except on this occasion; but I heard that the tumours increased with great rapidity; that the sensation of sinking remained most painfully upon him; and that he died on the 3d of April, six days after my visit.

I was present at the examination the next day, when the following appearances presented themselves.

The chest was perfectly healthy, but much encroached upon by the liver, which ascended as high as the space between the third and fourth ribs on each side.

On opening the abdomen, the liver was seen enormously enlarged by the presence of many large cerebriform tubera in its substance; so that the right lobe occupied the greater part of the central region of the abdomen, the left lobe being pushed under the ribs of the left side. The lower part of the right lobe was comparatively free from tubera, and the whole substance of the liver appeared natural, except immediately around the tubera, where the structure was somewhat compressed. Those tubera which were in sight were as large as small oranges; but on cutting into the substance of the liver, several were found, from the size of a small shot to that of a marble.

Immediately below the right lobe of the liver, and to the left of the umbilicus, was a large fungoid mass, of the size of a child's head, over which the omentum was finely spread, adhering to it in some parts. This large tumour was found, on further examination, to be firmly fixed to the side of the pylorus, so that it apparently arose from that part; it was likewise attached to the colon.

The other viscera were healthy.

Between this case and the last two there is considerable analogy in history as well as in post-mortem appearance. The disease in both had, probably, for some months, or even years, existed in a latent or greatly subdued state; for all three of these patients had been invalids, and suffering from abdominal pains for that length of time, and some with severe occasional aggravations; and in each, the attack which preceded death, and in which the hepatic tumour was first detected, was one of intense pain in the right hypochondriac region. They all died worn out by exhaustion and suffering.

The disease had, in each, shown itself by tubera of considerable magnitude; and in two, had shown a tendency to attack the glandular structures about the head of the pancreas and the pylorus; and had not in any case displayed itself by affections of the serous membranes, which we find very common in the most strictly scirrhous form of disease.

CASE 27.—*Tumour in the abdomen, from scirrhous tubera in the liver.—Peritoneum and other organs affected.*—April 3d, 1838, I was requested to meet Sir A. Cooper in consultation, in the case of a gentleman who bore all the marks of organic disease. We were told that he had formerly been an athletic and active man, but had been falling off about two years; one of the first signs of ailment having been occasional pain from food taken into the stomach, but never accompanied by sickness. It was not till about two months before I saw him that a tumour was discovered at the pit of the stomach, which a physician in Dublin, he says, considered in the stomach.

At present, we can most satisfactorily make out that the liver is beset with malignant tubera. We trace, at the scrobiculus cordis, the flat surface of the left lobe of the liver, with some flat tubera in it; and in the right lobe, one is detected about on a level with the umbilicus. The glands in the groins are rather enlarged; and one or two on the right side are as hard as peas. He complains of constant pain at the pit of the stomach. Tongue red at the tip; pulse quick; great emaciation.

23d.—There had been a gradual loss of strength, and occasional paroxysms of dreadful pain, chiefly in the upper part of the abdomen, followed by copious perspirations. Of all the anodynes we tried, nothing gave so great relief as the solution of muriate of morphia. In consequence of a slight serous effusion taking place in the abdomen, he had a little mercury; his bowels were regulated, and the stools appeared quite healthy. Urine generally dark coloured, and loaded with lithates. He had no vomiting, but great thirst. He was nourished on the mildest food. He died in a perfect state of exhaustion, on the 25th.

Sectio cadaveris.—On opening the abdomen, the left lobe of the liver was seen descending just in the seat of the chief hardness at the scrobiculus cordis, filled with innumerable scirrhous tubera; many of the size of a large filbert, a few larger, but the greater part of the size of a pea, or less. The small ones were nearly transparent; the large ones opaque. None of them were the least softened. The left lobe extended far into the left side, and the right into the right lumbar space; so that, during life, it had once suggested the idea that the kidney might be affected, though the mobility of the whole soon corrected this idea.

The stomach contained one very large mass of fungoid disease, of the size of an egg, flattened on one side, which occupied the small curvature of the stomach, and was obviously developed in the submucous tissue. The peritoneum opposite to it was vascular, and some slight adhesions had taken place between it and the liver. The mucous surface of the tumour was dark-coloured and flocculent, from a process of softening which was going on. The mucous membrane of the stomach was red, with several white spots, showing where malignant deposit had begun beneath the membrane. The pylorus healthy.

The peritoneum was throughout, both where reflected on the parietes and where covering the viscera, sprinkled with little malignant tubera. The small intestines were generally but thinly sprinkled with small tubera. The large intestines had more; and the sigmoid flexure and rectum were one hard mass of tubera of different sizes, from a grain of sand to a small bean. The mesentery was remarkably covered with these bodies, which were more about the insertion of the intestines than at the root; indeed, they formed like a row of flattened bullets, near the intestines. The vermiform process, and the portion of mesentery belonging to it, were covered with them. The omentum was corrugated, and, when unrolled, displayed a great many little white tubera, like seeds. The fundus of the bladder was covered with them, and so was the lower surface of the diaphragm. The whole peritoneum was red and vascular, and there had evidently been much action going on in it. There was nearly a washhand-basin full of serum, of a light sherry-colour, in the abdomen. The spleen, kidneys, aorta, and thoracic duct, healthy.

Pleuræ healthy; lungs somewhat emphysematous.

In this case, it is probable that the disease began in the stomach, where a large mass had gone on to a very advanced stage. All the first symptoms were referred to the stomach; and to such a degree, that, within three months of his death, a very eminent authority pronounced that organ the seat of disease. This was a well-marked case of the hard malignant tuber, which is often found pervading different structures, and very particularly the liver and the peritoneum, simultaneously with the mamma or with the stomach; in which, as in the present case, it forms flattened tubera, whose surfaces, going into a state of softening, bear the appearance of ulcers with enormously elevated margins. The hepatic tumours are characteristic, as being small and hard, and depressed in the centres.

CASE 28.—*The small hard scirrhous tumour of the liver, nearly confined to the left lobe. Peritoneum affected.*—John W—, æt. 62, was admitted into Guy's Hospital, under my care, February 2d, 1833; a tall man, of dark hair and sallow complexion; employed till the last two years as a sawyer, but since that time has supported himself as a general labourer; has lived in London for the last twenty-five years; and has been used to a glass of gin now and then, especially of a cold morning.

About forty years ago, when living in the Fens, had ague; but otherwise he has enjoyed good health. During last summer, if he worked harder than usual, he had pain where the tumour now is. About three months ago, felt a pain in the left side, just above the anterior part of the crest of the ilium, but recollects no swelling there; to this a blister and leeches were applied, and the pain ceased; but about the same time he began to be troubled with pain and tenderness over the whole abdomen, particularly the lower part; for this, very active purgatives were given, for about three weeks.

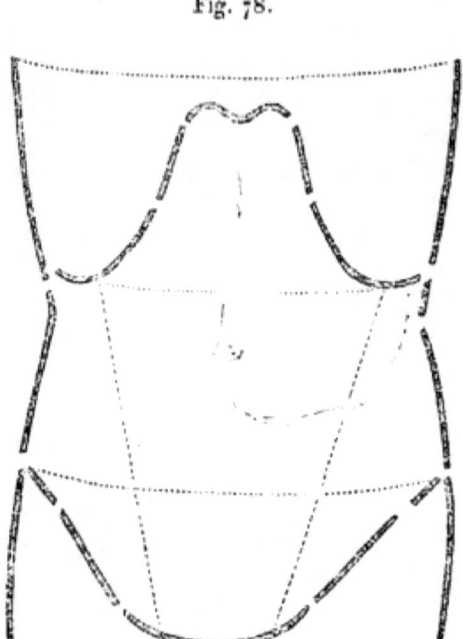

Fig. 78. Diagram, showing the portion of a tumour formed by the malignant enlargement of the left side of the liver.

At the time of admission, he complained of tenderness over the whole abdomen, which was very hard; with pain on that side on which he happened to lie. The lower part of the abdomen rather fuller than natural; and there is a hard, not very prominent tumour occupying the scrobiculus cordis, and extending up underneath the ribs. He has also a sense of oppression on the chest, but a deep inspiration produces pain in abdomen; bowels very irritable. He took a little tea last night, which produced vomiting; but to this he has not generally been subject. He is most comfortable when sitting, with his head on a table; but since he has adopted this, his legs have been œdematous. He is much emaciated, and has no inclination for food. There is an expression of great anxiety in his countenance. Tongue covered with a thin yellow crust.

February 3d.—Vomiting is very readily excited; but, by taking small quantities, he keeps down wine and sago.

4th.—An enema brought away a small dejection, deficient in bile. Pulse 96, small; urine very turbid, not bilious, a copious deposit of the purpurates at the bottom of the vessel.

On the 12th, his respiration became rather hurried; but he complained of no pain.

13th.—The house medicine, given him yesterday, induced vomiting; and therefore some colocynth pills were given, which produced a tolerable liquid, feculent motion. In the evening he appeared to be sinking fast. Pulse 130, feeble. Egg and wine was given, and remained on the stomach. At midnight he denied having any pain, and seemed inclined to sleep; but afterwards became delirious, and moaned and talked incoherently during greater part of night; at present in no pain, and seems better than he was yesterday afternoon. Pulse 120, feeble. The tumour is very hard, but not very prominent, and occupies the left of the scrobiculus cordis; and extends under the ribs, and downwards into the umbilical region, which it crosses, extending to the right of the mesian line, and about an inch below the umbilicus; he occasionally spits up mouthfuls of a dark grumous-looking fluid. He lingered on till the 20th, when he died.

Sectio cadaveris.—On endeavouring to open the cavity of the abdomen, the parietes were found closely adherent to the tumour on the upper part, which also was firmly and closely fixed to the diaphragm. The tumour was now evidently the left lobe of the liver, and its lower edge was not united to the parietes. This lobe was much enlarged, and of an almost stony hardness, and, on further observation, was seen to be diseased throughout, in a perfectly scirrhous state; the hard gristly scirrhus proceeding from centres to form circular bodies, which ran into each other, till the whole of the left lobe was nearly one continued mass of it. There were one or two separate tubercles, about the size of marbles, in the right lobe; and a few incipient deposits of the same between the acini, which had not yet fully assumed the circular form. The stomach was pressed upon, and the omentum lay congested and drawn up to the colon. The colon and all the intestines were very small and contracted.

The peritoneum was almost the only structure in the abdomen, except the liver, which was affected with this scirrhous disease, and that was most unusually studded. That portion which covered the diaphragm, and which adhered to the liver, as well as the portion similarly circumstanced which lined the parietes, bore upon it the marks of the white circular surfaces of the tubercles contained in the liver, appearing decidedly as if the morbid action had been communicated by contact. The peritoneum of the spleen was also covered with the disease, as was that covering the right kidney; the intestines were thickly sprinkled with it; and the small intestines were quite black, in the spaces intervening between the tubercles, from carbonaceous deposit. The peritoneum lining the sacrum presented a marked specimen of the disease. Throughout the whole peritoneum the tubercles presented somewhat the same aspect; they were scarcely raised above the surface, and assumed a somewhat circular form with broken edges, looking by no means unlike drops of tallow let fall into water; some were very imperfect, others of the thickness of a shilling. The tubercles on the surface of the intestines were smaller than the rest, and rather more round and projecting from the surface.

The liver was the only organ into the substance of which the disease seemed to have penetrated; but the kidneys were both unhealthy, particularly the left, which looked tuberculated; and on laying it open, it was found to be pervaded by many vesicles, which were filled with a yellowish glutinous substance, like transparent deep-coloured honey.

In the chest much mischief had been going on, chiefly in the left lung and the pericardium. The left lung adhered to the ribs, and its lower lobe was extensively excavated, and showed some peculiar appearance, which seemed to arise from the influence of the fungoid disease. The whole upper lobe of the left lung was hepatized.

For a more particular description of the structure of the tubera in this case, I must refer to the first volume of 'Guy's Hospital Reports,' p. 647.

CASE 29.—*Liver converted into a scirrhous mass, so contracted as to form no external tumour.—Uterus scirrhous.*—Eliz. B—, æt. 56, was admitted, under my care, into Guy's Hospital, October 6th, 1831, the subject of marked tympanitis, and slight serous effusion in the abdomen. In the whole of the upper part of the abdomen, as far as the umbilicus, and in both of the hypochondriac regions, the hollow tympanitic sound and elastic feel were very well marked; while in the lower part of the abdomen, fluctuation was felt. No hard tumour was discoverable. She looked a good deal worn by disease, and aged; but not altogether broken down, nor had she the slightest tinge of jaundice. She stated, that, a month before, she had first felt pain in the abdomen and back; and soon after began to experience difficulty in passing her urine, as well as a deficiency of the secretion; and she said that the quantity of urine passed was exceedingly small. The remedies which were recommended were combinations of diuretics, and such aromatic and tonic medicines as seemed likely to restore the tone of the large intestines by acting gently and regularly; while at the same time, by warmth of flannel rollers and friction, the external action was kept up: however, though the flatulent distension yielded a good deal, the serous accumulation increased; and on the 2d of December, seventeen pints of light straw-coloured serum were drawn off, which became rather opaque by standing, and coagulated moderately by the application of heat. The abdomen was only partially reduced in size. She bore the operation tolerably well; but in the course of a very few days the serum again collected; and, at her urgent desire, she was again tapped on the 20th, when fifteen pints of fluid, in which a few red particles subsided to the bottom, were taken away. It is evident, that after this operation she did not rally, but suffered much from pain and uneasiness of the abdomen, which gradually increased; sometimes the tenderness was considerable, sometimes sickness came on. She gradually sunk, and died about the 11th of January.

Sectio cadaveris.—Great emaciation, no yellowness of the skin; the abdomen contained about four pints of turbid serum, in which were floating some rather curious tissues, like fine vessels spread upon exceedingly thin membranes.

The omentum was corrugated, and contracted to the colon; and attached to it was a clot of blood, evidently arising from some vessels punctured in the operation of tapping. The colon, considerably inflated and thickened in its coats, lay across the upper part of the abdomen; while the whole of the small intestines were contracted and small. The liver formed a thick ill-shapen mass, in its ordinary situation, rather less than the natural healthy size, and covered with a honeycomb peritoneum. The whole of the peritoneum was covered with a false membrane, and was quite irregular on its surface.

On cutting into the liver, it was found to be of a scirrhous hardness throughout; so that it cut more like cartilage than any other substance, and was composed of innumerable small scirrhous masses, apparently originating from every part, and occupying the whole viscus. It looked almost like the semi-crystalline masses which collect at the bottom of the pots for fusing glass in glass-houses, where the crystallization begins at various distinct parts, increasing till they unite all in one mass.

The gall-bladder was with difficulty distinguished, and was at last found greatly thickened by a scirrhous alteration of its whole coats, and contracted around a biliary calculus, which completely filled its diminished cavity. There was, besides all this disease in the liver, a round white tumour near the convex surface; which, on being cut through, proved to be what appeared the remnant of an hydatid cavity, of the size of a walnut, which was filled with chalky matter and the remnants of hydatids.

The pancreas and spleen healthy.

The colon lay across the upper part of the abdomen, fully distended, though drawn in, in different parts, by the thickening of the peritoneum. The mucous membrane of the colon was abraded in several parts, and the feculent matter adhered to it. The fæces were moderately tinged with bile.

The uterus formed a large irregular mass, owing to its having four or five rounded tubera in its substance; which, though apparently in a completely quiescent state, were obviously of the malignant structure, and were each as large as a moderate-sized plum. A tumour of the same kind depended from the uterus. The whole mass made firm pressure on the rectum, and accounted well for the enlarged state of the colon.

The kidneys were small, but healthy.

Lungs healthy; heart unusually small.

The condition of parts sufficiently explained the symptoms of tympanites, and afterwards ascites.

This is by no means an uncommon combination; the colon loses its tone generally, in consequence of the imperfect secretion of bile; and this is, therefore, one of the first effects of that disease on which the ascites depends: but in the present instance, there is little doubt that the obstruction afforded by the disease of the uterus was one great cause of the distended state of the colon.

Case 30.—*Scirrhous tubera of the liver.—Mamma and ovaria diseased.*—Mary R——, æt. 45, was admitted, under the care of Mr. Morgan, with scirrhus of the right mamma. She was unmarried, of sallow complexion, and spare habit. Ever since she can remember, even when young, she had a small hard tumour under the right nipple, occasionally accompanied by pain. Menstruation always regular, to the present time. Within the last three years the tumour has increased, with more pain in the part, and derangement of the general health. The breast very hard, moveable, and, in some parts, seems to contain fungoid cysts. There is manifest irregular hardness in the region of the liver; and therefore no operation was admissible.

She shortly became the subject both of ascites and anasarca, and died March 6th.

Sectio cadaveris.—The liver was seen of great size, and universally pervaded by carcinomatous tubera, from the size of a grain of rice to that of a plover's egg. They all assumed a spherical shape, forming circular spots upon the surface, which, in most parts, touched each other, and in some, pressed each other out of shape, occupying a very large portion of the surface. The circular patches were of a whitish flesh colour, depressed towards the centre, and scarcely elevated at their circumferences, and marked with radiated vascularity, protruding from their centre. They were harder and more elastic than the surrounding liver, but could not be completely separated from it, as their edges, though defined to the eye, seemed to be not only strongly attached, but actually to amalgamate with the liver, as if the morbid deposit were insinuating itself between the acini. The liver itself was rather soft, of a light colour, and some parts stained with bile. The coats of the gall-bladder were about a quarter of an inch thick, somewhat resembling a scirrhous stomach, and very much contracted.

The left kidney had a fungoid growth upon its surface. In the left ovary was a well-marked apoplexy of a Graafian vesicle; in the right ovary, a fungoid growth. The lumbar glands partook of the malignant disease.

Case 31.—*Large irregular tumour, from melanosis of the liver.*—December 14th, 1839.—I was requested to see a lady affected with a great enlargement of the abdomen. She was a married woman, and had lain-in fourteen months before, at which time the abdomen was not discovered to be diseased; nor was it till eight months ago that the tumour was detected. Within the last week effusion had taken place into the peritoneum. I found her greatly emaciated; her complexion scarcely sallow, certainly not jaundiced. She was as large as a woman near the full time of her pregnancy. On examination I found a hard nodulated mass, extending quite to the pelvis, and pretty obviously continuous with the liver. The ribs on the left side rather raised, and percussion dull. Examining this extensive tumour as carefully as I was able, I could not satisfactorily account for one or two hardened masses situated in the left iliac region with the liver; and I therefore concluded that the disease had been communicated to the peritoneum or omentum. I entered in my note, that "I perceive one black spot, which I consider a small melanotic tuber, under the skin on the abdomen; and I suspect that the disease will be found of that character."

The swelling increased. The œdema of the legs was so great, that the cuticle gave way. She greatly emaciated; and sunk, exhausted, on the 11th of January; yet within forty-eight hours of her death she had been able to come down stairs and join her family.

Sectio cadaveris.—On removing the parietes, and opening the chest, the liver was seen, as a black mass, extending from the fifth rib to the pelvis and into both lumbar regions. This was everywhere pervaded by melanosis; in some parts assuming rounded forms, but more generally appearing to percolate between the acini, without attaining any fixed form, or being moulded by the cellular tissue in which it was deposited. Mingled with this black matter were many small white tubera of a scirrhous character; and in one part of the convex surface a space of several inches had the appearance of a porphyritic granite, from the intimate intermixture of the white and black. The gall-bladder contained but little bile; a few small melanotic glands on the mesocolon; the spleen and kidneys healthy. A few very small glands pervaded by melanosis were seen buried so deep in the integuments as not to show themselves on the surface. One melanotic gland on the pericardium; one small one on the heart itself. There was decided melanotic deposit in the cancellated structure of the sternum, about its juncture with the first and second ribs.

The upper part of the lungs was spotted with melanosis, in round spots, not resembling the ordinary pulmonary blackness.

In this case, a period of nine months alone was occupied in the formation of the enormous deposit in the liver, which extended so far into the iliac and pubic regions, that we were inclined to ascribe some of the more distant tubera to morbid growths upon the peritoneum; while a little more examination would in all probability have traced them uninterruptedly to the liver, and have shown, that when the liver was moved, the other parts followed its movements. The melanotic deposit in this case was very general throughout the liver, and took place rather in small granules than in rounded tubera, as you might imagine the black matter to dispose itself if poured out abundantly into the meshes of cellular membrane; and it was mingled with white malignant deposit, as I have seen in specimens of melanosis taken from the horse. The occurrence of some subcutaneous melanotic deposits formed almost a convincing proof of the nature of the internal disease.

CASE 32.—*Melanosis occupying the liver very extensively; very slight jaundice before death.*—(Fig. 79.)—James T—, æt. 62, was admitted into Guy's Hospital under my care, January 9th, 1830. He was by business a weaver, not intemperate in his habits, and had enjoyed good health till about four months previously, when his legs began to swell; and about two months after he perceived that

Fig. 79.

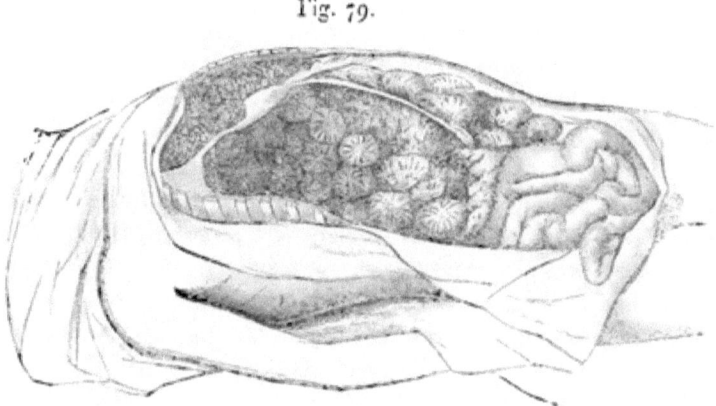

Fig. 79. The liver greatly enlarged from melanotic deposit.

his abdomen grew large and hard; and since that he has lost flesh rapidly. He has never had ague, nor has he been jaundiced, either during the present illness or before. The only malady by which he has been habitually troubled is a difficulty of swallowing solids, which he has experienced for at least two years. At the time of his admission, the legs were very œdematous; the countenance slightly sallow; the urine rather high coloured; the stools not very remarkable; and a large tuberculated swelling occupied the abdomen to such an extent, that it was difficult to ascribe it to the liver alone; indeed, some of the lumps of which it was composed were felt quite in the iliac region, on the right side. At that time there appeared to be no fluid effused into the abdomen; but on the 14th I could perceive that ascites had taken place, and his legs had become enormously swollen. From day to day his countenance became rather more dingy, and the conjunctiva very slightly tinged with bile; and at the end of the month, the urine assumed a deep bilious tinge, and the tongue became dry and partially red. It was always a great source of complaint with him that he passed his water in such small quantities. He felt his weakness daily increasing; and about the 3d of July he left the hospital. He survived, however, only three days; and on the following day, at the request of his friends, the body was opened.

Sectio cadaveris.—The parietes greatly emaciated; slight œdema of the arms and ankles. The whole surface, and the conjunctivæ, slightly tinged with bile. On the back and forehead were some small encysted tumours; and immediately beneath the skin on the chest a small black tumour was seen, which first suggested the belief that the tumour of the liver was melanotic. In the cavities of the pleura about two pints of fluid. The lungs were pervaded with much black deposit; and a few small tubercles of a deep black colour were seen on their surface. Heart small, but healthy; some melanotic matter in the cancellated structure of the sternum.

When the parietes of the abdomen were removed, the liver came into view, of a most enormous size, reaching quite into the left side, and low in the right iliac region, and ascending so far upwards as to force the diaphragm into the chest, as high as the fifth rib, and weighing fourteen pounds two ounces. Its general colour was a dark purple brown, and it was studded with tubera, some of which projected as a section of a sphere; but when they became large, and some, indeed, while yet small, presented a circular elevated margin, with a flattening or a deep depression in the centre, precisely in the same way as the ordinary fungus tuber, from which, except in colour, I could not perceive any difference. These tubera occupied fully three fourths of the whole surface; and though there were no red vessels upon them, as far as we could perceive by simple inspection, yet their whole mode of formation appeared precisely like that of ordinary tubera. The same was the fact when incisions were made into them in every direction; they appeared radiated from the centre, and divided by bands of cellular substance; the line of separation between them and the rest of the liver was quite distinct; and there was no appearance of the ordinary structure of the liver pervading any of the tubera, but they appeared a completely independent and new growth. The larger tubers were of the size of a small orange; and they varied from this to the size of a bean, occupying, throughout the whole mass of the organ, as great a proportion as on the surface. These tubera, when cut into, were of a soot colour; and when placed upon paper, left a deep olive-black pigment; their colour was uniform throughout, except the fine membranous bands, which were lighter. The intervening portions of the liver were of a dark olive colour, deeply tinged with black matter; but, both by their more spongy texture and their lighter colour, affording a decided contrast with the tubera.

The gall-bladder was very small, but was stained externally with bile.

The omentum was shrivelled, and the appendices epiploicæ small as shots. In the mesentery were a few black spots, hard to the feel, and larger than millet-seed, which were evidently of the same character as the disease in the liver. The pancreas quite healthy; the spleen rather small, externally natural, but internally of an olive-brown colour, decidedly peculiar. The kidneys had some vesicles externally, and one or two spots of melanosis, and deeply imbedded in the substance, particularly of the left kidney, a few tubera, of a black colour and hard consistence.

In this case, the form in which the melanotic deposit took place was decidedly different from that which was observed in the preceding case, and the progress of the disease appeared to have been even more rapid; for he could not trace his illness back to a period above four months before his death. In this, as in the last, the very extent of the hepatic disease led to a doubt, whether there were not peritoneal complication; but, as in the last, the peritoneum was but very slightly affected; indeed, no form of malignant disease seems so apt to affect the peritoneum as the true scirrhus. In this case we also had another opportunity of taking subcutaneous melanosis for our guide.

CASE 33.—*Extensive malignant disease, very rapidly implicating the organs both of the chest and the abdomen.*—John M—, æt. 35, admitted into Job's Ward, No. 22, on the 4th of March, 1840, under the care of Dr. Back, and died 28th March, 1840, at eight p.m.

A ship-rigger, light hair and blue eyes; always enjoyed good health till fifteen weeks since, when he experienced acute throbbing pain in the right lumbar region, attended by a swelling in that portion of the abdomen, but not extending in the course of the ureters; occasional vomiting and headache; acute pain; and a sense of heat on the inner side of the right thigh, and swelling of the right testicle, without retraction; urine passed in natural quantity, but of dark colour, depositing, on cooling, a substance like pus. Was bled from the arm, blistered on the right loin, and given various internal remedies. Under this plan of treatment, the pain continuing, and the swelling increasing almost to its present size, he applied to another medical man, whose treatment consisted in the application of leeches three times to the tumour, and in producing ptyalism. Receiving no benefit from these remedies, it was determined, in consultation, that the tumour should be punctured; this was performed with a common lancet, introduced to some depth, and the result was the escape of only a few drops of blood. This occurred five weeks before admission. The tumour has continued increasing, and the general health declining, up to the present time.

Recent Symptoms.—Appears much emaciated; right pupil more contracted than the left; pulse 112, small and weak; tongue dry and furred; skin hot and dry; bowels regular; urine dark-coloured, not albuminous; right testicle swollen; cough and hectic during the night; no pain in the tumour, except on pressure.

The tumour situated chiefly in the right side, extending from the ribs of that side towards the liver, and to the right iliac fossa, round the right lumbar region towards the spine, and also to the left of the mesial line of the abdomen, forcing the umbilicus somewhat to the right of the latter; percussion yields a dull sound, and imparts a feeling of indistinct fluctuation.

Right lung dull on percussion; respiration inaudible, except at its apex; left lung apparently healthy.

Ordered—Hydrocyanic Acid.

5th.—Burning pain in the inner side of the right thigh; urine scanty, turbid, and of brown colour; moderate heat renders it clear; but when raised to the boiling point, there is a copious white precipitate, which is dissolved by nitric acid: sp. gr. 1·031. Acid reaction.

Castor Oil and Morphia.

7th.—Passed a larger quantity of urine, which deposited no salts on cooling: sp. gr. 1·025. Acid re-action.

15th.—Has remained much the same.

16th.—Complains of pain in the posterior part of the tumour.

17th.—Pain and numbness down the outer side of right thigh to the ankle.

Omit Anodyne. Ordered Ext. Strammonii.

18th.—Much the same, suffered from a severe attack of dyspnœa, relieved by vomiting; skin covered with a clammy perspiration.

20th.—Suffered from urgent dyspnœa; pulse 120; skin clammy; tongue covered with a creamy fur; bowels open.

21st.—The pain in the throat, sense of suffocation, and dyspnœa returned last evening, and were present for some time, till relieved by vomiting; after which he slept for a short time; but, on the whole, passed a restless night, with great pain in the tumour, and a sense of shivering, not followed by heat or perspiration. He now complained of pain in the throat, and dyspnœa, with increased pain in the tumour, but none in the groin or thigh. Bowels open; urine scanty, loaded with pale lithates; tongue covered with a creamy fur; pulse 120, irritable; skin dry and hot.

Julep Magnesiæ cum Vin. Opii, ℳ viii, p. r. n.

23d.—Passed a restless night, being troubled with a husky cough, attended by a very slight mucous expectoration; urgent thirst and dyspnœa; pain in the tumour not extending to the thigh or groin; no vomiting since taking the M. M. cum Vin. Opii. Bowels open once; tongue covered with a creamy fur; pulse 120, weak and small; skin hot and dry; urine scanty, loaded with pale lithates; dyspnœa considerable.

Emp. Lyttæ scrob. cord.;
Mist. Camph. cum Mucilag. Acaciæ, ʒj;
Syr. Papav., ʒj;
Sp. Æth. Sulph. Comp., ʒj, sextis horis.

24th.—Blister acted well; passed a good night, without pain, dyspnœa, or sickness; tumour slightly painful; bowels confined; pulse 130, small and feeble; skin clammy; urine same as yesterday.

Rep. Pil., et Pergat.

25th.—Passed a tolerably good night, but was twice disturbed by pain in the tumour; no sickness; less dyspnœa; occasional pain in the tumour this morning; dyspnœa more urgent; abdomen tympanitic; tongue and urine the same; pulse 120, small and weak; bowels open once.

26th.—Passed a tolerable night, but coughed occasionally; no sickness; no pain in the tumour; bowels confined; pulse 146; skin clammy; urine as before.

28th.—Has passed a very bad night; dyspnœa more urgent this morning; breathing convulsive; profuse perspiration; pulse 136; bowels open. He continued sinking, and died at eight o'clock, p.m.

Sectio cadaveris.—The head was not opened.

On opening the chest, the diaphragm was noticed pushed up by the right kidney as high as the fourth rib.

Both lungs were everywhere firmly adherent by cellular membrane to the costal pleuræ, their structure was nearly everywhere affected by white rounded malignant tumours, many as large as damsons, and they contained only small quantities of air. The bronchial tubes were healthy.

The heart was healthy.

On opening the abdomen, nearly all the small intestines were noticed pushed to the left side by the tumour in the right kidney.

The structure of the liver was nearly everywhere affected by rounded scirrhous tumours differing in size from that of a walnut to that of a small orange.

The spleen was of remarkably small size, and fleshy.

The left kidney was healthy.

The right kidney was much enlarged; it was nearly eight times the healthy size, owing to a fungoid tumour (fungus hæmatodes) developed within its structure; the infundibula were enlarged, and were equal in size to small peas. The structure of the tumour was, in several places, of pinkish appearance; in others, very much like blood.

The mucous membrane of the stomach was much congested with blood; but the mucous membrane of the small and large intestines was healthy.

I have copied this case, which, however, I had myself an opportunity of seeing, both during life and after death, from the Clinical books, and the Inspection books kept in the Museum of Guy's, as a strong instance of complicated malignant disease, scarcely, from its extent, admitting of accurate diagnosis, and showing with what rapidity malignant disease is sometimes distributed throughout the whole body. A very valuable lesson may be learnt from this case; as it teaches us not to give too exclusive an opinion on the seat of disease, in this class of cases, when the symptoms seem incapable of being referred to the lesion of any single organ. In this case several opinions were given; but I doubt whether any embraced the whole of the diseased organs.

The cases and observations which I have thus thrown together may be considered as forming an outline of one very important class of abdominal tumours; and though many of them would seem to point out the difficulties of diagnosis, yet I trust, as a whole, they may rather serve as an assistance and an encouragement to our endeavours, in this essential pursuit.

INDEX.

	PAGE
ABDOMEN, exploration of	1
hysterical distension of	137
Abdominal organs, malposition of	259
Acephalocysts. See *Hydatid*.	
ADDISON, Dr., case under care of	118
on fatty disease of liver	241, 284
Ascites, with ovarian tumours	81, 131
BABINGTON, Dr., analysis by	254
discovery of urea in the blood by	viii
BARLOW, Dr., case by	101
Bile, accumulation of	270
retention of	271, 277
BOSTOCK, discovery of urea in the blood by	viii
BLACKALL, Dr., researches of, in dropsy	vi
Broad ligament, cyst in	58, 109
rupture of cyst in	109
Classification of tumours	2
Colon, communication with ovarian cyst	104
abscess in spleen	175
loaded, forming a tumour	243—250
Exploration of abdomen	1
Fallopian cysts	58, 59
Gall-bladder, the, forming a tumour	279
calculi in	280
Graafian vesicle, distension of	60, 63, 70
Hæmaturia, as a symptom	204
HODGKIN, case by	23, 29
Hydatid tumours	11
analysis of fluid	44
cases, in abdomen	13, 23, 30
diagnosis of	12
escape by intestines	49
escape of, externally	50
general observations on	52—55
microscopic examination	18

	PAGE
Hydatid tumours, organs affected by	11
ossification of cyst	38
paracentesis of cyst	41, 42
peritonitis induced by	38
post-mortem appearances	18, 26, 29, 33
remarks on treatment	55
rupture of cyst	44, 46, 47
various stages of growth of	22
See also *List of Cases*.	
Hysterical distension of abdomen	137
Jaundice, as a symptom	241
Kidney, tumours of	198
difficult diagnosis of	199
calculus in	217, 227
cystic disease of	208
disease of, frequency in children	208
general considerations	236
malignant disease of	220, 229, 232, 233
paracentesis of	229
suppuration of	210, 212, 217, 223, 224
tumours, different forms of	202
Liver, tumours connected with	230—237
abscess in	293, 297
cicatrices in	296
chronic hypertrophy of	280—284
and diaphragm, abscess between	257
displacement of, by empyema	255, 256
enlarged, from obstructed circulation in chest	264
fatty degeneration of	241, 284—290
form and size of	240
irregular tumours in	293—320
malignant tumour in	260, 291, 298—320
melanosis in	315
smooth tumours in	263—292
tumefaction of	263, 269, 277
tumours of, diagnosis of	242
Malignant disease of kidney	220, 229, 232, 233
mesentery	234
ovary	97
spleen	151, 184, 188
Melanosis of liver	313, 315
spleen	152
Mesentery, malignant disease of	234

INDEX. 325

	PAGE
Outline figures, use of	9
Organs, malposition of	259
Ovarian tumours	57
distinct forms of	57
frequency of	57
with ascites	81, 131
diagnosis of	64, 65, 139
diagram of growth	66
enlargement of the breast in	141
general considerations	139
inflammation of	76
malignant forms of	71, 75, 124, 131
prognosis of	141
paracentesis in	67, 107, 144
danger of	109
simulation of	137
solid and fleshy	146
treatment	142
cyst, communication with colon	104
analysis of fluid	73, 93
cysts, pathology of	61
rupture internally	118, 121
Peritoneum, malignant disease of	127, 129, 251, 305, 307
pendulous, malignant tumours of	130
Pleura, distension by fluid	255
Pus in the urine	206, 224, 227
Rees, Dr. Owen, analysis by	73, 93
Regions, division of	4
Region, epigastric	3
umbilical	5
hypogastric	5
lumbar	7
inguinal	8
Renal disease	198
See *Kidney*.	
Sigmoid flexure, accumulation in	243, 244, 246, 250
Spleen, abscess in	173
tumours of	148
bony deposits	153, 189
chronic enlargement	150, 172
cysts in	189
disease of, in fever	182
ecchymosis in	195

		PAGE
Spleen, enlarged, with diseased liver		171, 173, 177
with fatal diarrhœa		. 169
in ague		. 159
treatment of		163, 164
in children		. 165
fibroid deposits		. 152
fluid state of		. 179
function of		. 149
gangrene		. 151
tubercles		151, 180, 181
general considerations		. 196
hydatids		. 153
induration		. 150
inflammation		. 151
laceration of		154, 193—195
malignant disease		151, 184—188
melanosis		. 152
normal differences in size		. 149
peritoneal covering, disease of		190—192
remarkable distension		. 165
simple congestion		. 149
situation		. 148
sloughing abscess in		. 176
softening		. 150
suppuration		. 151
sympathy with skin		. 197
Splenic disease, symptoms of		. 156
tumour, diagnosis		157, 158
Spleens, supernumerary		. 154
Stricture of urethra		. 201
Uterus, fibroid tubera in		. 127
Urethra, stricture of		. 210
Urine, pus in		206, 224, 227
blood in		. 204
Viscera, normal position of		3—10
Wells, Dr., researches of, in dropsy		vi

www.ingramcontent.com/pod-product-compliance
Lightning Source LLC
Chambersburg PA
CBHW031851220426
43663CB00006B/578